WE WANT TO LIVE! *Expanded and Revised in 2005*

by Aajonus Vonderplanitz

"Revolutionary! This is an exciting book. An important book." Dr. Robert Atkins, M.D. Author of numerous best selling diet books

"...a revelation. It is one of the most impressive books I have ever read." Rob Strauds, Health writer/editor

"...an impressive addition to any health and medicine reference book collection." Wisconsin Bookwatch

"...fascinating...absolute dedication to finding answers... many, many peoples lives it will empower." Leslie Kenton, Author of New Raw Energy; Ageless Aging

"This isn't just about having disease and trying to heal, [but]...getting healthier. Marvelous! Scott Cluthe, KENR, Houston

Endorsements: Malibu Health & Rehabilitation Clinic, Monika Klein, B.H.Ec, C.N., Clinical Nutritionist, Member I.A.A.C.N., Dr. John Finnegan, N.D., Institute for Internal Healing, Kaumari Research Foundation, Dr. Gene Hummel, Leslie Kenton (Health researcher, writer, London), Dr. Stephen L. Sokolow

WE WANT TO LIVE!

Expanded and Revised in 2005

the PRIMAL DIET ™

Through this remarkable but true story of Aajonus' battle to save his son from life-threatening injuries following an automobile accident, we learn how Aajonus healed himself of terminal cancers, diabetes, bursitis and psoriasis. We learn how thousands of his clients have healed themselves of hundreds of "incurable" diseases. All of those miracles were accomplished simply by eating foods prepared in specific ways and in specific combinations. Aajonus shares with us the overall, fundamental premises and practical guidelines that created those phenomenal results.

At last, all of the disappointments and despair that people have endured because of failed medical treatments, "miracle-cure" diets and expensive "magic-bullet" supplements and drug-therapies can be understood and set aside. The revolutionary information contained in this book, culled from over 40 years of medical and naturopathic experience and experimentation, brings new hope and inspiration to anyone who has ever suffered from disease or physical decline, or who wishes to increase their peace of mind, physical and mental vitality, endurance, athletic skills, and happiness.

This book includes a remedy section listing hundreds of diseases and ailments, with specific foods and combinations of foods that people have used to cure themselves. Listed is everything from beauty tips, the common cold and infant problems, to aging, muscular dystrophy, HIV and cancer. Most people who applied the principles of the Primal Diet to their lives reduced their medical bills by at least 90%. Many people eliminated their medical bills entirely. Imagine living a life you control, as well as being healthy and feeling great!

ABOUT THE AUTHOR

Aajonus Vonderplanitz was a sickly and accident-prone child who also suffered autism that caused learning, attention and social disorders. At twelve he survived his first life-and-death situation from peritonitis that was misdiagnosed and treated as appendicitis. His health continued to decline throughout his adolescence. At twenty, he was diagnosed with blood and bone cancers and given less than six months to live. Medical therapies made him semi-invalid with three new "incurable" diseases, along with the medical death sentence of "three months at best".

His struggle with diseases drove him to pursue the boundaries of health. He studied and explored every alternative: physical exercise, psychotherapy, positive-thinking, metaphysics, religion, dietary regimes, and vitamin, mineral and enzyme supplement therapies. He obtained substantial results from certain diets.

After his health improved significantly, he traveled for three years on a bicycle laden with his sleeping bag and four saddle bags containing books on health, physiology and anatomy. He adventured the North American continent, living outdoors while studying the diets and healing methods of various cultural groups and animals. He discovered a dietary approach that changed his life and all of his diseases completely reversed. He outlives his medical death sentence now by three decades, and enjoys excellent health.

Mr. Vonderplanitz is based in Malibu, California, USA, and advises people on nutrition all over the world. Disney's *Epcot TV Magazine* featured him in an episode entitled "You Are What You Eat" (1983), FOX-6 News featured him in "The Primal Diet" (2005), and *Ripley's Believe It Or Not* featured him in the television episode "No Fear of Bacteria" (2002). He fostered nutritional education on several TV and radio talk shows and children's programs (1979-2005). People all over the world seek his individualized counseling. In 2002, he developed a companion volume of raw-food recipes with extensive scientific support for the Primal Diet entitled, **The Recipe For Living Without Disease**.

WE WANT TO LIVE!

Expanded and Revised in 2005

the PRIMAL DIET ™

Volume One

Out of the Grips of Disease and Death

(the story)

Volume Two

Healthfully

(the facts)

Aajonus Vonderplanitz

CARNELIAN BAY CASTLE PRESS
Los Angeles

Published by
CARNELIAN BAY CASTLE PRESS, LLC
P. O. Box 66663
Los Angeles, CA 90066

Jacket design by Aajonus Vonderplanitz and Niki Ng
Jacket photo by Julia Dean

Library of Congress Cataloging-in-publication Data
Vonderplanitz, Aajonus, 1947-
We Want To Live!; the PRIMAL DIET expanded and revised in 2005 /
the PRIMAL DIET; We Want To Live! expanded and revised in 2005 /
by Aajonus Vonderplanitz.
p. cm.
Includes bibliographical references and index.
Contents: v. 1. Out of the grips of disease and death --
v. 2. Healthfully
ISBN 978-1-889356-10-5
1. Vonderplanitz, Aajonus, 1947- --Health.
2. Naturopaths - United States - Biography. 3. Naturopathy. I. Title.
RZ439.7.V66A3 1997
615.5'35--dc20 96-34036
[B] CIP

Second Printing 2007
Expanded and Revised Edition, 2005
First Edition by CARNELIAN BAY CASTLE PRESS, 1997
Printed in the United States of America

CONTENTS

VOLUME TWO

Healthfully (the facts)

Expanded and Revised in 2005

Understanding the Primal Diet

DEDICATION

(In order of appearance in my life)

TO MOM, Dad, my brothers Donald, Douglas, David, my hundreds of relatives, especially Lanny Sims, to Ann Ergen, Claudia Fieglein, Ann Gablein, Jack Tepker, John Maloney, Mary Linder-Marshall, Margaret and William Linder, my son John Jeffrey, Steve and Elsie Sanico, Pauline Gerber, Steve Flanagan, Dore Freeman, Marvin Paige, Lurene Tuttle, Kathy Hill, Bruno Corigliano, Monica Lauren-Corueil, Terry Costa, Rení Rodriguez, Dr. Jim Rota, Louis Cangemi, Yomi Perry, Susan Stewart-Clark, Tony Plana, Myron Scheinhaus, Paul and Teresita Echaniz, my esteemed colleague Owanza di Mdina, Charles Berendt, Benjamin Stewart, Kathy Pattiz, Beatriz Cervantes, Laura Long, Mary Ivory, Véronique Bertier, Beth Duffy, all my clients throughout the many years, Kate Seitz and Debra Powell for their wonderful help editing this book so many times, Ruth Ross for editing this revision, and my dear friend Paul Kruhm President of Carnelian Bay Castle Press.

ACKNOWLEDGMENT

OWANZA'S knowledgeable and experimental contributions to diet over the years, and to the remedy section of this book, have enabled me to reach, affect and facilitate healing of many more people than I would have otherwise. Owanza thought of the simple food formula that alters coma. Not only is she wonderfully insightful, she has been one of the three most generous, kind and loving people I have known. My nutritional mentor Bruno Corigliano, and uncle Lanny Sims are the other two. Bruno and Lanny's examples showed me how to evolve to the extent that I primarily live free of anger, resentment and self-pity, except when drama is an element of teaching.

PROLOGUE

Three doctors declared that I would die at age twenty-one after I had received medical treatments for cancer. I began searching, experimenting and exploring other means to gain my health. I discovered that good health most often comes when one eats a diet consisting of foods that supply the most bioactive nutrients; they are mentioned throughout the following pages.

Since I was intent on sharing all that I learned, I became a nutritional counselor and learned more by helping others. The high point of gratification in my work in the health field is the saga that *We Want To Live; Volume One, Out of the Grips of Disease and Death* tells. It is the battle I waged when the doctors said that my son was on his deathbed.

WARNING / DISCLAIMER

This material has been written and published solely for educational purposes. The reader understands that the author and publisher are not engaged in rendering medical advice or services. The author and publisher provide this information, and the reader accepts it, with the understanding that each reader will act on it with full knowledge that, like everything in life, action is at her or his own risk.

The author and publisher shall have neither liability or responsibility to any person or entity with respect to any loss, damage or injury caused, or alleged to be caused, directly or indirectly by the information contained in this book.

If you do not wish to be bound by the above, you may return this book, unread and in perfect condition, for a full refund.

VOLUME ONE

WE WANT TO LIVE!

the PRIMAL DIET ™

Out Of The Grips Of Disease And Death

The story
Several names have been changed.

The efficacy of all of the dietary wisdom in this book is from experience, experimentation, trial and error and does not rely upon whether we chemically understand the phenomenon or not.

Although the author would like to, he does NOT imply or suggest that anyone interfere with medical procedure.

The Appendix contains biochemical, dietary and nutritional explanations that were too distracting to the story but they are important to those with inquiring minds. People have benefited the most by reading the story through to the end, and then reading the Appendix.

1

Friday, September 26th

"Hi, Mom," I say groggily. "Are you okay? We usually talk on Sundays."

I peer through the curtains above my bed. It's a clear early morning in Beverly Hills, California. I wonder what in the world - or in Cincinnati - happened to get Mom to call on day rates.

"Jeff was in an accident."

"How bad?"

"His car went into a ravine and he suffered severe brain damage. He's in a coma."

"No... I'll be on the next flight."

"The doctors say he won't live through another night," she hesitates. "There's no point in your coming...until it's over."

Why would Mom say such a thing? "If there's anything I can do I want to be there."

"Mary doesn't want you here."

"She actually said that?"

"She told me to tell you not to come."

"If Mary and I could have done what each other wanted we'd still be married. I'll call you as soon as I've booked a flight."

"Okay. We'll pick you up at the airport."

"Thank you. I love you."

"I love you," she replies sincerely and hangs up.

Oh, my God, I'm going to have to face the helplessness I felt when Jeff was an infant and I was seventeen. And the divorce with Mary at nineteen. I feel delirious.

I flip open my personal phone directory and punch in the numbers. The lines are busy. A recorded voice answers. I check my pulse rate. It's faster. Although my heart and mind seem a little frenzied, I notice my adrenals haven't triggered panic in my body. Is my body protecting me from the inevitable? Can't death just leave me alone?

I won't spend energy on that probability. Okay. Jeff will need lots of--

"This is Cyndi, may I help you?"

"Hi, Cyndi, what is your next flight leaving L.A.X. to Cincinnati? This is a life-and-death emergency."

I wonder how corny that sounds and how often she's heard that line.

"My son's been in an accident."

"I'm sorry," she says timidly.

I hear her computer keys clicking away. I drift into memory.

Jeff was one month old. He had my blue eyes and my fairness when I was his age with many of Mary's facial features. Mary sat in the rocker holding Jeff in her arms. Her thick, dark brown, wavy hair folded on to her shoulders. Her large brown eyes and full lips are flanked by high full cheek bones and jowls. Mary and Jeff rocked. He screamed. He pushed and twisted his face into the blouse covering Mary's breast. His scream pressed his lungs completely void of air, creating a vacuum. Then he desperately sucked in air as if suffocating. He released another blood-curdling scream and then gasped for air. He screamed again and again. Grieved and frustrated, Mary and I didn't know what to do for him.

"I'm still searching," Cyndi's voice rescues me.

But my thoughts keep churning. I remember Jeff screaming for hours, night after night. I turn my thoughts to life right after Jeff's conception.

Like normal teenagers in love, Mary and I adored each other. She was a senior at Finneytown High and I was a junior (she was older than I). Our parents were understanding and supportive, which surprised me at the time. We married in another state and hid it from everybody because the school didn't allow married or pregnant students. Mary did sit-ups, wore sweaters and blouses that hung to hide her pregnancy. She graduated with honors in her sixth month. Within four weeks after that her stomach bulged to the size of a basketball.

Jeff was born the first week of my senior year. Surprisingly, the school faculty changed policy for me. They encouraged me to attend as a part-time student, allowing me to take only the courses necessary to graduate so I could work and tend to my family. Very little in my life was happy until I met Mary more than two years before Jeff was born. All of a sudden, encouragement came from everywhere.

Margaret, Mary's mother, took care of Jeff while I was in school and Mary was at work. Margaret was strong, fun-loving, attractive and had reddish-blond hair. She hated to be called a redhead. Why, I still don't know. After school I'd get Jeff from Margaret. Jeff and I went home to our apartment in a lower middle-class suburb at a very small business intersection. We lived above a "Family Billiards" hall and I remember being comforted by the happy noises of people playing.

After settling Jeff, I'd usually prepare dinner for the three of us. I'd gobble down my share and rush off to work the moment Mary walked in the door from work. She was a prized secretary for the electric company. I breaded and fried chicken and French fries in a short-order restaurant.

I got home from work between twelve and one in the morning. Mary was often asleep in the rocker with Jeff fussing or asleep in her arms. I'd take over, hold him in my arms and rock. On a rare occasion I did some homework while I rocked him. Sometimes we alternated in one- to two-hour shifts, rocking Jeff through the night.

Everybody except Margaret insisted we were spoiling him. Fear of spoiling a child was the mindset back then. So several times we let him cry in his crib. One time he screamed for six-and-a-half hours until we picked him up. We knew his pain was more than a need to be cuddled.

We discovered our baby had severe colic. We gave him baby aspirin. They made him worse when the effects wore off. The doctors prescribed every infant milk formula on the market. None worked. Everything the doctors said and did did not help him. I wish we had known then that if a mother is on a healthy diet, breast-feeding would have resolved the problem.

The doctors steered us away from breast-feeding. The consciousness seemed to be that breast-feeding was unsanitary, primitive and disgusting. Consequently Jeff suffered for twelve months. We suffered with him. It stopped for no apparent reason.[1]

"The first available flight is 11 a.m. tomorrow," Cyndi's voice snaps me back.

"Who's going to Cincinnati in late September?!"

"You, sir," she quips.

I asked for that. "Please put me on your stand-by call list for all flights and book me on the first available, please. My name's Aajonus Vonderplanitz."

I spell it and Cyndi's keys clicking away takes me back to when Jeff

---

[1] *See* Appendix A, page 127.

was one year old. Mary was aloof. What was it about childbirth that robbed Mary of her ceaseless optimism, humor, joy of life and sensuality? That thought constantly perplexed me. I didn't understand that it was biological. Not knowing enough about anything, I thought it was merely psychological. I pressured her to desire me the way she had before. She couldn't. I said hurtful things to her. It made things worse. All the chores and responsibilities of family life didn't make any sense anymore. After work, I began drinking with work buddies until five or six in the morning.

During the days, I attended a breakthrough computer trade school. I got top grades in something other than art for the first time in my life. I began seeing one of the teachers after school. She was a single parent, divorced, eight years my senior. She was lonely for affection, too.

"Do you want to schedule a return flight?"

"Uh, yes. I have to be back next Wednesday late afternoon." What am I saying? Am I expecting a miracle in five days? I'll have to cancel my performance next Thursday. No. If I can't help Jeff I'll need the distraction.

"Okay, Mr. Vonderplanitz. We'll call you if a seat opens. You'll have about forty-five minutes to get to Los Angeles International Airport immediately after we call. So have your luggage ready. But for now your reservation going to Cincinnati is on flight___"

As I write down the information, I remember Jeff's first portrait-sitting. He was six months old. He sat on a cloth-covered table, clasping a small rubber ball between his chubby thighs. He laughed and giggled. The flash blinded him and he made a mean face. "Just like his father," Mary gibed. I was teasingly blamed for all of his "bad" behavior.

Jeff was a spirited, lively child once he got over colic. He was such a joy when he was feeling well. (But then, most everyone is.) When he got angry he would suck in his breath, puff himself up, turn red as a beet, clasp his fists at his sides and shake. "Just like his father," Margaret razzed. I enjoyed hearing the phrase, "Just like his father," although I never held my hands stiffly at my sides and shook.

Even Jeff's temper tantrums were cute, and ludicrous. We shared the same favorite word, ludicrous, and we gave it a clownish connotation. Actually, it was one of the few words he spoke. By the time he was two, when either of us tripped we'd laugh and say, "That was sure ludicrous, were you born yesterday?" He had a viable excuse.

Everything was cheerfully ludicrous, except the change in Mary after childbirth. I had never seen Mary violent and now she was spanking Jeff with a flyswatter and yelling at me. Often, I couldn't blame her for yelling at me.

I deserted them. We divorced.

I thank Cyndi and hang up the phone. I begin planning for the battle. The enemy is huge, shrewd and powerful. I must put the enemy at bay so I can use my nutritional expertise to help Jeff heal. The enemy - Jeff's body's enemy - is the medical profession's concepts and methods.

I get up, get dressed, eat and drive to a health food store to get the survival supplies I know I won't find in stores outside of California.[2]

I reach for a six-pound jar of unheated honey and place it in the hand basket. I know the glucose water that they are pumping into Jeff intravenously has no nutrients for healing. I know that his body is depleting the nutrients within himself, trying to heal. I've experienced that unheated honey has the nutrients to promote healing. I reach for another jar and a woman approaches me.

"Do you have a tribe of sweet tooths?" she flirts (or am I flattering myself?).

She is definitely attractive. Her upper lip is slightly larger than the lower and quivers sensuously, unconsciously, when she's quiet and curls when she speaks. What am I thinking about?! "Just two. My son and I."

"Oh... Have you been married long?"

Boy, is she fishing. I reach for a third jar and smile, "I'm divorced."

"Storing up for the fall and winter?" she asks merrily.

"I eat a jar or two a month."

"Aren't you afraid you'll get diabetes and your teeth'll rot?" she gasps.

Her persistence is charming, relaxing. "If I were to eat heated honeys I'd have diabetes again and dentures," I say.

"Well, whenever I ate Uncooked Raw honey it imbalanced my blood

---

2 *See* Appendix B, page 128.

sugar level. Like a roller coaster I was full of energy for an hour or two and then I was deep in depression or falling asleep," she says argumentatively.

Is she a lawyer? I want to turn this back into a conversation. "My name is Aajonus. Pronounced like homogeneous without the hum."

Caught off balance, she titters, "Aajonus? That's unusual. I'm Linda."

"That's not."

She finds it funnier than I do and laughs. She has a singer's airy rich laugh that makes us relax a bit more.

"I buy only honeys that are labeled 'Unheated', or that say something like 'We do not heat this honey in processing'. Honeys labeled 'Raw' or 'Uncooked' aren't the same," I clarify.

She furrows her brow and looks at me as if I were a simpleton. "What's the difference?" she asks.

I think of the many internal and external wounds I've seen heal rapidly with application and large consumption of unheated honeys. And how miraculously unheated honeys stimulate digestion. "Okay, honeys labeled 'Unheated' can't be heated over beehive temperature on a hot day - that's 92.8° Fahrenheit. On hot days, bees fan the honey with their wings to keep the honey temperature below 92.8° F. In the body, 80-90% of unheated honey turns into enzymes for digestion, assimilation and utilization. Whereas, honeys that are labeled 'Raw' or 'Uncooked' can be heated to 160° which they do to thin the honey for quicker filtering and bottling for more profits. 'Raw' or 'Uncooked' honeys mainly turn into radical blood sugar. 'Unheated' is the key word with honey. You can eat as much unheated honey as you want, as long as you have a taste for it."

"As one gets fatter and fatter," she scoffs.

"That depends on what you eat and what the honey helps you digest and utilize. There is nothing wrong with being fat as long as you are healthy. But do I look fat?"

"Your metabolism is different," she retorts.

"I used to get fat very easily and I would have to exercise four hours five days a week to stay as fit as I am now. I haven't exercised in seven years, so I can't take credit for my fitness. Except that I eat right for my body."

She looks at my naturally developed body disbelievingly.

"Linda, I have to go. I'll give you my card. I'll be tied up for a couple of weeks."

"Sounds like fun. Can I play, too?"

I must seem naïve because I'm turning red. I hand her my business card. She reads it and says, "Now I understand, you are a nutritionist."

"Yes. I've enjoyed talking with you but I must go, Linda. Bye."

"Bye..."

I walk over to the dairy section and remember that I'm supposed to speak at a group meeting tonight about my experience with cancer. I consider canceling as I place eight one-pound packages of unsalted certified raw butter in the basket. I decide to go to the meeting, so time will pass faster. The distraction could relieve some of my anxiety about not being able to get to Jeff sooner.

I glance over my shoulder and spot Linda watching me. As I walk past her she joins me.

"How much raw butter do you eat?"

I chuckle, "You don't want to know."

"Four tablespoons a day?"

"You asked for it. Eight to sixteen tablespoons a day."

She gives me an are-you-a-pathological-liar look and starts to say something but I intercede. "Like unheated honey, although the labeling requirements are different, 'Raw' butter hasn't been heated above a cow's normal body temperature. Raw fat, like raw butter, cleanses, lubricates, protects and fuels the body easily. Whereas heated and pasteurized fat often store as cellulite or other hard-to-use or non-utilizable waxy fat." I place the items on the checkout and pay. "Call me in a couple of weeks if you want to try my nutritional logic and see if it works for your body."

"I think you are out of your mind," she says utterly deadpan.

"Is that a compliment, Linda?"

Outside of the store, I punch in my voice-box number on the pay phone. It plays back a message, "Hi, sweetheart, I got your message about Jeff," Beatriz' voice says and pauses for the right words. "I'm sorry. Call me from Cincinnati and let me know how he is. I'll miss you. I love you. Bye."

2

I feel as if my muscles, like my thoughts, are stirred up. I can't sleep. I thank whoever invented flannel sheets. The softness feels comforting. The digital clock reads 1:02 a.m.

I rise and go to the kitchen. I pass by my packed luggage at the door. A tinge of fear rushes up my chest. The lonely luggage makes the unknown so foreboding.

I spread a slice of French bread with a 4 tablespoons of unsalted raw butter to calm me down while thoughts of Jeff keep coming.

It's been nine years since I've thought about Jeff this much. How little I know him. I left Mary for the second and last time a few months after Jeff's first birthday. For the next year, Jeff and I were together on Sundays, or for weekends.

I graduated from computer-programming trade school, and in September, two months after the divorce, I moved to Los Angeles to pursue a degree in architecture. I'll never forget the day before I left.

Jeff's second birthday was six days away. I had bought him a swing and slide set. Mary and Jeff were living with her parents in a two-bed-room house in a lower-middle-class neighborhood. Willy, Mary's father, and I were building the set in the backyard. Willy, or "Pawpaw" as Jeff called him, was about five-feet-four-inches tall with black hair receding on either side of his widow's peak. He was very shy, a gentle man. When he smiled with his large mouth, his head tilted shyly, playfully.

Jeff loved to swing and slide. He bounced, danced, laughed, shrieked and giggled around us because he couldn't wait for Willy and me to finish building the swing. Finally, when it was built, Willy, Margaret and I stood watching Mary swing Jeff. She pushed him too hard once and Jeff swung too high. His eyes opened wide, his arms stiffened, his hands gripped the chains tighter and his mouth made a donut shape. He lost his breath. When he swung back down he giggled, relieved he'd made it okay. He dragged his feet enough to slow himself down and took a deep breath.

"I guess that was too high for you, huh boogie?" Mary said.

Jeff nodded dramatically. He swung forward again and his mouth took on the donut shape fearing that he might sail too high. He didn't and he laughed. Mary did too. We all laughed. Mary and Jeff had similar mouths and they had the largest smiles, after Willy's. Once again I wanted to ask Mary to come with me to California but I knew she'd refuse. No one could guess which way I wanted things from one week to the next, especially me.

It came time to say good-byes and I stooped down to Jeff. "You're the man of the house now. You take care of Mommy, okay?"

"You be back, Daddy. Soon." He smiled real big.

"No, sweetheart, Daddy's going to the other side of the world, sort of. I'll only be able to see you about every six months or so. I'm going away to school in California."

He cried. I cried. Even Margaret cried. We all hugged and I left.

I didn't return for two years.

I rise from the dining table and return to the kitchen. I have a taste for something sweet. I get some unheated honey, fresh strawberries and cream to help my digestion and raise my blood sugar level to a happy balance. I take a drink of the raw cream, dip a strawberry in the honey and take a bite. I remember that Jeff and I had been together on only four separate occasions since the swing set and we rarely spoke on the phone.

I recall that the first of the four occasions was in August. Jeff was four. I had a form of leukemia called multiple myeloma (cancer of bone and blood).

I had already undergone surgery for an ulcer. Three months later I received radiation therapy because the scar was keloidal.[3] Four months after radiation I was diagnosed with leukemia. I was told that I would die by Christmas.

I was supposed to have begun chemotherapy that August. I postponed it until September because my family was having a reunion. I didn't want them to know about my illness because: back then most people were afraid that somehow cancer was catching like the Black Plague; Mom had a weak heart and had suffered a heart attack when I was ten or eleven (telling her I was dying could have killed her); and men in my family were expected to be strong and tough. Because I had always

---

[3] A keloid is an overgrowth of a scar, that is a fibrous tumor forming hard, irregular excrescence upon the skin.

been sickly, I put on a tough front.

The clan gathered in Cincinnati from all over the continental United States. I thought I was seeing everyone for the last time. I hid the radiation therapy burns under my clothes.

As I was driving to get Jeff to bring him to the reunion, I noticed a tall dark-haired father holding the hand of his golden-haired son. They walked along the sidewalk. Drops of joy filled my eyes because I would soon be holding Jeff's hand.

The father was a giant compared to his son but gentle. He carefully moved at the pace of the boy's little steps. I held back more tears. I thought red eyes would look unattractive and immature to Mary.

I arrived at the large apartment complex, parked and walked to Mary's apartment. She greeted me courteously. We both felt awkward. I was especially uncomfortable because I hadn't had enough time to adjust to the fact that Mary had remarried over a year ago. Mom wanted to protect me and had told me only a week ago. I blushed, facing Mary and thinking that several months ago I had asked her to move to Los Angeles so we could be together. Mary didn't tell me then she had remarried. I hid the pain, but, oh, God, I was wounded.

"Jeff'll be here any minute. He and Ben went for a walk," Mary said.

The door opened behind me and in walked the gentle giant and the golden-haired boy, Jeff.

"This is Ben," Mary smiled proudly introducing her husband, and Jeff's new father.

My heart sunk.

Ben must have been six-foot-four inches, dark, rugged-looking and very handsome. I felt like drab wallpaper.

Ben immediately let his head drop shyly, painfully. He left the room without a word. I could see the fear and hurt he felt with me coming to take Jeff for the day. Jeff called him Dad now. My presence was changing all of that. I felt like a schmuck.

"Do you remember him?" Mary asked Jeff as I crouched down to greet him.

Jeff's face winced as he tried to remember but didn't. I was crushed.

"Here is a change of shirt in case he makes a mess," Mary jested to break the awkward moment.

"No bag with diapers and bottles and all," I said playfully. I tried to appear unaffected.

"Yes, it's been a long time," she said somewhat scolding me.

But I could see she was relieved that Jeff didn't remember me. In my mind I could hear her telling Ben as soon as we walked out the door, "See? Jeff didn't even remember him." And knowing that Jeff's not-remembering me was going to mean some solace to Ben, gave me some solace.

At the reunion, I set Jeff free to play with several cousins, aunts and uncles. Then, when I thought I was emotionally detached enough, I played with him. We tossed a ball and frisbee. I tickled him. We giggled. I swung him around and laughed, until we were exhausted. It was time to drive him home but he wanted to stay. That made it a great day.

We parked in the lot outside Mary and Ben's apartment. Jeff wanted to get out with me on the driver's side. Just as he was about to put his arms around my neck for me to lift him, he said, "You helped Pawpaw put up my swing!" A wave of joy passed through me. He hugged me very tightly.

"It appears Jeff's head went partially through the driver's side of the windshield when his car flew down the ravine and hit a tree. The car spun and jolted him back inside. The car hit another tree and Jeff's head went through the passenger's side of the windshield. The car spun and hit the ground at the rear end, jolting him back into the front seat. Finally the car smashed into another tree on the passenger's side. His head went completely through the passenger's door window. His body was found draped over the car door," Mom's words echo in my head.

I lie down on the still warm flannel sheets. Will I be as unable to help Jeff as I was when he was an infant? Will I become hostile wanting to help but not knowing how? Will I be able to confront the medical professionals who'll think I'm a fanatic? Jeff is an accident victim! I haven't dealt with any serious accident victims. Yet, healing is healing, I remind myself. I know what the body needs to heal itself.

3

I'm in a tornado like Dorothy in "The Wizard Of Oz." Four doctors, who are circling around me, direct me to go with them. I sense I'll meet death. Their voices sound like the ringing of only one giant gong. The deep-echoing sound emanates from all four of their mouths, quadraphonically. It makes my heart pound until I think it'll burst from my chest. It's odd that the ringing doesn't disturb my ears and head, only my heart.

I refuse to go with the doctors. Suddenly they all wilt and die. I am happy I didn't go with them. But the ringing continues and my heart pounds. I become aware that the phone is ringing and I reach for it. I anticipate that the airline has an earlier flight. Then I realize it is already morning.

I lift the receiver. I remember my dream and the fear of death. I dread what the voice will say.

"Hello."

"This is your mother."

"Hi," my voice cracks.

"It's pouring here and I thought you should bring your boots and a raincoat. I have lots of umbrellas if you need one."

"Please! Mom, don't greet me with, 'This is your mother' ", I want to say. She seemed apprehensive, as if she were going to tell me Jeff is dead. It scared me! I take a deep breath and calm down.

I recall her umbrellas being flowered, bright and feminine. "Thanks, Mom, I'll bring a coat and my own umbrella." I take another deep breath, "Have you seen Jeff at all?"

"I'm waiting until you get here and we'll all go together. I called the hospital and talked with the head nurse. She said the doctors all agree his signs are worsening. Too much water has collected in his brain and there's no hope he'll pull through with this kind of brain damage." She takes a breath, "I just want you to be prepared. We'll see you this afternoon."

We say good-bye.

I have avoided Jeff since he was two-years-old. I have been afraid of getting attached and losing him again. Have I lost all chance to get to know him?

The alarm goes off and jolts me back to the physical world. I rise and go to the couch. I stretch and lean my head against the arm. I cross my feet tightly. I hug a pillow.

Okay, okay. Mom's a nurse. Like most nurses what she knows is what the doctors know. Whether from illness or injury, medical science believes that virus and germs, like bacteria cause disease. That is their "germ theory". They believe that germs are enemies of healing.

The standard approach is to attack virus and germs (bacteria and other microbes) with medical drugs and poisons to stop them. These drugs simultaneously attack, destroy and deteriorate the body. Drugs are like bombs, they most often kill, cripple, harm or destroy everything within their influence. They cause subtle or obvious mutations. The least harm that they do is create imbalances.

Medical science ignores that bacteria inspires healing and that drugs kill bacteria, and therefore, that drugs prevent healing.[4]

My approach is that bacteria, yeast, mold and virus are all part of a natural process for detoxification. Bacteria, yeast, mold and virus decompose body obstructions, such as dead or weak cells and tissue. When the body has too many obstructions, it has disease. The body encourages the detoxification process so it can cleanse itself of accumulated wastes that cause weaknesses, or damaged tissue in cases of injury. They also dissolve and eliminate foreign substances, like rust from taking iron supplements. That is, if the body is fed the proper nutrients during and after the detoxification processes.

For example, colds and flu are like changing the oil and flushing a car's radiator. If the body is allowed to take its course with colds and flu several times a year, or whenever necessary, an increase in health is the natural result. That is, if at the same time one feeds his or her body good nutrients. For instance, oranges and/or bananas blended with raw eggs, raw dairy fats and unheated honey; a smoothie. However, if these cleansing and renewing processes are interfered with or stopped by using medication, the body advances faster toward deterioration, aging and disease. I remind myself that instead of attacking the body, I

---

[4] *See* Appendix C, page 129.

nurture it.

I feel comforted that Jeff's doctors' prognosis isn't based on what I know. And that Jeff is still alive. I will work with Jeff's body to cleanse the dead and damaged tissues, and to regenerate new cells to replace them.

I am sitting at a window seat not far from first-class on this early morning flight to Cincinnati. I am facing the partition wall that separates the classes. It reminds me for a moment of the wailing wall in Israel. I feel a little claustrophobic. Will I celebrate life? Or will I be wailing for the dead? I have to stop thinking like that.

I feel excited by the gravitational pull as we climb. I notice outside the portal window that the smog isn't too bad on this golden sunlit Los Angeles morning. With amusement, I take it as a good omen. We loop over the Pacific Ocean. The plane levels off in the direction of our destination. The flight attendants push their carts down the aisles.

It's Saturday, four days from October, a time that marks a measurable decline of tourists in Los Angeles. The thought comes that I am a tourist visiting Earth. Whenever I talk to someone who doesn't know me about my view on health and my life-style, I'm considered bonkers.

I look around me and I see so much bodily suffering. I feel compassion for the people I see who aren't happy because they lack health. An unhappy-looking woman wheezes, then swallows three pills. At least seven people are already drinking or being served alcohol.

I recall when years ago I drank to relax and feel good. I couldn't go to sleep at night without drinking a bottle of bourbon or gin.

I was nineteen years old and had been living in Los Angeles six months. I was making good money. I yearned for Mary and Jeff, even though I knew I was too emotionally distorted to make family life work to anyone's benefit. So I partied a lot and enjoyed freedom from all responsibilities except work and child support. I wouldn't admit alcohol was affecting my work and studies and I ignored the symptoms that it was hurting my body. It relaxed my memories and guilt.

I think about Jeff being in the hospital and I recall my advent into cancer. It was a Sunday night in March, one month from my twentieth birthday. I had just returned from a weekend in Tijuana, Mexico, with friends. I was dizzy from drink. I stood over my toilet to urinate. I became dizzier and nauseous. As I collapsed to my knees I whacked my penis on the cold porcelain (I remember I had been accident prone as a child). A surge from my stomach curled my body and put my face in the toilet. Blood trailed with the vomit.

The doctor pointed to a very dark spot on my X-ray, "It's probably only an ulcer. You're too young and strong to have cancer."

"Don't let looks fool you. How do we find out?"

"It's an ulcer," he decided, "and we'll treat it."

After six months of drinking bottle after bottle of Maalox, I decided I should have stock in pharmaceuticals. Instead of being addicted to alcohol I was addicted to chalky Maalox. Maalox didn't have the good taste and didn't give me the feeling that alcohol did. I was sure that if I died a chalk factory would make a fortune with my remains.

In November, I was looking upward from an operating table. The ceiling was blurred and I was becoming unconscious from anesthetic, going into surgery to remedy my stomach ulcer. After "recovering enough" from surgery (the doctors had said), I received radiation therapy for five or six...or was it ten weeks. (My memory went into a slump during my year of cancer therapies and has never fully recovered.)

After returning from the August family reunion, I underwent chemotherapy for leukemia for my blood and bone cancers. With each chemo session I got sicker. Finally, after three months of the treatments I wouldn't tolerate it. That was eighteen years ago. I was only twenty-one but I remember as if it were yesterday.

"The cancer's not responding to the chemotherapy either. We'll try again in three weeks," Dr. Goldman said matter-of-factly.

"Doctor, I seem to be missing the point here. Let's retrace what's happened to me. I had a stomach ulcer. I had surgery to correct it. As a result of the surgery, I haven't been able to digest anything very well. Food seems to just sit in my digestive tract. I have lost my sexual drive. If I happen to have an orgasm it can be extremely painful. How in the world was my penis effected by stomach surgery?"

"I don't know," he said.

I thought for a moment and then continued, "I have terrible acne (the one common problem I have never had before). My waist line has gone from twenty-eight to thirty-four inches. And I have redeveloped very painful muscle spasms around my heart.

"Then I had radiation therapy to stop the keloidal tissue from growing. As a result of the radiation, I have burns that are mainly scar tissue. My spine is cauterized and I can barely turn to either side and I am always painful. I now have psoriasis and bursitis. I have inflamed, sore and bleeding gums. I have come down with chronic weakness, exhaustion and joint pains. I couldn't, and still can't even lift a large dictionary with my right arm because my shoulder and elbow ache so badly. My knees ache, too. They are always cold and numb--"

"We'll continue the treatments because there's always a chance we can stop the cancer from doing any more damage," he said.

"Please, listen, I'm leading to something. Then I was diagnosed with cancer of the blood and bones. I am receiving chemotherapy. As a result, I'm as pale as a ghost. I vomit no matter what I try to eat. I can't be away from a toilet for five minutes without a diaper. I'm bloated from head to toe. My acne is so bad that a film-director friend described my face as looking like raw hamburger. I have only a few sparse patches of hair and it's graying like I'm an old man. My teeth are rotting. My diabetes is worse. Homicidal and suicidal thoughts plague me--"

"Your anxiety and anger are side effects of the chemotherapy. It's normal," he interjects.

"Normal? Yesterday, I heard one of the biology professors say that radiation, especially radiation therapy, transforms certain body substances into toxins that are cancer-causing. Why would you treat keloidal tissue with a treatment that causes cancer?"

"It's like fighting fire with fire," he said smiling.

"Isn't that like burning down the forest to save the forest?"

"There is no other way to stop the formation of keloidal tissue or cancer. Disease is not nice, you can't treat it nicely," he argued.

"I also heard the professor say that for every one cancer cell that chemotherapy kills, at least one billion healthy cells are killed. I thought about that statistic and derived this analogy: If four humans were declared cancerous to the human race, the medical profession would be willing to kill four billion people - the entire population on Earth - in order to destroy only three or four individuals. That's an extreme and barbaric perspective, don't you think?"

"I'm trying to give you more time to live," he said, annoyed.

"Doctor, as a result, I have cancer. I didn't have cancer before receiving the cancer-causing therapies. I merely had an ulcer. I feel like the walking dead. Food doesn't taste good. Nothing pleases me anymore. Why didn't you tell me my quality of life and disposition would be miserable; that I'd be a semi-invalid as a side effect of the treatments? Why didn't you stress that the side effects would be a hundred times worse than cancer when you frightened me into taking your therapies? And now I'm going to die anyway."

"I'm sorry. It isn't possible to predict how anyone will react," he said belligerently.

"That doesn't make sense. Yesterday I studied the side effects in the Physician's Desk Reference and books on radiation research. All of mine and a hundred more side effects are listed. You never showed me any list. And the Physicians Desk Reference is right there on your shelf. Do you admit that the radiation treatment for keloidal tissue gave me blood and bone cancer?"

"Look, there's still a small chance that your cancer will respond to the chemotherapy."

"Did you hear what I just said?"

"I know how you must feel," he said.

Finally I realized that medical methods are barbaric. Surgery is butchering. Radiation is burning. Chemotherapy is poisoning. Why didn't it dawn on me before?

"Doctor, have you ever been cut and burned and poisoned to help you get well from cancer?"

"No."

I threatened to sue because the doctors didn't tell me that the therapies would kill much more of me than would any cancer. I would have taken my chances with cancer. Several attorneys said the doctors would all testify that I was dying anyway and that I had signed a release. How can they get away with that?! I wondered.

One month later, I discovered several successful alternative methods for healing cancer. All of them were pleasant by comparison. But because the doctors had said all the alternatives were hoaxes, I hadn't bothered to investigate them.

Education, religion, the media and government taught me to revere doctors. The doctors could deceive and frighten me, slowly and painfully kill me, get paid handsomely for it and go to heaven for "good" intent. It didn't make any sense.

Because I was left disabled, I couldn't afford child support. Ben adopted Jeff.

"Please fasten your seat belts. We are beginning our descent to Cincinnati Airport. Thank you for joining us and we hope__"

I ignore the pilot as I look over the rain-glistening, rich green landscape of Kentucky. I wonder why it is called the Greater Cincinnati Airport when it's across the river at Stringtown, Kentucky. I suppose that if it were named the Stringtown Airport no one would ever fly there.

The sun emerges through the passing rain clouds.

I'm so close to Jeff, a tingling rushes over my heart and into my spine.

4

Saturday afternoon, September 27th

I see Mom and Dad smiling, standing just beyond the crowd as I follow the procession through the terminal gate. Ever since Mom and Dad stopped worrying and began trusting me to make the right decisions for myself, I have been relaxed and happy to see them.

I'm surprised at how much they have aged since I saw them two years ago. Or does it seem more so because most of the people I see regularly are more or less on my type of diet? Raw diets slow down the normal aging process or reverse it altogether. (Gad, I wonder, would that have sounded pompous to anyone who hadn't experienced it?)

Or do Mom and Dad look older because I have been reliving my past and remembering them much younger?

Dad looks - and always has looked - inherently physically stronger than Mom. I imagine him as a child on the dairy farm where he grew healthfully with fresh food, raw dairy products and hard work. He is definitely healthier than his father, who was raised in Brooklyn in the mid 1800's when it was difficult to get fresh foods in large cities. Grandfather suffered crippling arthritis and strokes, and died in his sixties.

Amazingly, Mom's wearing slacks. This is the first time she's greeted me informally at an airport. I'm delighted she feels that relaxed. Looking into her eyes, I realize she has always had a stronger balanced will and more self-esteem than Dad. I deduce that's because, as a girl, she successfully raised six of her twelve brothers and sisters while Viola, her mother, tended their drugstore where Mom's father was the pharmacist.

Mom and I embrace and her hand automatically pats my back. I recall being an infant receiving that caring touch. Her perfume hides the nice smell of her body that I remember loving as an infant. Her salt-and-pepper Orphan Annie hair tickles the side of my face and I giggle. The hug ends and I become an adult again, instantly.

I turn to Dad and see that his wavy gray hair still has a trace of black remaining. Apart from his large stomach he looks fitter than most of his peers. We hug and his squeeze feels encouraging, different from when I was a child. But, then, I can't remember him hugging me after I was three. I was probably somewhat of an embarrassment to him. I think the first time he was unforgettably impressed with me was six years ago. He watched me give an eight-hour seminar on nutrition.

As we drive by downtown Cincinnati nothing looks familiar to me. I try to keep my mind from anxious thoughts about Jeff. I notice autumn settling in. The leaves are turning.

Ten miles farther, we pass the exit that would have taken us to Finneytown. I lived there from ages seven through eighteen.

I remember how grueling the cold weather was on me here. Like a hibernating bear, I would have slept through it if I could have. When I got a cold or flu, it lasted one to three months. Daily, I would fill two to five handkerchiefs until they were sopping wet. They made my pockets wet and me colder.

I realize how much I enjoy cold weather now that I am healthy. And when I get a cold or flu, it lasts only thirty minutes to three days.

"Is there a health food store on the way to the hospital?" I ask. "I'd like to buy some eggs, papayas and bananas."

"I don't know if they carry eggs," Mom says apologetically.

"Could we stop and see, please?"

"Sure," Dad encourages.

We do. They have eggs and the fruit I need.

Mom points to Mercy Hospital. It's a small modern four-story building alone near the top of a green rolling hill. We pull into the parking lot. In a matter of moments we will be facing Jeff. I seem to be ready for the battle ahead. Surprisingly, I feel calm and strong. Maybe it is my years. Also, because I no longer see doctors as my enemy. Doctors have not had power over my mind and body for one and a half decades. But they see Jeff's body as a battle ground. They are attacking it. I will defend him.

It dawns on me that Jeff is Mom and Dad's first grandchild. I look at them and they look rigid, like foot soldiers wearing armor. They are protecting their feelings. I wonder if my wisdom and strength are enough to protect mine.

I leave my blender and food in the car and we walk toward the hospital. The smell of wet grass and drying pavement remind me of the damp day I entered a hospital for my first traumatic stay. A chill passes through me.

It was early spring, the week before my twelfth birthday. I had had a near fatal reaction to my final polio vaccine.[5] The vaccine caused an acute intestinal infection, "deadly" peritonitis. The doctors misdiagnosed my condition as appendicitis. I underwent emergency surgery. The doctors found my appendix normal. They removed it anyway. "In case it would cause you problems in the future," the doctor said.

Now was the third night after my appendectomy. The doctors hadn't properly diagnosed my problem. They never did. I still had fevers of 104-106°. They packed me in ice - an agonizing process - to bring down the fever and prevent brain damage. I was in tremendous pain from the shots I received every three hours for infection or pain. Already I had had eight shots in each arm, seven high in the left gluteus maximus and

[5] *See* Appendix D, page 132.

eight high in the right.

I was sore on all sides. My front had surgery soreness and peritoneal pain. My left, right and back sides had the injection soreness. I wasn't able to lie on any side without severe pain. I couldn't sleep more than fifteen minutes before the pained area exceeded the painkiller's influence. I had to turn onto another side. My sleep was irregular and sparse. There was no escaping pain or the hospital.

It was 10 p.m. when the nurse entered with her tray and needle. She rolled me on to my right side. It hurt and I screamed. I pleaded for her not to inject me again.

"It's for your own good," she preached and scolded.

I watched the needle coming toward my bottom. I used every measure of energy I had to turn and knock the syringe out of her hand. The syringe hurled through space twisting and turning as if in slow motion. In my imagination I heard a wonderful crescendo of music. The nurse lifted the syringe, wiped the floor and left. I fell asleep only slightly more relaxed.

In deep sleep my hip began to burn and cramp. I remember thinking, I am not sleeping on my back, nor on that hip, why is there that much pain? The pain increased.

I woke and felt the last fluid of an injection entering my hip. I cried, "The medicines aren't working! You're killing me! You're making the pain worse and worse." The nurse gave me a disbelieving smile. She proudly put the needle back on the tray. I remember how amazed I was that this Florence Nightingale could be so proud of her insensitivity and ignorance.

"Have a nice night," the nurse said and walked out.

If I had had the strength at that moment to kill her, I probably would have. I wanted to. But instead I lay there crippled by pain. I cried for two and a half hours. I fell unconscious from pain.

In the morning I gave the doctors and nurses such a conniption that they didn't give me any more medication. Consequently, I got the sleep I needed. I faked being well enough for 24 hours. They let me go home the next morning.

Mom, Dad and I reach the elevator. It opens as if waiting for us. We enter and Mom pushes the third-floor button. We don't look at each other or say anything as it ascends. With the motion of the elevator I drift back into my experience in the hospital when I was twelve.

An intern stood towering over me. His manner was impatient and gruff. We had gotten off to a bad start two days earlier. He had asked if I had been farting. Since my puritan upbringing had taught me that the word fart was taboo, I was shocked to hear it come from a doctor. I stuttered and without judgment I asked if he meant did I pass gas. He thought I was a snob and turned malicious. I was afraid to try and rectify the misunderstanding because of autism and my experience that doing so merely compounded resentment.

"Sit up," he ordered like a sergeant.

I moaned in pain as I sat up very slowly.

"Don't pull that sympathy trick on me. I've seen too many appendectomies. I know the pain doesn't last more than a day and a half after surgery. You've been pulling this for four days now."

He pushed hard on my lower abdomen. I screamed in pain.

He smiled and said, "Look. Your buddy over here came in two days after you. He was up and running around the day after his appendectomy. He doesn't scream when I push on his stomach. And he's going home today too."

"I can't help it, it hurts. Even when I move."

It only made him angrier. He took my right arm which had the I.V. needle inserted in it. He gently pulled one end of each of the four strips of tape that held the needle in my arm. He took firm grip on those ends, looked me in the eyes, smiled, and ripped the tape from my arm. The roundness of the needle pulled my flesh until the force tore my skin. I cried.

"You act like a girl," he said.

I intuitively knew he wouldn't hurt me more, so I continued crying to release the pain and frustration while he put gauze and tape over the bleeding gouge to stop it. Two hours later I was out of the hospital and on my way home.

The elevator stopping sends a wave through my stomach. We step from the elevator and Mom leads the way toward Jeff. I feel nauseous. My heart misses a beat and then speeds up, pounding.

The halls are empty, except for a couple of staff personnel. We pass many doors. Only a few patients have visitors. The patients are all connected to machines. Of course this wing is eerie, I realize, this is intensive care, numb skull.

"Numb skull"? I haven't used that term in ages. Numb skull was something my parents called me. And probably what their parents called them. It never did help my self-esteem. Strange how old patterns surface when I'm back here.

Mom stops at room 317. Jeff is steps away. For the first time I visualize his cuts and bruises. I see him thrust and banged around inside the car. My adrenaline rushes. My heart pounds like a great symphonic drum sounding the battle charge. I take a slow deep breath and enter the room after Mom. I wonder if it would have been polite to enter before her.

We pass through a small dressing room-like foyer. It has a large picture window fixed with lavender Venetian mini-blinds. This is the room where loved ones wait and watch while emergency personnel work. This will be my supply room. On the wall is a locked medicine compartment. There is a counter and sink where I can put my blender to make food formulas for Jeff when he recovers from the coma. Am I deluding myself?

I see the end of the bed, the shape of Jeff's feet and legs under the covers. My blood rushes faster as the drumming of my heart pounds harder, louder and faster.

I see Jeff's arms and hands taped to boards so he can't bend them. Tubes run everywhere. A catheter empties his urine into a plastic container. An I.V. drips sugar water and chemicals into his right forearm.

I feel queasy. I want to stop for a moment to settle down. I keep trooping behind Mom. I remember Jeff's face from the last time I saw him when he was eighteen. His smile was big and his complexion ruddy.

The image disappears when I see two machines monitoring his body. Mary stands on one side of the bed, at the head, facing me. A nurse stands opposite her, obstructing my view of Jeff's face. They lean over him.

Now I see his chin. His mouth gapes open. His lips are gray-purple. Oh, my God, he looks dead. Oxygen tubes are strapped to his head and up the nostrils. His eyes are closed and recessed in unconsciousness. His skin looks waxy, ashen except where tubes enter his body, irritating him. Cuts spot his face. A long cut streaks his forehead. Another parts an eyebrow. The abrasions from the plunges through glass are swollen and inflamed.

I take it all in for a minute. I use positive thoughts to settle myself. I think: Jeff's not missing part of his head, brain or limbs. I'm thankful for that. My heart continues to drum frantically. I wish other instruments would join in so no one would hear it. It could expose my sensitivity. I want to look totally in control. The enemy will know that I'm not as strong as I want to be.

"Jeff! Wake up, Jeff! You've been asleep for six days now, wake up. Your mother wants to talk to you," the nurse shouts as if Jeff were deaf.

I guess she wants to shock him from his coma. Okay, I guess, if it works. But it doesn't. Jeff's head seems to roll slightly as if he were trying to tell her that her shouting hurts. Or is that my wishful thinking?

"Six days?" I whisper to Mom.

"Mary didn't call me until the night before I called you. You weren't home and I didn't want to leave that message on your answering machine," she says firmly.

"Why did she wait to call you?" I ask with a trace of anger. Fortunately, Mom does not take it personally.

"She figured there was nothing we could do. When they told her Jeff was definitely going to die, she called."

I wonder why Mary still hates me after twenty years.

"Jeff! Wake up!" screams the nurse.

He gives no response. I sense his coma is partially from medication. I know the shouting must hurt Jeff's ears. It hurts my ears and I'm eight feet away. I want to grab the nurse and scream in her ear to stop it. I feel helpless.

"Jeff! It's Mom. Wake up," Mary mimics the nurse but not nearly as loudly.

I look at Mary. She would not be considered cover-girl material but she still looks beautiful to me. She wears jeans and a plaid blouse. I realize I'm still attracted to her. I see she is strong-willed like Mom and compassionate.

"Hi, Mary," I say gently.

She gazes a moment, gropes and finally wields to our presence. She turns and looks over at Mom and says, "Hi, Doris," and then to Dad,

"Josef."

Finally, she manages to look straight into my blue eyes.

"Hi, Dick."

Oh, that nickname. All the reasons I changed to a Greece-Roman-sounding first name that I liked, flood my head. No matter how "Dick" was said to me, the innuendo was prevalent. It was like wearing a bright name tag with "scum" printed on it. My brothers, classmates, and some teachers often used it to patronize me.

"As you can see, Jeff isn't with us," Mary says bluntly.

I see the strain in her face and body. I want to hug and comfort her but that is out of the question. Instead, empathic tears fill my eyes. Seventeen years passed before I stopped dreaming about her.

Mary turns to Jeff. "Dick is here to see you. Wake up, boy," she says, trying to humor and ease her new tension because of my presence.

Oh, geezus , I'm going to break down.

"Jeff. Jeff, it's Aajonus," I say softly. My voice cracks.

He doesn't move.

"May I see his charts, please," I politely ask the nurse.

She is stunned and then derisive, "Are you a visiting doctor?"

Mary chortles and jokes, "No. He's from Los Angeleees, California." She gives it the sneering tone that she gave the nickname Dick.

The nurse chuckles, then settles, confused.

"This is Jeff's other father," Mary explains.

The nurse and I introduce ourselves.

"When is the soonest I can see Jeff's X-rays?" I ask kindly.

"You'll have to speak to one of his neurologists."

"How many does he have?"

"Four."

"Lead me to one of them."

"Dr. Braisley just left the floor and none of the others are expected until morning."

"Can we talk in the hall a minute, please?"

She scrutinizes my patient but determined stare. She realizes I could be trouble. She turns and we walk into the hall.

"Debra, I'm not here to make your job difficult. I'm here because my son is dying. I want to do everything I can to help him live."

"Are you a physician?"

My inclination is to mimic her patronizing attitude but that wouldn't be constructive, "I'm a nutritional counselor. And I'm Jeff's biological father. I have the right to see all of his records upon request. Would you be kind enough to make that as easy and as soon as possible? Please?"

"I can't do that. One of his doctors has to, and I don't know if Dr. Braisley is still on rounds," she says in a friendlier tone. "You'll have to wait until morning. Okay?"

"Would you give me his number, please? I'll have his answering service page him and have him call me here."

"I'll call his service," she relinquishes.

"One more thing? When he calls and you tell him my request, if he refuses please tell him I would like to speak with him. Will you do that for me and my son? Please?"

She relaxes, shrugs and snickers, "Okay, sir."

"Thank you. And would you pass the word to all the doctors and nurses that Jeff's biological father is here, that I will be taking an active part in his recovery?"

She is slightly impressed and amused but her reaction says she thinks my ego is larger than my brain. There are times when I would agree, but ego has nothing to do with this.

"The doctors all agree that Jeff isn't going to--" Compassion, I think, restrains her from finishing.

5

Finally, Mary and I are alone with Jeff. We ease into light conversation for a while. I mention that I am a nutritional counselor. I say a little about my nutritional point of view. I ask her if she would like to care for Jeff at home. She gives me a look of astonishment and absurdity. She tells me she wouldn't even consider removing Jeff from the hospital. She vacuums the mucus oozing into Jeff's throat so he can breathe without choking.

"The mucus is good. Through it, his body dumps dead cells and debris from the brain quickly. More will go to his bowels and dump there," I say.

"How do you know all of that stuff?"

"Remember when I said I was disabled from a car accident and couldn't pay child support? I had cancer. I didn't want anyone to know. I was disabled from the therapies. A kind, wonderful and intelligent man named Bruno tutored me for three and a half years in nutrition. I've spent most of the last seventeen years researching and experimenting with diets and health."

She frowns and looks at me curiously.

"I'll tell you about it later. Did all of the doctors tell you that Jeff's going to die?"

Mary nods, "They said if he hadn't responded by Wednesday, he'd die any time soon."

"I know you think I'm a California nut cake, but I'm asking you to put that judgment aside for Jeff's sake. Let me try nutrition."

"I know you mean well, Aajonus." She stops to take a deep breath, drained, then teases, "But he's not exactly able to eat."

"We can feed him under his tongue," I say handing her a canning jar. In it are equal portions of unsalted raw butter and unheated honey mixed together.

I explain its properties and I conclude by saying, "His salivary enzymes will dissolve it. Some will be absorbed directly into his blood through his mouth. The rest will drain down, soothe his throat and eventually, his stomach. In the blood, the nutrients from the butter/honey mix will go to his brain to protect living tissue and carry away the bruised and dead for elimination. I would like to put a teaspoon under his tongue at least every forty minutes."

A little hope sprouts and gives her strength. "Okay. If you think it'll help."

I am astounded. And relieved. Happy tears fill my eyes. I hold back though. Mary might think I'm weak. I must appear in complete control to defend Jeff.

I put some honey/butter mix under Jeff's tongue. I ask Mary if I may tell her about some of my nutritional work so she will know my perspective on nutrition versus medical methods.

"It beats just sitting here," Mary says.

"One day I arrived home at 9:30 p.m. from one of those exciting evenings in traffic school."

Mary chuckles, "Still speeding?"

"U-turn. I couldn't seem to comprehend that a residential-apartment-complex neighborhood was not a residential area. Anyway, it was a Tuesday in January, 1973. I was twenty-six at the time.

> I walked through the courtyard toward my Hollywood apartment. There were no lights on in the apartment. I wondered where Monica was. I took my keys from my flared-bottom jeans. I inserted one in the lock. My neighbor, Lien, heard me and came bursting from her apartment. She was panting, not from hurry but horror.
>
> "Aajonus! I took Monica to County General Hospital about two hours ago. She was having terrible stomach cramps. She came crawling over to my door, screaming. I, we, just panicked. I took her to Emergency."
>
> "She didn't say anything about her stomach four hours ago. What is it?"
>
> "They said it would take a while to do all the tests. But they thought it was appendicitis."
>
> I felt panicked. But I concealed it.
>
> Monica was still in Emergency when I arrived. I was relieved that she was not on an operating table. She laid on a gurney looking drugged and in pain. The doctor stood analyzing the lab reports.
>
> "Monica," I teased, imitating Bell Lagosi portraying Count Dracula, "let me take care of you at home, my dear. Your body probably won't like the chemicals they'll pump into--"
>
> "They haven't found out what it is for sure," she said, cutting me off.

The doctor stepped toward us and said, "If you're not a relative, please leave. Monica, you have peritonitis, which means that your intestines are infected, and possibly perforated and bleeding. It's serious."

"Excuse me?" I said. I feel badly about it now but I had little patience with doctors' scare tactics after my experiences. I mirrored his arrogant, patronizing attitude, and asked him, "Have you every had peritonitis?"

"No," he said as if my question were absurd.

"I have. Would that make me more knowledgeable?"

"I've treated forty cases of peritonitis and if she leaves she'll die," he asserted.

"How many of those forty patients died?" I asked.

The doctor stammered but quickly recovered, "Twenty-four."

I motioned for Monica to listen.

"So at worst Monica has a 60% chance of dying in here, is that right?"

The doctor nodded.

"That's something they won't normally tell you," I said to Monica.

"Without treatment she has no chance," he countered.

"How many cases do you know in which someone had peritonitis and treated it with wholistic methods?"

"None," he said firmly.

"Then how would you know that she would die without medical treatment?" I asked, putting him in checkmate.

"Common sense," he retorted.

"Do only doctors have this common sense?"

"These are ridiculous questions. If you knew the seriousness of this infection, you would be embarrassed."

"Excuse me? Which of the two of us had peritonitis?" I asked.

"I'm not answering any more of your questions." He turned to Monica, "Are you going to listen to this character and put your life in danger? Or do you have some sense?"

"Monica, he's trying to play you like an untuned piano inside a yoyo."

Mary laughs, "Did you really say that?!"

"Yes. Monica laughed but the doctor didn't. Then I said to Monica:

"According to R.B. Pearson's research and statistics listed in his book *Man's Correct Diet*, you have a 93% chance of living if you let me care for you nutritionally. Come on, honey, let's go home." I turned back to the doctor and said, "I'm sorry. I know you mean well but your logic is off."

Urgently, he raised his voice, "Don't you get it? If the infection isn't stopped she'll die."

Monica's drug-intoxicated state had the side effect of lowering her blood pressure and heightening paranoia. She was terrified. She looked back and forth between the doctor and me.

"Sweetheart, listen to his reasoning. He's going to treat you with antibiotics to kill the infection. That will also kill your intestinal flora. That will destroy your ability to digest food and synthesize your own proteins and B vitamins. If you can't properly digest the nutrients you need, you won't detoxify and heal properly."

"I'm warning you, if you don't stay here and stop the infection you'll die for certain," the doctor countered.

I wanted to suture his mouth. And I'm sure he wanted to suture mine. The fear on Monica's face advertised that the doctor's unsubstantiated scare tactics had won the debate. I was saddened. I was angry. But I decided that I should argue no further. I had been introduced to an ideal concept called unconditional love a few years ago. It meant respecting Monica's decision even if her life were at risk. It was her life and her will be done.

Twenty-four hours later, I stood looking down at her. On her arms and thighs were badly bruised dome-shaped swellings the size of quartered tennis balls.

"Monica, please take a look at the blackness around your sunken eyes, and your sallow complexion. They treat you not knowing how you'll react to chemicals," I cried out.

Drugged, she looked in a hand mirror and laughed, "Don't be silly. It's okay. I'm okay, really. I love you too."

I couldn't bear looking at her in that state and keep my mouth shut. I drove home.

The next morning she had two more bruised swellings on her

arms. Dr. Pine, the young intern assigned to her, looked over her chart.

"Doctor," I said gently, "Monica needs live nutrients including various strains of lactobacillus to aid her digestion. I'm going to take her home where I can feed her properly."

He shook his head and gave me a look that said, Oh, you're one of those misguided health fanatics. Then he said aloud, "Eating will exacerbate the infection. I'll give her a prescription for all the vitamins and minerals to be added to her I.V. Don't worry, we're taking good care of Monica."

"Why does she have these lumps and bruises all over her body?" I pleaded, and then added, "They aren't healing. They're getting worse by the hour."

"She was allergic to penicillin and three other antibiotics," he said.

"It took you seven shots to discover one she was not allergic to?"

"Yes."

"You just said not to worry, you are taking good care of her?"

"Now everything is under control."

"She has a hundred times more ailments to heal than when she came in here. Why are you saying you have everything under control?"

"Everything is okay now. I'll put the vitamins in her I.V. and she'll be fine," he said testily.

"She's betting her life on your expertise. Will you bet your expertise on her life?"

"We'll do the best we can for her. We can't promise anything," he said.

"Doctor, please, you just said you had everything under control now. Why won't you put your expertise on her life? I'll put my wholistic logic on her life. I'll even put my life on her life. Why won't you?"

"We're not miracle workers. Will you excuse me, I have many patients in this hospital who need my help," he said unnerved and briskly walked out.

I tried to convince Monica to leave but she was too intoxicated and drowsy.

In the evening of Monica's fifth day in the hospital, I stood over her. Her entire body was sallow with areas of black and blue. She had a milky stare that I had seen in animals just before they died. I realized I had to act.

"Monica," I pleaded, "you have to get hold of yourself. You have to become sober so you can examine yourself."

She was so drugged she didn't care.

"You have to refuse your sedatives and painkillers so you can make a clear decision about whether you are being helped or damaged. The nurse is due to give you your 8 o'clock shot. Refuse it, please. Just until the doctors get here in the morning. Please, baby, please."

She smiled. I placed in her hand a jar full of liquefied raw foods.

"This will aid and soothe your intestines," I said.

"What is it?" she whispered.

"I blended one raw fertile egg, one tomato, 2 tablespoons unsalted raw butter and two heaping tablespoons of unheated honey. It also regulates fever."[6]

"It doesn't sound very tasty," she whispered.

"Will you give it a chance?"

She sipped it. Then, I guess because it was the first food she had in days, she gulped it. My immediate thought was to stop her. But her gulping was instinctual.

I put the empty jar back in a bag. When I looked again, she was asleep. I stared at her frightful appearance. I remembered how beautiful her blushing color and pretty skin had been.

An hour passed and the raw tomato/butter formula had sobered her enough. She argued with the nurses against taking any more medication that night. And she won.

The next morning, I said to Monica, "Sweetheart, look at yourself." I pulled the covers down to her ankles and lifted her gown.

She looked at herself in horror, "Oh, my God, I'm going to die."

"Not if you let me take care of you." I wondered how I knew that.

"I'm scared, Aajonus."

---

[6] *See* Appendix E, page 137.

"I'm afraid, too. Yet, I'm certain that excellent health and raw (live) foods are as connected as falling and gravity. The doctor said if you ate anything it would make you worse. Your abdomen didn't swell and bruise from the raw food mixture. It has given you strength. God, I love you Monica. Don't die on me, please. Please let me help you?"

I explained the three different food formulas I devised to get her well.[7]

"Did you marry her?" Mary asks.

"No. We were together five years."

"Haven't you found anyone you wanted to marry?"

"It took me seventeen years to stop dreaming about you. How could I have stayed married while dreaming of you?" It's an awkward moment for both of us. I continue the story.

Monica agreed to go home. I gave her another jar of the tomato and butter mixture to drink. I went to the nurses and asked them to remove Monica's I.V. and catheter. They refused.

While I analyze how to remove Monica's catheter, three security guards, two nurses and three large male orderlies hurried into the room, stopped abruptly and stood watching me. If I had caught it on film it would have looked like one of those old black-and-white Buster Keaton films with that sudden stop-and-go motion. I covered Monica. Immediately following came three doctors with the same comical go-and-stop motion. One of them was the intern, Dr. Pine.

With the humor inspired by the moment I turned to Monica, "They're having a going away party for you. Isn't that sweet?"

"She can't leave here. I won't release her," said Dr. Pine.

The gall these guys have is amazing, I thought. I laughed, a short breathy laugh that was enough to insult him. That was not my intention but it happened.

I turned to Monica again, "Do you want his permission to go?" I knew I was irritating the doctor. I had mixed feelings about it. I

---

7 *See* Appendix F, page 138.

was still angry at doctors, in general.

"She can't leave this hospital unless I release her. And I won't." He turned to a nurse, "Call her mother right away."

"Dr. Pine. You've been really kind, and thank you. I'm leaving here now. So, if you don't remove this tube for me, Aajonus will," Monica said so diplomatically and maturely she seemed like a wise old empress.

Her manner affected everyone. They all turned to Dr. Pine. He seemed alarmed that his authority was being challenged.

"I won't release you. I won't be responsible for whatever happens if you leave this hospital," he said.

"I accept what you say. Now will you, or a nurse help me remove this, please?" Monica firmly implored.

Again everyone looked at Dr. Pine. He stood there staunchly.

"Help me, Aajonus," she ordered.

I pulled down Monica's covers. I looked around at everyone, "This is not a show." I started to lift Monica's gown but Dr. Pine stopped me, "Wait. A nurse will remove it. Let's talk about this. This is a life and death infection. Do you think some voodoo will save her?"

"Whoa," I said. "You thought throwing vitamins and minerals into her I.V. would help. It didn't. We will cure her with foods. That's all I have to say. If at some time in the future you are interested in what I feed Monica, I'll gladly tell you. Thank you."

Just then a nurse returned and blurted out, "Her mother says she is not to leave this hospital."

Her mother's voice rang through my head. I dreaded her intervention.

"Do I look underage, Dr. Pine?" Monica said growing angry.

Her mother's order had the opposite effect of what I had feared.

"Monica," Dr. Pine paused, "Please, take a few prescriptions I'll write for you."

Monica and I simultaneously raised our surprised eyebrows at each other; the fascist air had thinned.

"Give me whatever you want me to take," she said.

"You must take an antibiotic to kill the infection or you won't have a chance. I'll give you a painkiller to take as you need. Call me here everyday between nine and two and I'll do whatever I can to help."

The tension was still so high that the phone ringing startled all of us. Monica looked at me. We knew who it was.

"Hi, Mom. I'm just about to leave the hospital. Call me at home in about an hour, okay? I'm walking out the door, call me at home," Monica said.

She looked at me. She curled and twisted her smiling mouth, warning me. She tried to hand me the phone. Exaggeratedly, I shook my head and waved no. Monica laughed the way she did when I had been unintentionally acting silly.

"It'll be easier on all of us later if you can make some sense to her now," Monica said still laughing.

I was amazed at how much energy she had gained from the last tomato and butter drink. Reluctantly, I took the phone, "Hi, Ruth." Monica's divorced mother insisted I call her Ruth. It seemed to remove the generation gap. I liked that and we liked each other.

"It's you forcing Monica to leave the hospital, isn't it?"

"I've only fastened a chain from my car to her ankle."

"This is not funny."

"Ruth. You've seen Monica's condition since she's been in here. I'm certain she'll do better at home."

"The nurse said she'd die if she leaves the hospital." Ruth's blood pressure was rising.

"What would they say if she died in the hospital? 'The treatment was a success, we stopped the infection. We're sorry Monica's dead, and here's the bill.' "

Dr. Pine gave me a look.

Ruth argued parroting the doctor's every word although her concern was genuine.

"I understand that perspective but it doesn't make it right just because a doctor says it. You think lawyers are a big rip-off, right? Well, doctors are well-educated like attorneys," I countered knowing it was a cheap shot.

Dr. Pine and the nurse glared at me.

"If my daughter dies," Ruth paused. "I'll kill you."

"It's just something you say in a fit of passion," Mary says.

"It sent a chill through me because she meant it."

The nurse's voice announces through the intercom above Jeff's bed, "The doctor is on the phone about Jeff's X-rays."

I am delighted. I get up, feel Jeff's forehead and put some honey/butter mix under his tongue. I tell Mary a quick conclusion to the story. "Monica left the hospital in a wheelchair and was bedridden. I convinced her to flush the antibiotics down the toilet. Her mother threatened to skewer me on a clothesline. I fed Monica the mixtures. Within five days, Monica was on her feet and blending the food mixtures herself. In six weeks she was back in ballet classes. That was seventy-two weeks sooner than the doctors said she would if she survived in the hospital. I was so astounded by her rapid recovery that I vowed to eat only raw foods."

Mary seems impressed and hopeful.

The fear that I might let her down suddenly hits me. Even so, I must advance into battle or lose Jeff. "Jeff needs to be off medication. He needs to be conscious to eat and recover," I say.

Mary looks pensive and doesn't answer. I leave her to think about it.

6

I ponder as I sit waiting in Radiology about accumulated radiation emissions from X-rays being absorbed by everything. The lights, walls, floor, furniture and abstract paintings on the walls seem to glow. I feel a hyper-irritating sensation, as if my nerves and bones want to wear an ultraviolet shield.

I wonder if Dr. Braisley told the radiologists to make me wait here for the last two hours. Could he be punishing me for questioning his analysis and diagnosis? Jeff is upstairs needing the honey/butter mix. It's 11 p.m. and few patients have passed through this department and there's no backlog. Why is it taking so long?

I also wonder if the older radiologists are balding from exposure to these "low" levels of radiation. Is it absorbed into their skulls, gradually making the follicles impotent at producing hair?

"Mr. Marshall?" the white-uniformed, partially balding radiologist says as he approaches me.

I consider accepting Jeff's adopted name, Marshall, for the moment. I could avoid explaining my relation to Jeff. But I don't want Ben being mistaken for me, considering my radical presence in the hospital. I explain as the radiologist takes me into a room.

Aisles of open shelves full of X-ray files line most of the floor space. On one wall is mounted a row of backlit white opaque glass with X-rays hanging against them. They are of Jeff's head taken by CAT scan. I see three oval areas that portend severe brain damage. I see images of Jeff crashing through glass. I cringe and take a deep breath.

The radiologist points to the spots, "These are filling with fluids and creating pressure on Jeff's brain. The doctors are going to tap and drain them to prevent further brain damage."

I listen to the prognosis without comment. I visualize them assaulting Jeff's body as they drill into his skull. I know if I tell the radiologist that fresh raw green vegetable juices and no-salt-added raw cheese could help draw out the fluids without drilling into Jeff's head, he'd have me in a circus by day's end.

I have to get Jeff out of the coma so he can eat. I realize the next step is to eliminate consciousness-interfering drugs.

Wait, stop. I wonder if Jeff wants to live. I won't force his soul to stay in his body if it wants to leave. Somehow, I must get his permission.

I thank the radiologist and go back to Jeff.

Mary and a nurse wrestle Jeff's arms and convulsing body down. Jeff's subconscious has burst through and pulls out the urinary catheter. The bulb at the end is inflated. It tears his urethra. Blood spurts and spatters from his penis everywhere on him and the sheets.

"Can't you see his body doesn't want the thing in him?" I say.

"He'll be wetting the bed constantly and he's too big and heavy for us to be changing him all the time," the nurse says annoyed.

I know I am not going to be around every forty-five minutes to change a diaper and bed, so I don't say any more. Mary tells me, as if confessing, that Jeff had pulled the catheter twice before. I shudder.

I remember that after stomach surgery I had sharp, burning pain in my penis when I urinated. I felt as if I were being painfully electrocuted during orgasm, with the electrodes connected to my urethra. It still happens occasionally. Now I wonder if I had unconsciously pulled my catheter. Had I ripped the tissues and damaged the nerves? Is that what made my urethra so sensitive?

The nurse and Mary finish changing the sheets and Jeff's gown.

One nurse reinserts the catheter, the other leaves.

Mary tells me she's taking a snack break and goes. The last nurse leaves.

I lean close to Jeff's head. I give him entrancing suggestions. I repeat them until I see that he is probably hypnotized. I tell him I want to speak to his psyche (spirit). I ask him if he wants to live. I suggest the slightest positive or negative response. A vague movement up or down for "yes", to either side for "no", from his head or hands, or his eyes behind his closed eyelids.

He gives no response.

I assume that he has chosen death. A lump forms in my throat. I recall my near death experience of seventeen years ago when I was 22. I was experimenting with mind expansion to find specific answers about my health and reality. It was early Spring. I had already put my cancer in remission with diet but I still had multiple health troubles.

My youngest uncle, Lanny, who had been studying for his doctorate in psychology and worked as a Teaching Assistant at the University of California, Los Angeles was guiding me. We had consumed psilocybin (a manufactured chemical form of an hallucinogen) and smoked a mixture of hashish and marijuana.

At first, Lan and I had a wonderful experience communicating telepathically. Then the pleasant effects of the drugs had worn off and my mind was normal again. Then I realized I was having an extremely adverse reaction. My blood pressure was dangerously low. It was 86° inside my apartment but I was freezing. My lower back ached so badly I couldn't sit or stand comfortably. That was normal but this pain was approaching unbearable. I remember lying on the floor next to the floor heater.

"I'm still freezing."

"It's all in your mind. Imagine a fire," Lanny said.

I imagined sitting next to a fire. Then I imagined the fire inside my body. This provided a bit of relief but did not raise my blood pressure.

"I'm still freezing and my back aches."

"It's all in your mind," Lanny said.

I rose from the couch and turned the heater to the highest temperature. I stood on top of the heater in my tennis shoes. Lanny began to complain that he was suffering heat prostration.

"Isn't it all in your mind?" I asked.

He rose from the couch and left.

I noticed the hands on the clock pointed to 12:47 p.m. As I stood on the heater I was slightly more comfortable. I became aware that my skin was turning ashen. I was weakening. I fell back slouching against the wall. I thought I was losing consciousness but instead I turned inside out with a pop. I detached from my body. I felt free and whole. I knew this experience was not an hallucination and I became frightened. Then I realized there was nothing to fear and my fear disappeared. I left my body. I hovered above it, circling. My body was still propped against the wall, dead.

Of all things, I was leaving my body with fresh pizza stains on my shirt. What would Mom think if she knew I died with pizza stains on my shirt?

Suddenly, I drifted upward through the ceiling. Through the upstairs apartment. The roof. And into the sky. I flew into the stratosphere and glided through it. Everything went dark as if it were a moonless night, except the stars, which were clear, and the Earth, which glowed.

I traveled backward toward the Sun, faster until the Earth became pea-sized. Suddenly I realized that I had an invisible form. I felt an intense brightness penetrating me from behind. It was the Sun. I turned inside out to look toward the Sun. After I turned inside out this time, I saw in all directions at once. I sped into the Sun. It seemed like a bright white tunnel. Inside the Sun I turned inside out again. Pop. I seemed liquid now. I swelled like an invisible balloon. I had become the Sun.

I wondered how that was possible. The answer came instantly; it was simply the nature of that reality. Then my stratosphere - my skin - dissolved. Like water I seeped through all of creation. I experienced an infinite sense of oneness and I was all that is.

I enjoyed eternity briefly. The ultimate oxymoron, I thought. I laughed and every particle in creation laughed. Although so obvious, I realized that laughter is an expression of joy. Joy is the appreciation of Creation, of beingness. I realized that without joy a sense of separateness ensues. And then fear. Beingness loses its sense of love that unites everything. Joy is more important than I had ever imagined.

Then I formed into a tornado-like mass. I focused my consciousness in the calm center. I watched lives swirl around me. In that whirlpool of lives, I saw that I had been a Sun, many lives on many planets, and other existences that I can not describe. I relived each of those lives from birth to death with tremendous speed, yet I seemed to understand more. Emotions were the gage of experience here, that is, what I and everybody felt and thought as a result of my actions was all important. The importance of these lives was creating joy/love. Unconditional love.

Finally I glimpsed a lonely, unhappy, unloved and sometimes unloving life in this whirlpool. It was full of resentment. It was my "Dick" life.

I relived that life. I felt sick, weak and angry. I realized that for my life to be happy I had to love myself completely. I had to heal my instincts and intuition. Through instinct my body communicates with me. Through intuition my psyche (soul or spirit) communicates with me. I knew that every decision should be a trilateral agreement between my psyche (intuition), body (instinct) and mind (reason). In that order.

I saw that health and happiness in my Earth-reality started at the most basic level, my body. I saw that my body cells were loving, feeling and intelligent. I should have loved them more. Listened to them. Helped them enjoy life. My cells wanted to experience so much more with me but they were strained, exhausted and deformed from environmental and dietary adulterations. I realized that I had wanted to love my cells all along. Their love was evident, trying to help me enjoy life. I wanted them to enjoy being part of me, with as much effort I wanted to love my cells as much as they loved me. But conditioning and education confused my instincts and intuition. I had been forced to mistrust myself.

Now, I thought, if I had it to do over again, I would take better care of my cells, to heal my cells. I saw that the cells in food were alive, loving, feeling and intelligent also. I saw that cooking food kills most of its vitality that we would receive if we were to eat food fresh and raw. I saw how much disease, pain and unhappiness comes from eating dead toxic food. I realized that my body cells could have gradually transmuted to magnificent health in several decades of care if I would have eaten raw foods. Also, I realized that I had chosen the diseased state, my diseased life, to learn about and create health. I felt excitement growing. I felt overwhelmed with compassion. I wanted to return to Earth. I would literally reverse the direction of my life from the inside out. Instantly a change came over me.

I became a black hole and I traveled at many times the speed of light. I realized that my desire was sending me back to Earth. I felt whole again - loved and loving; recharged with vital loving purpose.

I traveled through the psychic umbilical cord – a black hole - to my pitiful dead physical body on the heater. I exploded into my body, turning outside in. My body bolted upright. The power of my love started my heart beating again and warmed it. My blood began to move again sluggishly. I was still ashen.

I smelled burning rubber. With tremendous effort, I opened my heavy eyelids. I was looking down at my tennis-shoed feet on the heater's grill. I noticed the maroon telephone cord had melted black and was about to catch fire. I couldn't control any part of my body, except my eyes.. I felt a bit panicked. My adrenaline rushed.

The hands of the clock pointed to 4:17 p.m. My body had been dead three and a half hours. Slowly my body began responding to my thoughts. I flipped the telephone cord off but it fragmented, melted onto the grill. I tried to step off the grill but my tennis shoes were melted to it. I was exhausted and sick. I forced myself to pull hard. Finally, my shoes released.

I went into the kitchen and grabbed a barbecue fork. I returned to the heater. I removed the grill with the fork. I trudged with it to the back driveway and put it down.

I felt the warmth of the Sun on my body and I relaxed. I felt more alive every second, many of my cells were returning to life.

The thought of delicious, heavily buttered garlic bread came to mind. I knew it was instinct, my body telling me what it needed to raise my blood pressure. I went back into my apartment and ate a little crushed raw garlic with fresh raw unripe pineapple, lots of raw unsalted butter and a little French bread. I hadn't eaten bread in 13 years.

Except of a little digestive difficulty from the cooked bread, within moments I felt better, satisfied. I decided from then on that at least 70% of my diet would consist of raw foods. I remember that that was 2½ years before my experience with Monica in the hospital.

I went to bed. I fell asleep knowing instinctively and intuitively that sleep is where I would do most of my healing.

I become aware that I am in the hospital at Jeff's side. I touch his cheek.

"Do you want to live, Jeff?" I ask again.

I watch him intently for an eternal minute, anticipating, hoping for any indication from him.

"Good-bye, son. I wish you happiness wherever you've gone."

Suddenly, Jeff's voice surges loudly and clearly past the tubes, "Live!"

7

Willy, Mary's father, enters looking burdened and disgruntled; the opposite of my memories of him. I haven't seen or talked with him since we erected the swing set for Jeff's second birthday 20 years ago. He ignores me.

"Any change?" he whispers to Mary.

Mary shakes her head no. She says, "Good night, Dad," ignores me and leaves. Willy and I sit uneasily.

After five minutes, I break the silence, "Hi, Willy."

He nods without looking at me.

"Remember how you, Margaret, Shirley," - his older daughter - "Mary and I used to play pinochle for hours? Before that I'd never experienced adults enjoying children for more than several minutes. Thank you. That helped turn me from cynic to skeptic," I say jokingly but meaning it.

"Well, you broke the bubble, Dick. You and Shirley's ex-husband, Bill. You two screwed up my daughters and then dumped them. Neither of you deserved them, that's for sure."

"For everyone's sake, it was better that I left. I was so difficult. I was confused, frustrated and enraged."

"You have to learn how to discipline yourself," he says disgustedly.

"Not when it was at Mary and Jeff's expense. My body had developed biological habits from so much fear, anger and violence caused by my jealous brother Doug, and my father's brutal punishments. Either my blood sugar would drop, causing depression, or my adrenaline would soar and I couldn't control my excess energy, causing manic behavior, or blood sugar would drop while adrenaline soared, causing irritability and sour disposition. When I first went to California my Uncle Lanny gave me some cognitive self-help tools. I learned to control myself. I mainly handle it through diet, now. If ever I've had angels in my life, one would be Lan," I say still feeling ill-at-ease.

"I never met Lanny."

"I think you did. Of my mother's twelve siblings he is the youngest - only eleven years older than I. Lanny was the witty one. He was more like the understanding brother that I had wanted."

"Do you have any idea, the hardships you caused everyone?"

"I can imagine."

He sits back, defeated, "Imagine? My daughters screw up with two bums who abandon them, move into my small two bedroom house with two infants, and I'm supposed to trust their choices," he says.

"I know saying I'm sorry won't change the past, but I am," I say as guilt swells. "I was so afraid of being hurt and taken advantage of, I desperately and sometimes maliciously tried to get control of things. I had been taught that a man had to be mean and callous, deceitful and ruthless to be in control of body, relationships, spirituality and economy.

"I even thought 'Leave It To Beaver' was all Hollywood hoopla because I rarely experienced people who were understanding. Compassion wasn't normal. Goodness was an ideal that eluded me. I was always prepared for life to knock the wind from me. I couldn't learn to trust myself in an untrusting world. I couldn't trust and appreciate Mary as she deserved. I didn't realize that with that attitude I often forced people and experience to crash in on me. I rarely find myself a victim of my past anymore. I've worked hard to change. I'm not perfect by any means but I'm here to help. That's something I couldn't do very well back then."

"Whatever you can do."

"Do you still repair machines or have you retired?"

"Retired a few years ago."

"Do you and Margaret still live in that nice little house?"

"We been separated a long time. Along with my cynicism, I developed a taste for alcohol. I threatened her with a gun once. I was drunk."

"Was it loaded?"

"Course not. I just wanted to scare the bejeezus out of her."

"I'm sorry."

He nods but his look is too bitter to be forgiving.

I had been holding on to my memories of his family as proof that family life could be happy. Now I know I was very responsible for his family breaking up. I feel miserable. But I wasn't aware of any self-help tools at the time. Self-forgiveness is my only appropriate action now.

I place honey/butter mix under Jeff's tongue. Willy and I sit quietly, uncomfortably.

"You making a living with your health stuff?" he breaks the silence.

"At times. I'm taking a break from working exclusively with illness. I paint murals, motif, trompe l'oeil and faux finishes in homes, mainly in Beverly Hills. I do some acting on the daytime soap 'General Hospital'. I make just enough to stay in business, afford my research and survive. As long as I'm healthy, doing more than one thing, and what I enjoy, I'm happy. How about you?"

"Just gettin' along, I guess," he sighs. We sit quietly, a little more at ease.

Sunday, September 28th

I awaken from napping in a chair and notice it's almost 8 a.m. My first morning in the hospital. Willy leaves the room. I place honey/butter under Jeff's tongue. He seems more settled in that calmer state. Looking somewhat rested, Mary walks in followed by Ben.

Willy returns and says good-bye. Everyone seems laconic. They are probably exhausted from six stressful days.[8]

I go to the anteroom for some raw pistachio nuts. A nurse enters, unlocks the medicine cabinet and removes a small bottle. I eat as I follow her over to Jeff and she hands Mary the bottle.

"What's that?" I ask.

"Medication," says the nurse.

"Yes, but what is it?"

"Dilantin," she says, "Keeps him from having seizures."

"But it keeps him completely drunk and unconscious."

"Would you rather he have seizures and die?!"

Mary pours a half teaspoonful of the thick medication into a spoon and into Jeff's mouth. It looks like the raw custard I make when I use reddish Mexican papayas - like the ones I bought on my way here.

Jeff's mouth fills with saliva and drains into his throat. He chokes. The nurse takes a thin flexible plastic tube and vacuums his throat.

"May I," I ask the nurse.

She hands me the vacuum tube. I lean close to Jeff's face, blocking everyone's view of his mouth. I vacuum his throat. Then I suction the diluted pool of Dilantin around his tongue. I press the tube to his tongue and gums. Another pool of saliva forms. No one will notice the medication is gone. I notice the nurse returning the bottle to the medicine cabinet. A sense of relief passes over me.

An attendant comes in with a food tray for Jeff. I give Mary a curious look.

"We eat it," Mary says.

One of Jeff's neurologists arrives on morning rounds. We introduce ourselves. I suddenly realize my blood sugar is very low. My brain doesn't have enough blood sugar to remember his difficult name from

---

[8] *See* Appendix G, page 138.

the instant it leaves his mouth. I go back to the anteroom and get some nonsteamed dates and raw butter to elevate my blood sugar.[9] I return and eat while I watch the doctor examine Jeff's stomach where there is a very long stitched incision.

"What's that?" I ask.

"Dr. Japtur performed exploratory surgery, searching for internal bleeding. But there was none," the doctor says.

I look over Jeff's abdominal area, hips and lower back. I see no bruises that would have indicated there could possibly have been internal bleeding.

I open Jeff's eyes. Using Iridology as a diagnostic tool, I search for blood spots in his irises.[10] Fading blood spots would indicate that there had recently been internal bleeding. There is none. My adrenaline rushes. Sadness fills me. The invasive surgery is another problem for Jeff to heal. I am angry that his life has been more endangered. I wonder if Dr. Japtur, believing Jeff was going to die anyway, performed the unnecessary surgery to make a house or swimming pool payment, or pay for a daughter's braces.

I remember the first remarkable experience I had after studying Iridology for two years. My New Zealander girlfriend, Susan, and I were making love. Her blond head was arched back and her hazel eyes were open. I suddenly noticed a blood red spot in her right iris. The spot was near the area relating to the peritoneum.

"Sweetheart, are you spotting?" I asked.

She laughed, "You don't have to worry, I'm not going to get pregnant. I have an IUD."

"That's not my concern. Do you have pain in your stomach or uterus? Are you spotting?"

"Well, yes, and yes. The pain only happens when I move in particular ways. When we're making love it hurts once in a while, just a little. How did you know?"

"Iridology."

"You see something that alarms you?!"

---

[9] *See* Appendix H, page 138.

[10] Iridology is a science using the patterns and discoloration in the irises to diagnose the body's condition without expensive dangerous X-rays or exploratory surgery. Each tiny area relates to a body part or system.

"Please, don't be frightened. I'm no Iridilogical expert, but I think we should get you to Cedars-Sinai Hospital. You might have a little problem that could become a big problem."

"But you don't believe in doctors."

"Disease is a natural process whereby the body cleanses itself of accumulated toxins that it hasn't been able to eliminate. Most often the body just needs good nutrition and time. But I think your IUD is causing problems. It's a foreign object that requires a mechanic to remove it."

Susan laid tensely on the examination table with her legs spread and feet in stirrups. The doctor (in his early thirties, as I was) pulled his scissors clamp from her crotch. In its clasp was Susan's IUD string. It had become disconnected from the IUD. Her tissue acids had dissolved the end like cat gut.

"Susan's IUD punctured through her uterus and floats somewhere in her abdomen," the doctor said. "We have to perform emergency surgery. It could cause peritonitis, which can be fatal. You may lose your uterus."

Susan looked as if the wind had been knocked out of her.

"Doctor, can we take this one step at a time?" I asked. "Since infections are the body's response to foreign or toxic substances, when you remove the IUD you will eliminate the primary cause for severe infection (if Susan has one). Then her uterus will heal."

"If I get inside and find an infection that I consider dangerous, I will have to remove her uterus."

"Couldn't you give her body a week to see if it heals first?" I asked.

"If it looks bad, I'll remove it."

"I don't like taking this attitude, but you leave me no choice. If you remove her uterus without giving her body a chance to cease the infection, we will file suit against you and this hospital. Please, be clear that this will be personal against you because your treatment of Susan is personal. When she signs the release for surgery, there will be a clause stating that you are not to do anything other than remove the IUD and possibly stitch the tear in her uterus, if necessary."

"We refuse to operate at all, then."

"Since we are in agreement that Susan needs emergency surgery to remove the IUD, why can't you just do that?"

"I'm not going to go inside her with shackles on. I need the freedom to do what I think is right."

"May I remind you of your oath. If you or any other qualified surgeon here refuses to perform the agreed upon necessary surgery, anything, anything from peritonitis to pneumonia to death that happens to Susan from this moment on, I will see that you and this hospital are swamped with litigation. All I'm asking is for you to give her a chance to heal with the IUD removed. You can always remove her uterus tomorrow or the next day if her condition gets serious, correct?"

He looked deep into my eyes. He must have seen inside me and knew I meant it because his attitude changed.

"Yes, sir," he said respectfully. "Administration will give you a release. I'll accept it with your limitation clause."

"I'm sorry I felt it necessary to be so aggressive. Maybe I should have been more patient."

"No. You haven't been unreasonable," he said.

I sat in the lounge while Susan had surgery. The doctor approached me. He smiled and said, "Susan is fine. We easily found the IUD and the infection looks as if it will go quickly. She has an inch long incision at the base of her belly button that is hardly noticeable."

My eyes filled, "Thank you, doctor."

Standing over Jeff, I realize that I have to let go of my anxiety about his unnecessary abdominal surgery. But I wonder, Why is it that doctors don't use Iridology as a safe diagnostic tool? Is it because it would not generate great profits? I can't think about that now, I must concentrate on what will benefit Jeff.

"Doctor," I say, "my son is much more likely to recover from his coma if we take him off medication."

He looks terrified and says, "That is not possible. He will have seizures and infections without medication. Then everything we do for him will be for nothing."

"I am feeding him enough unsalted raw butter to prevent seizures," I say.

"You are feeding him what?" he asks.

"Raw fat prevents seizures. I put it under his tongue every twenty to forty minutes. We have to take the chance or he will remain a vegetable or die."

"No," he says and looks to Mary for support.

Looking frightened, Mary says to me, "I appreciate whatever you can do, but the doctors know more about this than you. Please."

"Remember Monica? How is Jeff going to recover from his coma and eat if he's drugged unconscious?" I ask.

"Please, Aajonus, don't make things more difficult for everybody," Mary says firmly.

I remember the Dilantin looking exactly like the raw custard. I will sabotage the medication.

I go into the anteroom, unpack my blender and food. I make a thinner-than-usual raw custard.[11] I sit and eat some, waiting for everyone to leave.

Finally, I am alone with Jeff. I want to increase Jeff's thirst for juices, so I turn down the drip-speed of his I.V. I remind myself that the honey I am giving him eliminates his need for sugar water. I wish I could remove the I.V.

I lift a fork from the food tray and bend back one prong. I return to the anteroom and stick the bent prong in the medicine cabinet's lock. The lock is loose and seems broken. I jiggle it until it turns and opens. I wonder if this act is a crime. Could I go to jail for trying to save my son?

Trembling, I empty the contents of two bottles of Dilantin into the sink. It has such a strong odor, anybody who walks in might be suspicious. I rinse it down with cold water. I take a Dilantin bottle and pour in the custard. The bottle neck is small and the custard so thick it spills all over. I am so nervous I can barely manage tapping the bottle on my palm to get the custard to enter and settle.

One finished, I lift the other bottle and fill it with custard. I wipe both bottles and cap them. I hear someone in the hallway. I return the bottles to the cabinet and close it just as the nurse enters. She doesn't stop or say anything. I wipe the sink so she won't notice me trembling. I hope she doesn't notice the cabinet isn't locked.

She walks to Jeff and injects a syringe into the catheter on his I.V. She notices the I.V. speed is slow. She turns it up. She empties only half a

---

[11] I blend 2 raw eggs, 4 tablespoons unsalted raw butter, a quarter of a fresh papaya (skinned and seeded) and 2 tablespoons unheated honey.

cubic centimeter into his blood and leaves the needle inserted. I join her.

"What's that?" I ask.

"It's too strong to put more than a little in his blood at a time. I'll be back every ten minutes until the syringe is empty," she says, walking out.

I turn down the I.V. speed. I wonder why she didn't answer my question. The drug is probably to keep Jeff's blood pressure low. Low blood pressure in his condition interferes with healing. And if Jeff is anything like me, he could die from low blood pressure.

I remove the syringe and empty its contents into the sink. I refill the syringe with a solution of Evian water and a drop of honey. I tremble again. I have barely completed the task when the nurse returns.

I watch her squeeze the syringe. A little water/honey mix enters the I.V. and Jeff's veins. A wave of relief passes over me. She notices the drip is slow again. Looking puzzled, she turns it up and leaves again.

I turn the I.V. speed down. I return to the anteroom and insert the bent prong into the cabinet and lock it.

Realizing I have done all I can for awhile, I leave.

As I drive to Mom and Dad's for some rest and relaxation, I realize I am not afraid of harming Jeff. In life and death situations in the past I have been afraid that something I did would go wrong. This is the riskiest and most dangerous circumstance I have been in. Yet, I feel undaunted, fearless.

Have I lost my friggin' mind? What am I doing?!

8

I steer the car into my parents' driveway. Their home is a few miles from the hospital and near a hill top overlooking the autumn-colored valley. The neighborhood is slightly more urbanized than the hospital's.

"Hi," I say as I enter the house. Mom, Dad and Doug sit at the dining table.

They all say hello. Mom stands and clears their early luncheon dishes while Doug finishes eating.

"Any change?" Mom asks.

"Not that I could prove," I say.

It is a surprise seeing Doug here. I have forgiven him for the sixteen years of his brutality when we were children. I can't forget it. Doug and I have not been able to relate as loving brothers in all of these years.

"Glad you came," Doug mumbles. "Sorry about Jeff."

I give him a hug. It is awkward for both of us. It is the first sincere hug of our lives. Optimists see benefit in every calamity; cynics see calamity in every benefit. Which is this?

I sink into the shallow modern tub. I wonder what happened to old-fashioned deep tubs, where you could immerse your entire body and bathe in luxury. As the water slaps the sides, my thoughts drift to Jeff. What if he is crippled for life?! He may never be able to take a bath when he wants. He may never be able to do anything by himself. Would he rather die?

I remember wanting to die. It was midsummer on Jekyll Island, Georgia. My girlfriend, Owanza, and I were walking to the beach a block away. I spotted a patch of beautiful white mushrooms in a neighbor's yard. (I had identified and eaten mushrooms in the island's woods from the time I had arrived six months earlier.) Because these mushrooms resembled a poisonous amanita, I cleared the ground at the base of one of them. I searched it for a cup-like lip that the similar-looking amanita forms. I didn't find one, so Owanza and I shared a tasty mushroom the size of my fist. I ate two thirds and she ate a third. I remember she had had breakfast, I hadn't.

We talked and strolled the north beach where few people were that early hour, along the sudsy ebb and flow where sandpipers dashed in and out spearing the sand with their long thin beaks. The shrimp boats just beyond the sandbars tooted. Two hours later and three miles up the beach, Owanza vomited again and again. She had had terminal cancer. Becoming weak and vomiting was common for her back then. All of the mushroom and part of her breakfast seeped into the sand or washed into the ocean.

We walked a short distance to the road hoping to see someone we knew to give us a ride home. Then I began feeling shaky, dizzy and exhausted. I realized we had eaten a poisonous mushroom.

I wondered why I hadn't felt nauseous. Why hadn't my body reject it as Owanza's body had? Of course, the vagus nerve to my stomach had been severed in the surgery for my stomach cancer. My body's ability to defend itself from such a mistake had been damaged. I felt an ominous sensation, like I was about to enter the twilight zone.

I waved my arms to stop a car and the couple took us home. At home I began to vomit. Nothing spilled but saliva and hot acidic gases that burned my throat, sinuses and nostrils.

Within another half hour, muscles in my feet and legs began to cramp. I fell to the bathroom floor. The cramps traveled to my head. Every muscle, including my facial muscles, was in a lumpy knot. Pain was excruciating. I twisted into a fetal position.

Owanza tried to help but when she touched me the cramps worsened. I couldn't speak. I moaned and tears streamed from my eyes. Owanza began to weep. My muscles, locked in knots and started to spasm. The next twenty minutes seemed an eternity. I fell unconscious from pain and exhaustion.

I awakened about twenty minutes later, tired and very thirsty. I got off the floor. Immediately, my feet and legs cramped. I fell to the floor. I asked Owanza to get me some water, fast. I guzzled a quart just before the cramps reached my hands. Again, I laid in a painfully twisted fetal position for fifteen minutes and passed out.

I awakened twenty minutes later thirsty and having to urinate. Cautiously, I moved my hands and arms to see if movement would initiate cramps. My limbs felt foreign, detached, but I had no cramps. I carefully flexed my toes. The cycle of cramps started again.

"I'll call your mother," Owanza said trembling.

"No! She'll put me in a hospital and I'll be dead within days. People die from mushroom poisoning because they dehydrate and the poisons in the mushroom dissolve their livers. Please get me some water, quickly."

I realized that the slightest flex of any muscle from my toes to my crotch initiated cramps. I crawled on my belly, using my arms to pull myself around the house. I urinated into a bottle while lying on the floor. I carefully and slowly hoisted myself on to the toilet to defecate - as if I were paralyzed from the waist down - after which I was exhausted. Breathing was exhausting.

Unless I accidentally flexed my lower extremities or grasped either of my hands too tightly, the cycle was every hour. Like clockwork, twenty minutes conscious taking care of myself, twenty in excruciating cramps and twenty unconscious. My liver was in constant pain, sometimes mildly, other times severely.

By the fourth day I had consumed six pounds of unsalted raw butter, two dozen bananas, two dozen raw eggs and eight gallons of water. Yet I was twenty pounds lighter. Now I could move my lower half, slowly, without causing cramps. The cycle jumped to once every four hours.

I went to the neighbor's yard and dug deep under one of those mushrooms. I found that it had a cup-like lip one and a half inches below the dirt's surface. I wondered what had caused these mushrooms to deform. I figured it had been a chemical fertilizer or weed killer.

I had eaten the mushroom nicknamed "Death Cap". Several books claimed that every person on record who had eaten a half thumb-sized amount of the mushroom had died. I had eaten fifteen times that. One book stated, "Death usually comes within ten days and it is welcomed."

I thought that I would get used to the pain, but I didn't. On the tenth day, the cramps diminished to as few as four a day. Now Owanza could touch me. She rubbed my feet often, gently and kindly for hours at a time. It was the only thing I enjoyed.

The cramps continued for ten weeks. I had come almost full circle to where I had been after my cancer therapies: semi-invalid. I developed chronic fatigue syndrome again. If I walked two miles, it took me two weeks to recuperate. Many days, simple tasks like brushing my teeth took an act of God.

I lost most of my pleasurable sensations. Before, when I walked in the woods I had felt a connection to every living thing, like feelings one has for loved ones. It was comforting, invigorating. Before, I was moved by colors the way music evokes feelings. Now, I felt nothing from colors or the woods. I was dead and in hell. Most everything smelled repulsive. Noise drove me crazy. I remember a hyperactive mockingbird that hung around for weeks. It was all I could do to keep from buying a gun and shooting it. The sound of barking instantly drove me into panic and fury. I constantly forced myself to be kind and understanding although I felt destructive and chaotic. I had to eat every two hours to keep a semblance of equilibrium but I was never hungry.

After being that way for over three years, I feared I might remain that way for life. I worked hard at being optimistic. But often I wanted to die. I experimented and learned that a little cooked starches in combination with raw fat and fresh fruit could control my depression and rage. (This experience inspired me to ponder about how much violence is a result of ill health. I speculated that most is.) Now, almost six years later, I am mostly happy again. I triumphed over death, against all odds again. And I healed without being crippled.

As I fall asleep in the warm bath I wonder, again: How will Jeff fare? If he lives, will he be completely paralyzed? Will he be happy?

Mom and I walk back into Jeff's hospital room at 4:45 p.m. (twenty-four hours after my arrival). I carry a small cooler of food. A nurse stands at one side of the bed, Ben sits at the other. Margaret and a volunteer stand at the end of the bed. Everyone has more energy. They seem optimistic and more relaxed. I feel relieved.

As I pass behind the volunteer, I see that Jeff's eyes are open. He sees me and his eyes widen. His left eyebrow rises and his mouth opens in a left-sided laugh. He lifts his left arm, greeting me. Ben smiles but looks hurt. The nurse looks shocked, and says to no one in particular, "Who's he that gets such a hello?"

"Jeff's lucky, he has two fathers," Ben says with a tense smile.

No wonder everyone is more cheerful; Jeff recovered from his coma!

Within moments Jeff falls asleep. We say our greetings and Mom cuts the tension with light talk. After the nurse checks Jeff's vital signs, I put honey/butter under his tongue.

Another nurse escorts Dr. Braisley into the room. She nods toward me, smiles wryly at the doctor and walks out. Dr. Braisley approaches me. We formally introduce ourselves.

"Can we talk in the hall?" the doctor asks Ben and me. We follow him.

"I know it's a miracle that Jeff's out of the coma but it may not be a blessing. His brain damage is extensive. Although the body can repair the brain, brain cells don't reproduce like other cells. Jeff will have very little control over his body."

"Last evening, I watched him yank his catheter out. It took his mother and two nurses to wrest him still," I counter.

"That was an unconscious body response. He will have no conscious control. He won't be able to take care of himself, even feed himself," the doctor says and pauses.

"His brain is cleaning and healing. When I walked in today, he smiled and raised his entire left arm and waved at me (even though it looked more like a Nazi salute)," I say, hoping humor will lighten the tension. "And he hasn't seen me in four years! For his brain to assimilate and respond on that data in that manner he can hardly be considered a vegetable."

"He did?" the doctor asks looking to Ben.

Ben nods, yes.

"Two-year-olds recognize their parents. They can wave, smile and even laugh, but Jeff will never be normal. He will not have control of his right side. He will never walk."

I look at Ben and see in his face the memories and hardships that he and Mary experienced with their daughter who had been paraplegic. She did not properly develop hip bones. I remember seeing a picture of her with black hair, sprightly look and kind demeanor. I recall Jeff and Mom telling me that she was always cheerful and sweet. She died on the operating table when she was six years old. Although that was ten years ago, the thought of Jeff being crippled seems to regurgitate those feelings in Ben. I feel angry at the doctor for his hopeless prognosis.

"The fluids that have built up under Jeff's skull are putting pressure on the brain and causing further damage. We are going to operate in the morning and drain them."

The idea of them drilling panics me. I take two deep breaths slowly. The doctor assumes that my pause is agreement, so I blurt out, "It will only create more problems for Jeff to heal."

They look as if I've punched them. The doctor regains composure and says, "I understand your concern but I will drill small holes from which we can draw out the fluids as they build. This kind of procedure has risk but much to gain."

"You told everyone he would die, no question," I say. "The fluids that are in his brain supply healing nutrients and cleanse dead tissue. The raw fats I have been giving him have made that natural process possible, and he recovered from his coma. With the concentrated raw fat, his body will not call for more fluids than the areas need to cleanse and heal. We need to supply the proper nutrients, be patient and let his body heal. Jeff will get better."

Ben's face shows shock and fear. I don't believe he had ever heard anyone refute a doctor.

Smiling patronizingly, the doctor says, "As I said, it is a miracle that Jeff is out of his coma, but the water on his brain is a fact. We have to remove it."

"Let me share my position with you," I say getting in his face. "You don't know the logic of Jeff's healing, so you call it a bizarre miracle. But it is a natural miracle. You know disease and how to attack the body. You drill it, pound it, poison it, sedate it, trying to eliminate symptoms and not causes. This may be over-simplification, but the point is infallible: Are people hyperactive because they're deficient in sedatives? Do diabetics' pancreases stop producing insulin because they're deficient in insulin? Do people have pain because they're deficient in aspirin? Jeff's brain isn't swelling with fluids because he needs holes in his head. Jeff would not be in this hospital if it weren't for Mary and Ben's wishes. But be very sure that I will use whatever power I have to stop you from performing any more surgeries on Jeff."

Ben, cringing, remains silent.

Dr. Braisley, flabbergasted, says, "Very well, then. If we are going to treat Jeff with diet then we will tube-feed him."

"If we get him sober he can eat," I say.

"If he isn't eating solid food within twenty-four hours we will tube-feed him! I will at least do that," the doctor says, turns and leaves, ignoring my hint about medication.

"Give him a chance," I say after the doctor.

I know that the foods they will tube-feed Jeff will be too deficient in nutrients for healing but I say no more.

"Relax, Ben, that was a victory for Jeff."

Ben walks away without saying anything.

I walk back into Jeff's room. I put honey/butter under his tongue. A repairman comes into the anteroom. He checks the medicine cabinet. I watch him replace the lock. I wonder if I'll be able to get back in there. After the repairman leaves, I make Jeff ten ounces of raw custard.

"Jeff, buddy. Wake up and eat. You will heal properly and more easily."

His eyes open and his mouth drops. I place a half spoonful of custard on his tongue. I close his mouth and bring his head level so he won't choke. I gently glide my fingers downward along his Adam's apple encouraging him to swallow. He swallows it!

I give him another half spoonful, rub his throat and he swallows. I give him another and he swallows but coughs a little. His cough grows violent. He turns red choking.

I take the vacuum hose and insert it deep into his throat. Globs of mucus with the food flow through the tube. Jeff chokes on the tube as if he will vomit, but I finish clearing his esophagus and he doesn't. I give his throat muscles and nerves several minutes to relax.

I feed him another half spoonful. I gently stroke his throat. He swallows. He coughs a little and settles. I give him more. He coughs violently and chokes. I insert the tube deep and suction the mucus. He produces mucus faster than I can feed him. If I suction his throat before every other bite I'll prevent mucus from blocking his throat, I realize. But right now I'd better let him relax for four or five minutes.

I see that feedings will be long and painful for both of us. But he is eating!

Ben and Margaret return with coffee. They stand over Jeff watching him sleep. Jeff looks exhausted but more relaxed.

"Jeff kept down about three and a half ounces of custard," I say. "He choked a lot, but he kept down that much."

Ben and Margaret seem encouraged. Ben wipes the sweat off of Jeff's brow. Jeff would love to be aware of this. He has always resented Ben's aloofness.[12] Ben strokes Jeff's head again affectionately. He sits and stares at nothing. Should I try to talk with him? No, I don't want Ben to feel comfortable enough with me to counter my wishes with the doctors. I feed Jeff a little honey/butter to alleviate pain and to continue cleansing

[12] *See* Appendix I, page 139.

his internal wounds.

"Would you like to get anything to eat?" Margaret asks me.

"I brought food, thank you."

"How about some hot chocolate? It has milk in it."

"It would make me hyperactive, jittery.[13] But I'll go with you if you'd like."

"Yes, that would be nice," Margaret says and stands.

We walk to Intensive Care lounge without saying a word. I realize that I haven't seen Margaret since the day Willy and I built Jeff's swing when Jeff was two. The lounge is empty. We sit. I fear I'm in for a lecture.

"So, how's California?" she asks.

"I've moved away four times but I keep going back to Los Angeles. So, except for pollution, I guess it's still the promised land for me, for now."

"I hear you're on quite a strict diet."

"Very politely put, thank you."

"I want you to know that I never gave up on you. Some things just don't work out."

"And all these years, like Mary, I thought you despised me. You have every right to, you know."

"Believe me, I know," she says laughing.

We have a pleasant talk and I repeat a few of the stories I told Mary.

9

Monday, September 29th

Mary's arrival wakes me. I reposition my numb and sore bottom on the chair. It's 7 a.m. She and Ben go for coffee. Rather than awaken Jeff, I put honey/butter under his tongue. An attendant brings in a food tray. The nurse checks Jeff's vital signs.

---

[13] Chocolate has theobromine and caffeine - two nerve irritants called stimulants.

Mary returns without Ben and immediately assists the nurse. Mary inserts a straw in a carton of orange juice. I cringe because I know this juice is pasteurized and much more acidic than fresh. All of its enzymes and at least 50% of its vitamins are dead and some radical,[14] and the minerals are unstable and radical. It will give Jeff very little with which to heal and will burn his throat.

"Jeff! It's time to eat something. C'mon, drink some juice," says the nurse waking him.

"Jeff, welcome back, boy. Help us out here. You need to get your strength up. Sip a little, now," Mary says.

Jeff sips and immediately chokes violently. Mary vacuums his throat.

"That was a good try," says the nurse.

"Try again, Jeff," Mary says.

Jeff sips and instantly chokes again. Mary vacuums his throat. I can't stand here and keep my mouth shut, so I go to the anteroom. I juice several oranges.

I return to Jeff's bedside and exchange orange juices. Mary and the nurse give me looks.

"Which would you rather drink?" I ask.

They raise their eyebrows in agreement and feed Jeff the fresh juice. I go for a walk.

Forty-five minutes later I reenter the room. Mary sits on the bed talking to Jeff who mumbles incoherently. She seems to understand a little but I can't understand a word. Jeff dozes off.

"I guess Ben told you the doctor said Jeff will be a vegetable," I say.

"Yes," Mary says with her eyes filling.

"It doesn't have to be that way. The doctors' prior prognosis was that he'd definitely die, no question. They say his brain is permanently damaged. That's not necessarily so.

"For example, nine years ago a man named Louis came into Aunt Tilly's Too, the health food store where I was the nutritionist. He was a thirty-two-year-old man with a masters degree in Library Science. He

---

[14] A "radical" vitamin or mineral means that the structure has become brittle and/or sharp, and/or the chemistry has become dangerously acidic. Radicals irritate all types of cells, including blood.

approached me. It took him four and a half minutes to ask a simple question.

"At first, I thought he had a severe stuttering problem. But he didn't stumble consistently on consonants. Sometimes he stumbled on vowels. Mostly he stumbled trying to articulate thoughts. Among his many problems, all of his glands were overactive. His nervous system could never keep up with them. He had low blood sugar and protein levels. As a result, I assessed he had severe delays between the analytical, decision-making process and motor response. So his problem was complex. Just like Jeff's.

"After a fifteen minute conversation that took an hour, I presumed that Louis had been this way most of his life. His condition was so normal to himself that he had little awareness of his difference from others. He wondered why he had no real friends. I thought to myself, who has the time or patience?! I did.

"First, I suggested he eat all raw foods and eliminate all of the vitamin, mineral and protein supplements that he consumed."

"You don't believe in vitamin supplements?" Mary asks shocked.

"I suggest eating fresh foods that are rich in balanced bioactive enzymes, vitamins and minerals for optimal health rather than consuming supplements.[15] Anyway, Louis showed immediate results. Within six months, a fifteen minute conversation took only forty minutes."

"When did you develop all this patience? My God, I'd go crazy if I had to listen to someone take forever to have a conversation," Mary says.

"Look back at the patience you had with your daughter. My patience came with better health."

Mary nods. "How's Louis now?"

"Patience. I realized that Louis must have had synapse, axon and/or ganglia damage or mutation. I deduced that if he ate fresh raw ocean fish and raw organically raised free-range fowl, his body could regenerate and rebuild those nerves."

"Yuk," Mary says.

"An aversion to flesh food is either conceptual or you're an herbivore. Herbivores have hooves. I don't remember you having hooves."

Mary smiles wryly and says, "It's the fact that it's raw!"

"That's what I said, conceptual. Although Louis only ate raw fish or

---

[15] *See* Appendix K, page 140.

fowl twice a month, within a year he managed a fifteen minute conversation in thirty minutes. That was half his original time. If we feed Jeff raw meats while his body focuses on healing the brain, he should be able to repair himself in less time than Louis."

"What about worms and salmonella?" Mary says alarmed and repulsed.

"Intestinal worms do not thrive in healthy cells. When an intestine becomes excessively toxic and massive tissue degenerates, worms can thrive. Parasites actually help eliminate dead, weak and dangerous degenerative cells. They consume these damaged cells and break them down into substances that the body can most easily eliminate.

"Or the body can produce virus to dissolve the toxic degenerative tissue, or it can produce a bacterial infection to consume organic degenerative tissue, but those processes usually take more time and are more exhausting. Parasites are always the best and quickest the body can do to cleanse. Jeff's irises indicate he is not in danger of parasites.

"Now, regarding salmonella and similar bacteria. Normally, foods that naturally contain these bacteria produce a putrid odor when the bacterial count gets high. If you worry about bacteria, when meat stinks don't eat it. The bacterial count in cooked meat and eggs will grow as much as sixty times higher than in raw food. The waste products from bacteria that feeds on cooked food is 10-100 times more toxic than the waste products from bacteria feeding on raw rood. That's why in our advanced society, bacterial food-poisoning is from cooked, packaged or restaurant food. I will not feed Jeff stinky meat."

"I must be as crazy as you. If it works, do it," Mary says.

"May I ask you something?"

"What?"

"Why didn't you want me here? After all these years, why do you still hate me?"

Mary looks straight into my eyes for a moment. "When Jeff had his tonsils removed, I submitted the Teamster's insurance forms that you sent when you worked as a dispatcher for that trucking company. I waited months. The Teamsters said they sent you the check because it was your insurance. The check had been cashed. How could you do such a thing?"

"I remember receiving insurance checks regularly for all my medical bills back then. I automatically sent them to the doctors. One of my doctors got a hearty, undeserved tip. Why didn't you call me? I could have looked into it. I had no idea. Mary, I would never purposely do anything like that to you and Jeff."

She looks at me, then touches my hand. "You trying to live forever?"

"How long isn't all that important to me. How healthy and happy I am while I'm alive is important."

She looks at me pensively and smiles.

10

I am in a lush tropical rain forest. I hear Jeff groaning. He sounds far away. I awaken from a dream to find myself in a chair at Jeff's bedside. He thrashes about. With his left hand, he pulls at the boards binding both hands and arms. I look around. Thank God no one is here to see this.

"Jeff, please. If you pull your tubes and all, the nurses and doctors will sedate you. Or they'll give you a paralyzing drug. You won't be able to eat to get well. It's okay to thrash about if only I am here but please don't pull your tubes."

He continues thrashing but stops pulling at the boards.

"Great, that's good exercise."

I place my fingers in his left palm.

"Can you grip my fingers? Squeeze, let me feel your strength."

His grip is shaky with little strength but he does it.

"Terrific, you're controlling some movements! Now squeeze my fingers with your right hand."

His hand doesn't respond. He furrows his brow despondently.

"It's okay. Give it time. Your car won't recover but you will." Should I be telling him that, I wonder. Do I know enough to help Jeff get through this?

When I didn't know as much as I do now, I was not always successful with my nutritional advice. Failing Lanny was a disappointment to me.[16] In his late thirties Lanny became severely schizophrenic and depressed. He had been to doctors and they told him that cures were rare and that a lifetime of medication was his only solution. Several years later doctors convinced him that thyroid removal might help. It did briefly. Then he was labeled incurable and forever dependent on thyroid hormones and antidepressants.

I failed Lanny before doctors convinced him to let them remove his thyroid. I was still a diehard fruitarian/vegetarian. I had encouraged him to fast and follow a raw fruitarian/vegetarian diet. His digestion improved. He felt better. But he was prone to low blood sugar (hypoglycemia). I didn't realize then - I was this ignorant - that a fruitarian or vegetarian diet is often rapid debilitation for people with hypoglycemia. Fasting - starving the body - is rapid debilitation for almost every body. Nor did I recognize at the time that hypoglycemia and protein deficiency are the main cause of depression.[17]

My suggestions were more harmful than helpful to Lanny. Lanny has not been open to my suggestions since. He continues to suffer terribly unless heavily medicated. With or without medication, the most he can do is take care of his basic needs. He cannot work. I miss his vitality, intelligence, compassion and humor.

"Awwwsssooot mmaaaph," Jeff groans and releases me from my misery.

"Jeff, how about eating some custard?"

"Uhhheeeuuhnnn," he says and I take it as a yes.

I make a raw custard in five minutes. I raise Jeff's bed so he sits erect as possible.

"You have been having difficulty swallowing. I have had to vacuum your throat a lot. But be patient with yourself. You are doing very well. The doctor said it is a miracle that you are recovering. It is. A natural miracle that depends upon you eating these wonderful live foods that give you their life. In time you won't have any difficulty swallowing. But right now, accept it as a challenge. Okay? I love you, Jeff. I've always wished I could show you that. Lanny said that if I really wanted

---

[16] Lanny was not a client but I had encouraged him toward a dietary solution.

[17] *See* Appendix L, page 141.

to, I would have. I suppose that may be true but I've been focusing on getting myself well all these years. Open a little wider, kiddo. This isn't a baby spoon."

He chews a little and swallows on his own. I give him another spoonful. He gets it down easily. I feed him another. He chokes. I vacuum his throat. We start again.

Tuesday, September 30th

I open the shades and see the sunrise over the autumn trees on my third morning in the hospital. The parking lot is filling with employees arriving for the next shift and early callers paying visits to loved ones before they go to work. Mary sleeps peacefully but looks uncomfortable sitting in a chair with two blankets wrapped around her; one around her upper body and one around her lap and legs.

"Aashama, aamaa sirsa," Jeff says awakening Mary.

She approaches him, "Did you say you're thirsty, Jeff?"

"Yyyeeehhhsss."

"You understood that?!" I whisper to her.

"We've known each other for awhile."

"I know, stupid question," I say as I reach for Perrier water.

Jeff's left leg moves.

"Did you see that?! He moved his left leg a little. And he's conscious."

"I didn't see," Mary says. "Jeff, can you move your left leg? Try."

He lifts it. He looks at it. It drops.

"Hey boy, you did it! All right!" Mary says.

"Siiirssa!" Jeff grumbles.

"Just a minute, kid, give us a break here. Maybe you're not impressed that you moved your leg, but we are," Mary says.

I pour some Perrier water into a cup.

"Siiirssaaa!" Jeff grumbles.

"Chill out! Aajonus is pouring you some water right this second."

I hand Mary the cup of water with a straw.

"Don't you think the bubbles will make him choke more?" Mary asks.

"He needs as much oxygen to his brain as possible. Natural carbonation somehow increases nitrogen in the digestive tract and oxygen in the blood. Also, the high natural mineral content will bind with toxic substances and neutralize them. It will reduce water-on-the-brain. Sip just a little at a time, Jeff."

He sips. He swallows and coughs a little.

"Good, sweetheart," Mary soothes. "When you're ready just sip."

Jeff lifts his head toward the straw, sips and coughs violently. I vacuum deep into his throat. He gags and spits up.

"Let's elevate him higher so he sits erect. He'll probably be able to swallow more easily," I say.

Jeff reaches for the cup with his left arm and spills it on himself and the bed.

"Wait a minute, Jeff," Mary says admonishingly, but delighted by his enthusiasm for water. "Aajonus has to raise the bed. We'll pour you some more."

Jeff looks down at the wetness.

"We were gonna change your bed anyway. You get a bath every morning right here in bed," Mary consoles. "I have to go to work for a change, but Ben, Aajonus and the nurses will bathe and shave you very soon."

Just as she says that, Ben arrives. He walks over to Mary and touches her shoulder. She hands him the cup.

"Jeff's demanding like his old self again," Mary tells Ben. "I told him you'd help with his bath. I need to go clean up for work. Call every couple of hours, would you?" Ben smiles and nods, towering over her. "Don't cause too much trouble, kid," she teases Jeff. She says good-bye and leaves.

"Aaaterrrrrr!" Jeff grumbles.

Ben sits on the bed. He gives Jeff a sip of water. Jeff swallows. He takes another sip and coughs violently. I vacuum his throat. Ben gives him a couple more swallows.

The nurse enters and announces, "We're taking Jeff down for a CAT scan."

It is several hours after the CAT scan. Dr. Braisley approaches me in the hall on my way to Jeff's room, "The water on Jeff's brain has diminished. But his progress is as good as it's going to get. If he makes it out of intensive care, think about a long-term facility where they can care for him properly. Call my office and someone will supply you with names of facilities that handle chronic invalids." The doctor gestures toward the nurse beside him, "We will begin tube-feeding him."

"Excuse me, you said that only if he weren't eating solid food would you tube-feed him. He's eaten custard with eggs, mashed potatoes and butter," I say.

"He's not getting any protein."

"Correct me if I'm wrong, doesn't science consider eggs protein?" I ask.

"He's not eating enough. He's almost skin and bones."

"That's an exaggeration, doctor, and you know it. I'm sorry, you cannot tube-feed him. Swallowing is good exercise for his head and brain. Tube-feeding will cause more irritation and damage to his throat. Yesterday, Jeff wasn't eating at all. In the last twenty-four hours he's consumed six ounces of custard which consisted of three eggs, 2 tablespoons of butter with one ounce honey. Plus he's eaten two ounces of mashed potatoes with butter," I say.

"By tomorrow, he'd better be eating twice that much or we will tube-feed him," the doctor says and walks away.

The nurse gives me a disparaging look and walks away.

I remind myself that Jeff can make fast progress. I recollect how quickly Ray's wife responded in a crisis.

Ray was slender, well-educated and a gentle man. He came into Aunt Tilly's asking about supplements for his wife. He told me that she had a malignant tumor wrapped like an octopus around her brain stem. The doctors thought that the tumor had been forming for years. They told Ray that his wife would not live more than a few months. That the only chance she had was an operation to cut away the tumor and scrape the brain stem. They said her chances of surviving the operation were remote.

I suggested that Ray refuse the surgery and feed his wife a blend of fresh raw tomatoes, stone-pressed wheat germ oil[18] and a primary yeast[19]

---

[18] A chemically unprocessed, completely cold-pressed (under 86 degrees Fahrenheit) refrigerated wheat germ is what I recommended and Ray used, but

three times daily. And as much fresh carrot juice as she wanted.[20]

"I don't know about calling off the surgery, but I'll give your suggestions a try. Thank you for your help," Ray said. He turned in the aisle and walked toward produce.

Four weeks later, Ray returned, looking forlorn.

"I guess my suggestions didn't work," I said.

"On the contrary. The day I talked with you the tests showed that the tumor was solidly adhered to her brain stem. She ate what you suggested and ten days later, when the doctors removed the tumor, it had 'miraculously detached' (their wording). But they scraped the brain stem anyway, fearing metastasis. She's been in a coma for weeks. They don't expect her to come out of it."

Back then, I didn't know anything about how to help someone recover from coma, so I wasn't able to help her further. But just as Ray's wife had responded quickly, so could Jeff. I won't let Dr. Braisley confuse me. I'll trust my intuition that everything will be fine.

Again, I stand looking at the locked medicine cabinet. I have a fresh custard sitting on the counter. I insert the bent prong of the fork into the new lock and turn. "Please, please open," I chant to myself. It opens more easily than the broken one did! I remove the fresh bottles of Dilantin and close the cabinet. I dump the drug into the sink, wash it down the drain with cold water and fill the bottle's with raw custard..

I sit close to Jeff's bedside reading and memorizing the play I am to perform three days from now.

"Maaarroowssiss fouuunigh," Jeff struggles.

"I'm sorry, Jeff, I can't understand you. Mary's gone for something to eat. She'll be back in about an hour. Are you hungry?"

"Yeaaahsss."

---

is no longer available. An unheated stone-pressed or granite-pressed olive oil is equivalent.

[19] Grown on the whey of raw milk without ever being heated above 96 degrees Fahrenheit.

[20] *See* Appendix M, page 143.

"Would you like to try something more solid? You will have to chew more to turn it liquid enough to swallow. It will help you regenerate tissue quickly and easily. Shall we give it a try?"

"Yaaahhss."

I remove two small canning jars from the side table. In one is a combination of room-temperature raw fish, raw beef and unheated honey that I had made into pâté in a food processor. In the other jar is 3 tablespoons of unsalted raw butter. I immerse both jars, lids tight, in the sink full of hot water (only as hot as my hand can take). While I wait for the butter to melt, I raise the bed so Jeff is in a sitting position. Then I pour and mix the melted butter into the pâté to help him swallow.

"Okay, my boy, here we go. I'm going to put only a small amount in your mouth first, to see how you handle it. Okay?"

Jeff's eyes nod and his mouth opens.

"Open just a little wider, please. Thank you."

I sweep the pâté into his mouth by passing the spoon over his upper teeth and lip. He sits there in a stupor. "It won't go down if you let it sit there. You have to chew a little - or suck - to mix saliva with it." He does both. "That's excellent. Stay calm and swallow only when you sense it will go down easily. Okay? Good. Great! That's terrific! You did it! Okay. Would you like another? Good."

I place another half spoonful in his mouth. He goes into another daze.

"Jeff, you have to chew each time. That's it."

He coughs. The cough graduates to choking.

"Don't panic, you are not going to choke to death." I vacuum his throat. He settles.

"I'll tell you what, I'll vacuum your throat each time before each bite, so mucus will not block your throat and make you choke."

An hour later, Jeff sleeps peacefully and I sit memorizing the play. Mary returns and I tell her, "Well, he did it. He ate the food that will start repairing his brain quickly and completely."

"You got him to eat raw meat?" Mary says fearfully.

"He swallowed about three ounces before he got tired."[21]

"Did he choke much?"

"No more than usual."

"I guess we'll discover soon enough if it kills or helps him."

"The first time I ate raw meat, I thought it would kill me, but here I sit," I say knowing Mary has no idea how literally I meant that.

11

5 a.m. Wednesday, October 1st

"Aaet meeyout. Thaaa aaeeieesiint mi. Aaaeet meeeyooouut! Aaeeieesiint meeee! Aaaaeeet mmeeeeyooouuuss!"

I leap from my chair, startled awake, "Easy, Jeff. No one is going to hurt you. I'm making sure of that."

"Aaaaaaat mmeeeeyooouuuut!"

"Jeff, it's okay. If you get too unruly, they'll drug you. And then, I don't know if I would be able to feed you so you can heal properly and quickly. Thrash around, if you like. It's good exercise. But don't pull your tubes or make too much noise, please." I seem to have said that fifteen times in the last four days. "Listen, I would like you to think about eating as much custard and meat as you can today. I'm leaving for Los Angeles late this afternoon."

"Aaeernn yoouu ooonna sthaaayy!"

"I'll be back tomorrow night or Friday morning. Tomorrow, you'll be getting a full injection of a drug I've been sabotaging. You need to eat a lot of custard so the raw eggs will prevent the drug from creating too much havoc in your body. I don't know if your mother will feed you the meat while I'm gone, so it would be beneficial for you to eat as much as possible now. That way you'll continue healing your brain while I'm gone. Okay?"

---

21 *See* Appendix N, page 144.

He lifts his right arm as if he were intending to gesture with it but it drops.

"Hey, you moved your right arm! Was that a choice?"

"Iiii sssothhnnn't knnnowww."

"What the heck, try it again."

His brow furrows. His mouth twists. He exerts tremendous effort. Finally, his right arm raises slowly and rests on his stomach.

"That's great! Can you move your right leg?"

He moves his left leg fairly easily.

"No, your right leg."

His right leg doesn't respond.

"Try one more time."

Again, he moves his left leg.

"That's your left leg. Try the other one. I'm touching your right leg, can you feel it?"

He looks bewildered. I pat his shin. He nods.

"Terrific! Can you move it?"

He twists the muscles in his shoulders, neck and face. He bites his lower lip. He rolls his head back. He does all of this to help himself lift the leg. It raises an inch at the knee! He lets go, exhausted.

"You did it, you moved your knee a little! That's a start."

"What's this I hear, you moved your right leg?" says the nurse behind me, startling me.

"He moved his right arm even more."

"Can I see?" asks the nurse. "Jeff, will you move your right arm for me?"

He tightens the muscles in his shoulders and face again. The arm doesn't move.

"I know it's difficult, try again," says the nurse.

He tries with all of his might. He lifts it an inch and drops it.

"That was pretty good. I put two of my fingers in your right palm, grip as tightly as you can. Try real hard."

Jeff's eyes look around but not at anything outside of himself. He seems to search for some connection to those fingers. He doesn't find any.

"You can't?" she says more as a statement than a question.

"That's okay, Jeff. Yesterday you couldn't move your right arm at all. Maybe tomorrow you'll move your fingers. No problem. It's just a matter of time. Okay?" I turn to the nurse and ask, "What time do Jeff's doctors usually come on Wednesdays?"

"Sometime between ten and two. Usually."

"Be sure the doctor reads on the chart that Jeff ate five ounces of hamburger between yesterday and this morning," I say without mentioning the words raw and fish, "Therefore, please, enter on Jeff's chart that I formally refuse tube-feeding."

"Are you leaving us?!"

"I'm taking a day's rest," I say because I don't trust that my wishes will be followed if the hospital staff and doctors know I will be gone.

"You certainly deserve it," she says and turns to Jeff, "Are you ready for your bath, young man?"

"Aaahhh thhhhon thiii iiit."

"What was that? I didn't understand you."

"He says he doesn't like sponge baths," I say.

"That's what he said?"

"More or less."

"Well, okay, we'll postpone it for awhile. Okay, Jeff?" She strokes Jeff's hair off of his forehead.

"Sssaaan yooouuu."

"My Lord, he didn't swear at me, did he?"

"No. He said thank you."

"You're welcome, Jeff. I have to check your blood pressure and temperature, okay?"

Jeff nods.

"Good. Thank you."

"Bath time?" Mary asks as she enters.

"Ssssh, don't mention bath. Jeff doesn't like them today. So we're putting it off for as long as we can," says the nurse.

"You mean for as long as we can stand him. You want to stink us out, boy?" Mary says. Jeff gets upset.

"She's teasing you. You know how mothers tease," I say and take Mary aside. "I'm leaving for a day and a half. I have a rehearsal tonight and a performance tomorrow morning. I was wondering if – I know I'm asking for a long shot, but-- Would you consider-- Please think about it before you answer, okay?"

Mary says straight-faced, "Is your name Louis?"

"Funny. That was good. Would you be willing to feed Jeff the unheated honey/butter mix, make some raw custard and feed him some raw meat while I'm gone? I'll leave everything you'll need in the cooler here."

"I don't know about the raw meat, but the rest I can handle."

"I have to go buy some eggs, papaya, oranges and bananas for Jeff. I don't feed him the honey/butter mix by itself too often. I mash banana and mix it in. It relaxes his muscles and is better at relieving pain."

"You really have all this nutritional stuff down."

"I'm always working on it. I rely on myself and not doctors for good health. I learned a long time ago that going to allopathic doctors is like playing a state lottery. A handful of people will benefit and millions lose. Regardless, the medical business gets rich. That's just the way it is. Our society makes too many choices based on economics."

"Have you ever met a doctor you respect? Do you think anything they do is beneficial?"

"I respect Dr. Robert Mendelsohn. He's a doctor who realized the medical search-find-destroy methodology is futile. He's written several books about it. And yes, I think that doctors who put disfigured accident victims back together and relocate broken bones are wonderful. But the way doctors treat infection and disease, and conditions like Jeff's, assaults the detoxification and healing processes."

"I don't think I would care to have your view."

"Dr. Mendelsohn once said that the poor are fortunate because they can't afford doctors."

12

As I park my car, I feel like I've left a dream. I take another deep breath and realize the air quality is bad. Here I am back in Los Angeles after a long day at the hospital, an hour's drive to Cincinnati Airport (in Kentucky), a five-hour flight with a two-hour nap, a taxi from LAX to home in the slums of Beverly Hills and the drive to Hollywood for rehearsal.

I exit my car and approach an old-style Spanish apartment building. I knock on the door and wait a few moments.

Lorain, the director, opens the door and smiles with wide eyes, sparkling, "You're here!"

"I left a message from the airport that I'd be thirty minutes late, you didn't get it?"

"Yes, but I'm just excited that you are here."

"Thanks," I say and wonder what would it be like to always be greeted that way? Hmm...

Lorain, about thirty, very attractive with an educated and relaxed grace says, "I'm happy your son is improving, Aajonus, but I really feel awful that you left him."

"Sixteen to twenty-four hours a day in that hospital has been intense. I couldn't think of a better way to release my tension than doing this. Thank you for your concern."

"I'm glad you're here too. I'm Faye," says the thirtysomething, lean and fit actress with whom I will be working.

"Hi, I'm Aajonus. You look great for the role," I say sincerely.

"And you look great for yours," she says as she flips her short red hair back.

"I know you're tired, so we'll make this rehearsal as brief as possible," says Lorain to me. She shows us stage blocking as she moves agilely around her lovely Spanish-style living room. "These chairs will be the park bench on and around which you will work."

"Before we go any further, I have a reservation," I say, "When I auditioned, I didn't know my character was fighting in the Golden Gloves. I had no idea he was twenty years old. I'm one of those actors who would like to think he can do almost anything, and will try. But, my God, my son's that young."

"Good actors are excused of some imperfections, so don't worry. This is just an exercise for directors to better learn their craft," Lorain says.

"Just wanted to admit that I know I'm physically too old for this character."

"Up close you look like you're twenty eight or twenty-nine. The audience is going to be at least ten feet away; you'll look twenty, no problem. You're perfect or I wouldn't have cast you."

"Okay," I say.

"The two of you are taking a walk together and you come to this park bench, stop and talk. Faye, flirt with him. You've been with your stuffy boxing manager boyfriend too long and this young man is refreshing. Aajonus, your character is naïve but loyal. So even though you are aroused by her, you would never make a pass at your manager's girlfriend. All right? Let's do it," Lorain says.

9 a.m. Thursday, October 2nd

Standing in the hall in my apartment, I am on the phone, waiting, dressed for the performance: 1950's slacks and knit short-sleeved shirt.

"Intensive Care Unit," says a female voice.

"Hi. May I speak with the head nurse, please?"

"One moment, please."

"This is Mrs. Baine, how may I help you?"

"This is Aajonus. How is my son, Jeff, room 317?"

"Marshall... Oh, you'll have to ask his doctor, I can't give out any information."

"You know how difficult it is to track down a doctor. I'm not going to be around a phone where anyone can reach me for four or five hours. Please, just tell me if Jeff is stable, improved or worsened since yesterday afternoon."

"He's not with us anymore."

"He didn't die...?!"

"He was transferred from intensive care. You will have to call admissions for his room."

"My son's out of danger! Thank you, thank you. He's not in danger! Have a fabulous day, Mrs. Baine."

10:40 a.m. at the American Film Institute

I watch forty directing fellows applauding Faye and me enthusiastically. This moment, at the end of a performance, is the only time I allow myself to notice the audience.

Professor Dorn stands and says, "Yes, it was very good." She waits another moment for everyone to quiet, "But each scene has to be more than that. The actors were interesting. Believable. We could relate to them. But what was missing? Film is visual. Let's give them action, something to do within their characters. Aajonus is playing a viable contender in the Golden Gloves, right? Aajonus, I would like you to practice your foot and fist work during the scene. Let's do it again. Actors take your places."

Ten minutes later.

Faye, in character, rises from the bench, approaches me and says. "I just think you should be careful of Tom. Watch your back."

I give my imaginary opponent a succession of quick jabs to the stomach then dance back. I duck an imaginary punch to my right eye. I come back with a barrage of jabs to his face. "Don't worry, I can take care of myself." I stop shuffling and jabbing the air. I'm breathing heavily but not winded. "I have to get back. I'll see you later."

"Cut," Professor Dorn says.

The room fills with whistling, howling and applause.

"You see how exciting it was after adding action appropriate for one character? Let's give Faye and Aajonus another thank you and that's it for today."

They applaud. Faye and I bow and leave.

10 p.m.

Just having awakened from a nap, I lie in Beatriz' bed watching her undress. Her athletic Latin body is covered with lightly tanned satin skin and accented with rich black hair.

"What are you thinking about?"

"How a nap a day gives me more waking hours in a day and how much better I think and function. Why, were you thinking I was making love to you while you undressed?" I tease.

"Yes. I'm embarrassed."

"Don't be. I was also admiring your beauty."

"Would you mind if we didn't make love right now, sweetheart? Can we talk?"

"Sure. What's on your mind?" I ask.

"I spent three of the five days you were gone staying with Owanza. She shared all the wonderful things you two did together. And how you saved her life. She's still very much in love with you. I don't know if I could love anyone as much as she loves you."

"May I ask a few questions? Answer aloud only if you want. Would a rose look to a gardenia for how a rose should grow? If the rose were able to produce the chemicals to breakdown the soil, absorb the nutrients and recreate them the way a gardenia does, then, would the rose be a rose or a gardenia?"

"A rose would probably go crazy trying to behave like something it wasn't," Beatriz says.

"Okay, then. How can you know what you personally feel about anything if you are immersed in Owanza's thinking and feelings? Is it important for you to judge your thinking and feeling by hers?"

"Sometimes. If I don't like the way I feel. Or the results of what I'm doing. That's what education is all about."

"True, other peoples' experience can be inspiring. But if you were to try to feel and think the way anyone else does, then aren't you like the rose trying to be a gardenia? If anyone did that in school, wouldn't they be admonished for plagiarism?" I ask.

"This is getting too confusing."

"Sorry. What's your favorite color?"

"It varies, but mostly rich reds."

"Why?"

"I don't know. I like the way it makes me feel."

"Do you think that Owanza's passion for pink makes your passion for red less or wrong?"

"I get the point. And you're absolutely right. But I feel so much empathy for her. She wants you to be her lover again and I feel like I'm the reason you're not in love with her. I feel like I'm taking you away from her."

"I guess I'd better start from the beginning. Owanza and I met on Jekyll Island, Georgia. The couple who owned the local health food store referred Owanza to me. When Owanza came for her first appointment, she was frail, trim and pallid as a corpse. She trembled. Her skin on the back of her arms hung like an elderly person's. She was allergic to everything but fresh self-squeezed grapefruit juice. She had been diagnosed as having terminal cancer; sixteen malignant tumors in her liver, thirty pea-sized tumors in her spine, six in her uterus, and innumerable tiny nonmalignant tumors in her brain. She was given as little as one week to live."

"How old was she?"

"Thirty-four. Owanza and I sat and talked about her diet."[22]

"And she really had only one week to live?"

"She was in danger of suffering a stroke at any moment. And when you're down to one food in liquid form and you can't even drink water without getting maddening hives, the end is very near. But I was optimistic. Right then and there, I gave her a selection of foods to eat in combination.

"She was afraid to eat any one of them alone, so the idea of eating them all together terrified her. I asked her what she had to gain and lose. She ate for two and a half hours while I explained my theories and conclusions about diet. She didn't get one hive. She was elated. Since then, she gets hives only twice a year for two-week periods - when she goes through a lymph detoxification.

"I also instructed her to get more sleep because most healing happens in the sleep state. She had her own gift shop and worked an eight- to twelve-hour day there. I insisted that she tell her husband and son to fix their own meals, do their own laundry and tidy after themselves. Her husband had a fit because she wouldn't be making him any more stuffed mushrooms. She divorced him."

"She told me the same story. She said you nursed her back to health. You're her angel."

"Her body, with the proper foods and sleep, healed itself. I didn't. I helped her discover what foods were right for her body at any given

---

[22] *See* Appendix O, page 145.

time (which she does very well on her own now by following her instincts and intuition). Anyway, her cancer went into remission immediately, but her body will be discarding those tumors, particle by particle, for years to come.

"When her husband left and she had to surrender the gift shop, she couldn't handle all the bills on her own and get well too, so we rented a house together. We fell in love.

"Several months later, I ate the poisonous mushroom that killed every feeling I had but pain, empathy and my sense of smell. And everything smelled awful. I lost my sexual drive too. I had been the picture of health and overnight I became as sick as she had been most of the time. Owanza and I went from making love three to five times daily to zip. That was difficult for her. She said she had never experienced the passion we shared.

"We took turns nursing each other, and yes, I nursed her a lot more, but we did what was compassionate. We loved and cared for each other. We still do. But, basically, the romance ended when my senses died with the poisonous mushroom.

"When my sexuality returned five years later, it was not for Owanza. Until a few months ago, when you and I met, that kind of affection was something I thought had ended for me. I can't transfer my passion for you on to Owanza. It would be debilitating and fruitless to try to be a bird of paradise if what I am is a sunflower," I joke.

"Hi, sunflower. Do you want to shine on me?" Beatriz says, leaning on me and nibbling my ear.

"Can you take the heat?"

Beatriz wets her lips and kisses me with her mouth open while pulling me down on top of her.

13

The next day, Friday; Back in Cincinnati

I am feeling sprightly after my two-hour nap on the plane. I amble down the hall to Jeff's new room. I enter, "Hi, kiddo, it's Johnny! Direct from Los Angeles," I say imitating the Johnny Carson Show. The room is empty of visitors. "Now that you're in a regular room, no one stays with you?"

"Hhii. Tthheirrr kkiillinn' meee. I gauttaa get oouutta hheeere. Tthheirrr kkillinn' meeee, daadd. Tthheirrr eeevviil," he pleads.

The right side of his face is still predominantly paralyzed. I find it hard to look at him. I will get used to it again. "I used to get paranoid when they gave me medication that lowered my blood pressure. I thought the sky was falling on me. I knew this would happen to you, so I slowly melted some unsalted raw butter and blended in some fresh garlic and mixed it with some raw pâté that I made. All before I boarded the plane."

Jeff slowly moves his left hand to my chest, grasps my shirt and pulls me toward him. I am just noticing that neither of his arms are taped to boards.

"Tthheirrr ttrryyiiinnn' tooo kkkkkiiilll mmeee."

"I'm back, and I assure you, they won't get away with it."

"I wwon't ccaaarrre wwhhhennn I'mmm deaddd."

"Wow, you really have improved. Jeff, what I meant was, I'm not going to let them kill you. I think the fear you feel is biological. Your blood-pressure is too low. Open your mouth and eat this. The danger you are feeling will pass. Chew or mix it around in your mouth so saliva will thin it. It will be easier to swallow. Are you conscious enough to do all of this without me talking you through it?"

Jeff shakes his head no.

"Then I'll talk you through it when I see you distracted, okay?"

He nods.

"The hospital personnel are not purposely trying to kill you. They simply don't understand the subtle disasters that lowering your blood-pressure causes. What they normally do is counter danger-symptoms of fear and panic with a drug that'll dope you. I had been sabotaging that drug before I left. I'm sorry I couldn't get here an hour sooner or I could have sabotaged the injection again. But the flight was late. If they see you panic like this, they'll drug you more and you won't be able to eat."

"I'mmm ccollld. Fffeeeezzinn'."

"Before I give you another bite I'll put some honey in the pâté. If the body needs its temperature raised, unheated honey with raw meat and/or raw butter will raise it. It'll be about twenty minutes before it takes effect. So please be patient. I'll get you another blanket. You want to hear a joke?"

"Yyeess."

"Since you'll be getting out of here soon and coming to visit me, I'll tell you a traveler's joke."

"Iii'mmm ccuuummmiiinn' ta vviisssit yyyuuu?"

"I was hoping you would want to."

"Yyeesss."

"Great. The passenger walks up to a ticket agent and says--"

"Whaaat tiiicket aaaggennnt?"

"I'm telling you the joke. The passenger approaches a ticket agent and says, 'Send this bag to Hong Kong, that one to Honolulu and the last one to Fiji.' 'We can't do that, sir. You're only going to Los Angeles.' 'Well, you did the last time I was here. And I had no luggage when I got there!' "

"Oooooohhh. Ooowww."

"I know, it only hurts when you laugh. No more jokes for you."

"Ooowww. Ooww. Ooohh."

An hour passes and Jeff is completely calm and warm.

A stout woman enters, says, "Hi, Jeff. I'm Adele. I'm your speech therapist. We'll be working together until you're well enough to leave the hospital and go to a rehabilitation facility. We'll start off working thirty minutes or more. Or until you become too tired." Adele seems annoyed with my presence and says to me, "Jeff and I need to be alone, would you be so kind? Thank you. Jeff, I want you to say the word day."

Feeling a bit insulted I leave and walk to the anteroom.

"Tthhaaaaa."

"That was pretty good. This time put the end of your tongue on the roof of your mouth, not at the back of your teeth. The roof of your mouth. Day."

"Dthaaaa."

"Better. Put your tongue a little higher on the roof of your mouth. And this time, close your mouth a little at the end of the word to round off the 'A' sound. Day."

"Daaay."

"Excellent. You know, you may never be the fast talker you were before, but that'll be kind of sexy. Be patient. I have to be, so it's only fair you be patient with me. A deal?"

"Yyyeaasss."

Adele looks over at me in the anteroom, rises, comes over, gives me a look, closes the lavender mini-blinds and walks back to Jeff.

Wow, she doesn't like me. I feel hurt and I don't even know her!

An hour later I return to Jeff's room, "Did Adele wear you out?"

"Yyyeass."

"Hi, Jeff," a voice comes resounding from behind me, startling me. I step aside. A large African-American gentleman in a hospital uniform passes me. Owning the room with his presence, he says to Jeff, "I'm Harold. I'll be your physical therapist while you're here. Looks like your easy days of lying around are over. You ready to get that body back to doing something?"

"Would you like me to leave?" I ask.

"I'm Harold, who might you be?"

"I'm Aajonus, like homogenous without the hum. I'm one of Jeff's fathers. The biological one."

"What did you do, become a father at seven years old?!"

"Seventeen years old."

"What is your secret?!"

"You don't want to hear."

"Gotcha. Jeff and I'll work an hour or two a day. If you work some with him, it's better you do it right. So watch and learn."

"Thank you, I appreciate that. We'll have Jeff dancing from this hospital," I say.

Harold gives me a distressed look. Then he looks to Jeff and says, "Your nervous system has been badly damaged, Jeff. So, we are working with limitations. We'd all better come to the realization right now that you'll probably never dance. But we'll get you moving as much as we can. We might even get you on a walker some day. Maybe. We'll just do the very best we can. So try real hard. Okay?"

"Yyeass."

"Harold, if I sound offensive, understand and forgive me. Just let me take one minute to tell Jeff about Oscar (one of my clients)."

"Go for it."

"Jeff, Oscar was twenty-two (your age) when he came to me. He had knee injuries. He was a ski instructor and loved skiing. The doctors said that he must have surgery or he would have a lot of trouble and pain for the rest of his life. They told him that with or without surgery he would never ski again. Oscar refused surgery. I suggested a diet that was heavy in raw eggs, raw meat with unsalted raw butter, no-salt-added raw cheese, avocado, raw milk, and a little raw fruit and raw germinated grains." Harold gives me a strange look but I continue, "Within nine months Oscar was back to skiing like a mad man. Within eighteen months he won two ski ribbons in Switzerland. Oscar healed. You can heal too, Jeff. Your muscles don't have to atrophy like normal brain-damaged accident victims. You'll regain connection to your muscles as quickly as you heal the damaged nerve connections. Okay, Harold. Thanks."

Harold swallows an impulse to call me nuts. He looks at me pitifully. He looks at Jeff, "Let's see what you can do. Move your right arm." Jeff's arm doesn't move. "Keep trying, it may take a while before enough messages get to the motor center and down to your arm." Jeff clinches his teeth and buckles his chin to his neck, trying. But he can't do it. "That's okay, don't get discouraged," Harold says.

"He lifted it an inch two days ago. Twice."

"Let's see the left arm move," Harold says. Jeff easily curls his left arm. "Good, my man. With a little work, looks like you could play hard ball with that one. Now turn it back and forth. Twist at the wrist," Harold continues.

14

Next afternoon, Saturday, October 4th

I walk down the hall past nurses, orderlies, patients, visitors and doctors on the way to Jeff's room.

"Aajonus," the nurse calls.

I stop and approach the nurses' station.

"My shift ends in about thirty minutes. Did you forget to tell me what Jeff ate last night and so far today?"

"Oh, yes. Three ounces of fish, four ounces beef, half cup of potatoes, 8 tablespoons of butter, four ounces of honey, cup of custard, six ounces fruit juice and six ounces of water. He still coughs a little but I only had to vacuum his throat twice."

"Very impressive. Word's around that you're feeding him raw eggs and meat," she angles.

"I would have to say...that is very true. Raw, or should I say, live foods, are what have made Jeff's progress impressive. Potato is the only thing I've fed him that's been cooked."

She glares at me without saying anything.

"Is there something else you want to know?" I ask.

She smiles wily and I get a bad feeling. She gestures no.

"Excuse me, then. I'm going to see if Jeff needs anything. I've been gone several hours. Have a pleasant evening. Are you working tomorrow?"

"My husband and I are going to my mother's for dinner," she asserts.

Why is being friendly often considered a come-on? To make my intention clear, I say, somberly, "I wish you and your family a wonderful day off together, Mrs. McCauley."

"Thank you."

As I amble into Jeff's room, I take a playful ape-like posture to amuse Jeff. I see a pretty, petite young lady with light hair sitting in Jeff's room. I straighten up, embarrassed. She looks familiar. She stands as I come closer. I notice Jeff sleeping.

"Hi, I'm Stacey," she says with a fraught smile.

"Jeff's fiancée!" I say, remembering her from the picture Jeff sent me of them at Stacey's prom. "I'm Aajonus. I'm happy to meet you. Does Jeff know you're here?"

"Yes, but he fell asleep."

"He's pretty drained," I say.

"Jeff talked a lot about you."

"He did? I wonder from whom he got his information."

"That's true, you certainly haven't been around for him to get it first hand," she says playfully.

"I'm Ralph," says a young man, who stands to greet me, "Jeff and I were best friends."

"Jeff is no longer considered dead, so I assume you're still best friends," I say jovially.

Ralph gives Stacey a noncommittal look that frightens me.

"Jeff hasn't had a relapse in the last six hours, has he?!" I dart over to Jeff. He sleeps quietly.

"No, he's doing okay," Stacey says.

"Have you talked to him?" I ask.

"He's hard to understand but he recognizes us," Stacey says and hesitates, "But I think he's completely forgotten what he did."

"What do you mean?" I ask.

"You don't know?" Stacey asks rhetorically, wishing she hadn't mentioned it.

"What do you know?" Ralph asks.

"He lost control of his car and went down a ravine."

"Did you know he was carrying a loaded revolver when it happened?" Ralph asks.

"No."

"Maybe we'd better sit down," Ralph says empathically. A chill runs up and down my spine.

Stacey begins, "The night before the accident, Jeff and I got in a fight about something that happened a few days ago. The three of us had been hanging out at Ralph's house. Jeff and I were fooling around inside. Ralph was by the pool. Jeff was drinking a lot and getting crazy. He went into one of the bedrooms to sleep it off. I went out to the pool. I gave Ralph a harmless, friendly kiss. Jeff saw us and snapped, got crazy jealous. Accused Ralph and me of having an affair. I was engaged to Jeff and Ralph was his best friend!"

Then Ralph says, "We tried to reason with him. He said he'd been watching Stacey and me together for a long time. That we were getting along too well to be just friends. Accused me of <u>fucking</u> Stacey. I was his best friend! Called her a slut. She was his fiancée!"

Stacey resumes the story, "An hour or so before the accident, I called and told Jeff that I'd filed a police report against him for hitting me. He just kept saying things like, 'You're fucking Ralph, aren't you, you whore? I'll kill you. You can't do this to me, you bitch.' I told him he was insane and I hung up."

"Then he called me," Ralph says, "and he said, 'I'm comin' to kill both of you!' Next thing we knew, his mother called to tell us he had had an accident. The police called to ask how much he'd had to drink, about some drugs and the loaded gun."

"Wow," I say.

I remember my jealousy. If Mary were even ten minutes late, I imagined that she was screwing around with a salesman at work. I reasoned that the salesman had more education, intelligence and money than I and could easily seduce her. I trembled with fury. I never had the guts to talk to anyone, even Mary, about my ridiculous fears and jealousy. Thank my lucky stars, I didn't become an alcoholic until after Mary and I separated. Although I was a happy drunk. I was nasty only when I was sober.

I feel disoriented, fearful, angry and sad. How am I going to put this in some compassionate and practical perspective? Is an accident all that separates my son from being a murderer? It doesn't matter, Jeff has not killed anyone!

"Sstaacyy! Iii llovvve yyuuu. Ddad, tthiss iisss mmy ffianncee."

"Yes, we met," I say.

"Hii, ssweeethhheart."

"Hi, Jeff," Stacey says sympathetically.

I can see whatever romantic feelings she had for him are dead now. I wonder if she will be able to tell him.

"I have to go now," Stacey says and turns to me, "It was nice meeting you."

"Thank you. Me too. Take care, Stacey, and I hope you do whatever is right for you."

"Thanks for understanding."

"Ssstaaay," Jeff pleads.

"I have to go," Stacey says.

"Thhaannkss forrr cuummin'. Cuuumm baaack lllaterrr."

She gives him a kiss and leaves without answering him. Jeff knows that something is very wrong. Sadly he watches her go. Tears fill his eyes. He crossed the line. It is over and he knows it.

15

Next day, Sunday, October 5th

"I ii donn't wannt taa usse the bed pan. Iii cann go ta the toiiilet," Jeff says as he sits up. He slides his legs to the side of the bed. Margaret and I help Jeff position himself on the edge. We take him by the arms. We get ready to move him to the wheel chair.

"Iii cann waulk," Jeff says.

"No, Jeff!" Margaret says.

"Iii haave taa go ta the baahffroom."

"Jeff, now you stop it. You can't do it. Please, sweetheart," she says.

"Let him try," I say, knowing very well that he has only slight movement in his right side. "If you think you can walk we'll help you. You are just planning to walk the two steps to the wheel chair, aren't you?"

"Iii cann doo it on my ouwn."

"No, Jeff!" Margaret says.

"Gra'maaa, Iii cann doo it!"

"But you can't!"

"Let him. He won't know unless he tries. You never know," I say allowing for a miracle. And my skeptical side assumes that if he falls on his face he will know his limitations. We won't have to wrestle and argue with him. I am sabotaging his medication, so he is not drugged and he will remember. Jeff lifts himself by pushing with his left arm. I help balance him on his feet. "Can you feel both feet on the floor?" I ask.

"Yeesss," he says with more air than voice. He has that look infants have when they first try standing on their own. I can see he is convincing himself that he can do it. "Okaaay, le' go."

"Just to be safe, can you step forward with your right foot?" I ask. He slides it forward very slowly and shakily. "I'm impressed! Now can you put your weight on it while you lift your left leg forward?" He gives me a frustrated look. "I know, people can walk very well until they're asked to think about it. But I'm just trying to help you explore your strength, or lack of it."

"Le' meee go, nouw!"

"Okay, we're letting you go very slowly," I say.

Jeff stands on his own, shakily. I reach for a pillow to throw under him in case he falls. He bends his left knee. He shifts his weight on to his right side and collapses. He crashes to the floor before I can get the pillow under him. His reflexes are so slow his arms don't brace the fall. He lands hard. I cringe. A lump forms on his brow as fast as my ego shrinks. Margaret and I lift him up. We put him into the wheel chair.

"Iii ccaann't doo it," he says embarrassed, grieved and humbled.

"It's okay. Now you know for sure. Take your time, work with the therapist and you'll be walking in no time. The doctors say you will never walk again. Take what they say very lightly. They don't know what we know," I say.

"Whhat do wee knnoww?" Jeff asks with surprised innocence.

"We know what foods in what form will help your body heal."

"Aamm Iii eeating them?"

"Better and more than I imagined."

"Thaaat'ss goood."

"That's wonderful! I'm going to wheel you into the toilet now. You won't mind if we help you on to the toilet, will you?" I ask.

"No, Iii neeed ya taa hhelp mee, plllease."

"Such a polite cripple."

"Ii'mm nnnot a crippaalle!"

"I'm teasing you. I'm sorry. That was in bad taste, I know. I was trying to lighten us up. I want to talk to you about something and I'm afraid to. But here it goes. I hope the anxiety from your accident will inspire you to take better care of yourself. Avoid drugs, including alcohol. Sermon said and done, I put it to rest, okay?"

"No, yoo arre rriiight."

"Shall we go to the toilet, or would you rather use the bedpan?"

"Toiiilllet."

"Let's wheel you in."

Next afternoon, Monday, October 6th

A gray-suited, gaunt, thin, austere, somewhat anxious man enters Jeff's room and looks around. I have a bad feeling about him. "Jeff has gone to physical therapy. Are you another doctor?" I ask with trepidation that he might be.

"I am the president of this hospital. You are Age-ee-nees?"

"Hi. It's Aajonus." I extend my hand. We shake hands. He furtively wipes his hand on his pants. I surmise that he is terribly germ phobic. Either his immune system is very low, or he has allergies or he's just paranoid.

"I understand you have brought raw meat and eggs into this hospital," he says confrontationally.

"Is there a problem?"

"Raw meat and eggs carry disease. They don't belong anywhere in this hospital, except the kitchen. In fact, for sanitation, no meat or eggs come into this hospital raw. Everything but fresh fruit is processed," he says with pride and authority.

"Hospital food is the most processed and denatured. Is that something to be proud of? Does it have any life to give sick people?"

"I want you to remove all raw food from the hospital." He waits glaringly for my acceptance.

"May I say something about the disease theory?"

"Those bacteria show up in lab tests."

"All of us have the syphilis germ within us, like meat has bacteria. However, active bacteria are distressing only when they feed on toxic substances, like in cooked, processed and chemically grown food.[23] The bacterial count in cooked meat and eggs will grow sixty times higher than in raw meat and eggs before it produces a putrid odor. The waste produced by bacteria feeding on cooked food is extremely toxic. That's why bacterial food-poisoning in this country is from cooked, packaged or restaurant food. I could not find one laboratory test that proved bacteria living on raw meat caused food-poisoning in animals who ate it."

"Are you going to remove what I asked?"

"Would you stop doing something for your son that has been helpful and working because I asked you to?" I ask.

"Not likely."

"Then may I have a little latitude, please. Decades of research documents and photographs held by the Price-Pottenger Foundation in La Mesa, California, prove that raw meat, raw dairy and raw foods in general create excellent health, free of disease. That's the Price-Pottenger Foundation, in case you want to research the raw issue before you make that decision."

"Shall I call security?"

"Fresh raw meat promotes cellular reproduction, good health and vitality."

"I'm not going to argue the issue. The facts as I know them are that raw meat and eggs cause disease. Now, if you don't remove those items, I will have security come and do it. And you with it."

"Please. My son's life is at stake. The doctors said my son would be a vegetable, living off machines. When Jeff's progress shattered that prognosis, they said he would be paralyzed and have the mind of a two-year-old. Look what the raw meat and eggs have done. The raw foods continued to heal him and have made that prognosis obsolete."

He raises his voice, "The medication and everything the doctors and nurses have done in this hospital have saved your son!"

I can't tell him that I sabotaged the medication. And arguing that all the hospital has done was to house, butcher, radiate and drug Jeff, would get me thrown out.

"Shall I call security?"

---

[23] *See* Appendix Q, page 151.

"Let me ask one more thing, please."

He shakes his head disgustedly but lets me talk.

"How would it look if the media got a hold of this miracle story and it said that the president of this hospital risked a young man's life by changing what had been working? How many people would be willing to come to your hospital?"

"Don't threaten me."

"Actually, it was intended as a wake-up call," I say trying to lighten the air.

"Don't try my patience any longer. Take that raw food out of my hospital!"

I am pissed but I know that more argument would be detrimental. "Take it easy. I'll take it to the car," I say knowing very well that I will sneak it in later. I lift my cooler and carry it from the hospital.

Two hours later

Jeff and Harold have just finished physical therapy. Harold leaves. Mary, on a long lunch break from work, sits reading a magazine. Jeff watches TV. I read a book. How much more typical can we look.

The nurse enters and examines Jeff. Her face curls comically from Jeff's body odor. She playfully says, "Now that you're doing so well and you've had your exercise, how about a shower? We can give you a thorough scrubbing."

"That sounds good. Les go," Jeff says with a big smile.

"Wow, you're speaking so well already," she remarks.

"I know," Jeff says, now sounding a little like John Wayne - slow-talking and gravel-voiced. "Isn't it amazing?"

"I'll say," she says.

"And the hits just keep comin'," Mary says mirthfully.

"We'll have to wait for an orderly to take you to the shower; you're too heavy for me," says the nurse.

"I'll help," I say.

"Then les go," the nurse says. We help Jeff scoot to the side of the bed.

"Do you want to try walking the two steps to the wheel chair?" I ask wryly.

"Are you crazy?!" Jeff says. Tears come to my eyes. "Are you all right?" he asks.

"I'm just happy you're healing so fast."

"So am I," he says.

I move the wheel chair back a few feet and say, "Okay, the nurse and I will get under your arms so you can simulate walking; just to give you the sensation, okay?" The nurse and Mary give me wry looks. "We'll take two small steps, all together we'll turn around, take two small steps backward and sit you in the chair. Ready?" We move like a slow and clumsy chorus line but we all feel exhilaration.

Ten minutes later, I lift and carry Jeff from the wheel chair into the shower stall. I place him on a stool with his left hand at the bar-handle on the wall. "Can you hold yourself up?"

"No problem," Jeff says.

I remove his gown.

"Is this like an automatic car wash, or are we gonna get wet?" I ask.

"We'll get soaked," the nurse says.

"You may have other clothes here but I don't. Therefore, I'm getting naked. If a healthy naked man bothers you, I can wash him alone."

"I'll see you later," she says with a wry salacious grin. She gracefully turns and walks out.

"You keep this progress going and you'll be home in no time," I say as I remove my clothes.

"I'll do the best I can."

"I'm sorry, I didn't mean that to rush you. I meant to be encouraging."

"I appreciate it and all you're doin' for me, Dad."

He seems to like calling me Dad as much as I like hearing it. I have no illusions about it, with all due respect, Ben has been his father.

The next morning, Tuesday, October 7th

Jeff sits in bed nonchalantly eating a bowl of raw ground beef with butter only. I realize I should have put honey in it when all of a sudden his eyes widen and his mouth twists.

"This is raw!" he says.

Mary and I exchange looks and break into laughter. Jeff puts down the bowl.

"I can put some honey in it to make it more appealing."

"But this is raw."

"You've been eating that for seven days. It's what has helped you heal so well and quickly."

"I'm not eating that raw! That's *raw* meat. I'm no savage."

"Would you please keep it down. The hospital banned me from bringing raw meat in here," I whisper, still laughing. "I would not force you to eat anything that isn't appealing to you."

"I appreciate that."

A nurse comes in and I go for the bowl of meat. "I'll clean your bowl," I say and furtively pass it by the nurse. In the anteroom I put the meat back in the jar and inside a sack. I return to Jeff and see the nurse leaning over him. She arranges something I can't see. Jeff strokes her bottom and says, "You're very nice to me, thank you."

"Jeffrey Marshall!" the nurse says shocked, pushing his hand away.

Mary and I exchange looks.

"That boy is definitely okay, now," Mary says. "Jeff, you don't do things like that!"

"Why not? It feels good," Jeff says innocently.

"You don't touch people unless they want you to touch them. All right?!" Mary says.

Jeff looks at the nurse and says, "Can I touch you?"

"Absolutely not," she says.

"How about a kiss?" he teases.

"You know what this means, Jeff?" I ask.

"What?"

"When the nurses have to put up with your sexual harassment, your ass is on the way out of this hospital. Unless you want them to give you a drug to make your sexual organ limp."

"They'd do that to me?!"

"Without the bat of an eye," says the nurse. "Tomorrow or the next day, you'll be sent to Good Samaritan Hospital where they have a terrific physical rehabilitation unit."

"See?" I say. "Listen, everyone, I'm outta here. I have to get back to work or I might not have a roof over my head next month."

"You have to go?" Jeff asks.

"I've done all I can. Do you want me to stay just to watch the nurses slap your sweet face? I'm leaving you two six-pound jars of unheated honey and four pounds of unsalted raw butter. Remember, they will help you get well, so eat lots of them. The honey helps you digest, utilize and assimilate nutrients and the butter will minimize infection, cleanse dead cells and other waste and make what you have strong. Raw meat, if you ever eat it, will help your body replace the cells killed as a result of the accident. Eat them together or with whatever you like. Just don't cook or put them in or on food that's hotter than your touch can take. You got it, kid?"

"Yes, sir," he says comically.

"Good-bye, Mary," I say and hug her. I may be imagining this, but I think her eyes are tearing up. I turn and go to Jeff. I give him a hug and kiss on the cheek. "Call me anytime. If you need anything I can help you with, especially your health, call me. Take care of yourself. I love you."

"I love you too. You take care."

"Thanks. Bye." I leave feeling satisfied. But I also feel guilt that I am leaving him again.

16

Four-and-a-half months later
in Beverly Hills, California

Beatriz and I stand in our cantaloupe- and honeydew-colored kitchen. We drink a blend of orange juice we have just squeezed, raw egg and raw cream. I notice it is almost 2 p.m. We watch Jeff on the sofa bed in the living room. He is just waking from fifteen hours of sleep. He moves as if acutely intoxicated, literally moving in slow-motion, wearing only baggy briefs. The right side of his body is retarded, including his face slightly. He straps a small electrical device to his right hand and wrist. It sends mild currents to stimulate the dormant nerves.

He attempts to stand. He falls back on to the bed. He does this six times. Finally, with tremendous determination and effort, he moves to his feet. He stands wavering in slow-motion for three minutes. Then he gets somewhat sure-footed. He realizes he can't move with the hand device strapped on. He removes it. He scuffles across the hardwood floor toward the bathroom. He moves as if he were a hundred-year-old man in a young-looking body. He disappears into the hall.

"I expected him to be so much better, the way you described his progress in the hospital," Beatriz says.

"Me, too. The few times we talked on the phone he must have been at his best. He always talked slowly, but I had no idea. Healing has reduced to a crawl if at all. He's been here five days and I can't get myself to talk to him about his condition. He has improved a little since he's been here, eating the raw custard and raw foods. But I need to talk to him about meat and his medication. I feel like a father who doesn't deserve to be a father. Yet I can't watch him flounder through life like this. I must sound like someone who needs a shrink. Am I being selfish, wanting him to be better?"

"You always care just enough about everybody. But you nag me about my diet a little too much."

"I know. I'll work on trusting that you can manage your life by yourself. Sometimes I have difficulty watching people hurt themselves. Not that they have to care for themselves the way I do. I just want them to take care of themselves. And it's really none of my business. But I'm going to try with Jeff, anyway. He has to be taking medication for him to sleep this much and move around like a drunk trying to be sober. Here I go." I take a deep and gather courage from within myself. I march to the bathroom. The door is completely open. Jeff stands wavering over the toilet, urinating. Now I know why the toilet and all around are wet so often. I halt and wait for him to finish. He doesn't even realize that I'm only seven feet away. Now, that's intoxicated!

"Can we talk?"

"Sure."

"Here's a blend of orange, raw egg and cream to get some fuel in you. It'll help wake you."

"I sure sleep a lot," he says with slow speech and a coarse voice.

"Are you taking medication?"

"Dilantin."

"For how long?"

"Ever since the accident."

"Jeff, I know I haven't been there for you. Except for a few flashing moments. But I want to help you get well. To be normal again."

"I want to be normal again."

"I can help. If you want me to."

"I want you to help me. However you can. Or want to."

"First, I suggest you stop taking medication."

"The doctors said I would have seizures and I'd have to start all over again. Or die!"

"If you will eat lots of raw fat every day for a month, then at least every other day for six months more, you will never have to worry about seizures. If you will also eat raw meat at least twice weekly for one year, I figure that you'll be completely normal again. It could take less time but you've been taking Dilantin for four and a half months. Drugs interfere with healing. They are often just toxic enough to usurp most of the blood nutrients without causing trauma. So no one is conscious enough to realize the harm they do. Very few people respond well. And even fewer don't have side effects from medication. Medication is the Great Risk."[24]

"Aajonus, I don't want to have a seizure."

"Do you think you will ever drive again?"

"If I can."

"The risk of you getting in a car and having an accident on your way to get a six-pack is astronomical compared to the remote chance that you would have a seizure if you would eat as I've suggested."

"The doctor really got on Mom's case about making sure I take the Dilantin. He said one seizure and it's all over again."

"You know the saying, 'Get a life'?" I ask playfully. Jeff smiles. "If

---

[24] *See* Appendix R, page 153.

you get tired of sleeping fourteen to sixteen hours a day and not having a life, take the chance. If you do it while you're here I will monitor you. I guarantee that that isn't necessary. But if it will put you at ease, I'm here for you.

"Let me tell you about a client with a similar circumstance. Barbara was a talented singer who had been diagnosed as incurably manic depressive and schizophrenic. She was suicidal unless medicated. I think she was twenty-seven when Owanza and I began counseling her. She had been on medication for nine years and hadn't been able to work in all that time. Her parents supported her. I really didn't get the point of her medication because she was still extremely depressed. Maybe it disoriented her enough to keep her from killing herself. I would have preferred death to a life like that. Jeff, I see you suffering and I ask myself, 'Will you hate me for helping to save your life if you don't get any better than this?' "

Jeff ponders the question. He doesn't comment.

"Anyway, since Barbara had been on medication for so long, Owanza and I suggested she wean herself off it over three months. First, she cut her dosage in half for a month. Then in half again for another month. And in half again for the final month. By the end of her first year off medication she had written five hundred songs and was recording a few."

"But I'm different, I have physiological damage."

"On the correct diet for your body, it can heal. I won't be a nag about it, so I doubt I will mention it more than twice after this. After that, you'll have to ask me. And I'll help you, without any I-told-you-so. Just ask. I love you, Jeff."

"I'll think about it. I'll probably do it but I need to get my head in the right place first. I'll be here a little over three more weeks. Will that be enough time?"

"Easily. I'll wait three days before I mention it again."

"Thanks. How many days do you think I have to eat the fats before I can stop taking medication?"

"Three to five days. You are already there. The unsalted raw butter and raw eggs I've been putting in your custard and banana smoothies have already prepared you. Now it's up to you."

"Good. Can we go to the store and get me a steak? I don't care for ground meat too much."

"Whatever you want. I have a porterhouse steak in the fridge. Help yourself."

"Thanks." Jeff pauses, then says. "I would like us to get to know each other. Talk about what we've been through."

"I was going to suggest something like that. But since a lot of my past is unpleasant, I'd prefer talking about what we like and don't like. See what we have in common."

"That sounds good," he says fading out. He looks barely in touch with this world. He sways like a palm in the wind as he sits down on the toilet, exhausted.

"The orange juice, egg and cream in your hand will bring you back to life if you'll drink it," I tease.

"Oh, yeah," he says chuckling. He drinks it.

"I'm speaking at a cancer support group this evening. Would you like to see what your old man really cares about?"

"I'd like that."

"Be aware that most of these people are suffering and not too happy."

"I can relate to that."

17

In the evening

The soft lighting sprays warm highlights and shadows on the thirty-three faces before me. I feel this loving mood has been set to help everyone forget about death for the next few hours. Everyone has terminal cancer except Pamela, our host, who is in remission. I can barely see Jeff sitting back in a corner in the shadows where he felt he wanted to be, alone.

All eyes are riveted on me while I'm being introduced. I feel comfortable with it; the prospect that I might be helpful is exciting, especially with Jeff here. I look into everyone's eyes.

"Please, welcome Aajonus," Pamela concludes.

I stand and receive their warm applause.

"You may sit. We like everyone to feel at home," Pamela says as she sits to my left near the stone fireplace. The fire burns low. Her living room is decorated with antique furniture and knickknacks.

"I'd prefer standing for awhile, thank you. First, I would like to introduce you to my son, Jeff. We've been separated for most of his life. Please stand, Jeff."

He stands somewhat uncomfortably.

"Jeff is recovering from a near-fatal accident. What I mean by that is, four doctors said it was impossible for him to live because of the brain damage he suffered. But here he stands due to good nutrition. So there is more hope for health than doctors know about. Thank you, Jeff. Sorry for embarrassing you."

"It's okay. It seems like it could be helpful," he says and sits.

The room is so quiet I can hear people breathing and the gas hissing as it passes through the pipe before it burns in the fireplace.

"When I was dying of cancer seventeen years ago - actually, I was dying from medical treatments for cancer - I met a man who drank the juice from carrots. Can you imagine?!"

Almost everyone laughs or chuckles.

"He told me about a woman who'd cured herself of cancer with carrot juice. She had written a book about it. I scoffed at the idea. I mean, anyone who could drink carrot juice, I thought, couldn't have everything in her head in place."

There are more laughs.

"I hated cooked carrots, and I'd never eaten one raw. Eventually, he got me to taste the carrot juice. It was delicious. Something clicked in my head with that sip. Instantly, I linked health and diet together. Within weeks I went to a health food store and purchased eight books that had some reference to cancer and diet. I didn't get--"

"This is hoopla. Carrot juice. If it were that easy these people wouldn't be here!" a skeptical voice from the far side says.

"Gabe, you agreed to keep an open mind. Do you have any answers? No, you don't. If you want to leave, leave. But don't start," says the woman next to him.

"What's your name, Ms.?" I ask.

"It's Mrs. This is my husband, cynical Gabe here. I'm Sarah."

"If you want to deck him, it's perfectly okay with me. I'm just kidding, Gabe. You have a right to be cynical. We've all been conditioned to depend on doctors for our health. They've failed us. As I said, the carrot juice incident got me to link diet and health together. I didn't cure myself with carrot juice alone. I don't know how many people here can heal themselves with the diet-logic I've devised. But it has been my experience that it works for everyone who does it. For as long as he or she stays with it."

The tension dissolves. A hand from the darkest shadow next to Jeff rises and I call on her or him.

"My name's Jill," a teenage girl's wounded voice says.

"Hi, Jill."

She leans forward and I see her face. The tension is extreme around her eyes. I recognize that below her baseball cap she is bald from chemotherapy, which has also made her puffy and pallid with large dark circles around her sunken red eyes. I also see traces of radiation burn. Seeing her brings back my image after I had had devastating radiation and chemo therapies.

"I'd like to know why I got cancer so young. Do you know why you got cancer so young?" she asks.

"I avoid remembering."

"But don't you think burying it causes cancer? I mean, some people say it does," Sarah asks very sensitively.

"Not necessarily. My experience has been that stress usurps massive amounts of nutrients. As long as we eat enough live raw nutrients, stress will not weaken our bodies."

"Your stress must not have been as great as mine, then," Jill says.

"That may be true. But does that negate what I just said?"

"Why don't you want to get it out? Doesn't it eat at you?" demands an elderly woman to my right. She has black circles in her sunken eyes and is bone thin. She wears heavy make-up and an elegant scarf covering her baldness. Again, I recognize the effects of chemotherapy. The sight of her brings me to tears.

"Talking about it won't change my past. I've made peace with it and I move on from here. When I was young I was always sick. Now I'm healthy. What more is there?" I ask.

"I think if you'd let it out you'd be even healthier," says a man confrontationally. I see the fresh burns on his neck and face from radiation therapy. I cringe. I remember how sore and tender my flesh was after radiation treatments.

"I would agree, if I were bitter about my past. But I'm not a victim anymore. The past was. My present is mainly what I make it," I say.

"If you made your peace with it, it shouldn't bother you to face it," Gabe mocks me.

I notice Jeff and Pamela getting angry for me.

"I'm sorry, this isn't going well, Aajonus. What's the matter with all of you? He's come to give us what he has to offer. Please," Pamela says anguished.

"How can he look so healthy and have had blood and bone cancer? I want to hear the whole story," Jill, the teenage girl, demands.

Pamela rises and stands in front of the fireplace, "Aajonus is going to leave if you--"

"It's okay. I'll give you some highlights as I remember them. I was born in a pile of shit and wherever I went, if there was another pile within fifty miles, my feet found it."

Everyone laughs except Gabe.

"By the way, Jill, where did you get all that information about me? You seem to know more about me than I do."

"One of your clients told me," Jill says.

I pause. I take a deep breath bracing myself. "I feel like I need to hold a flash card that says: Some people may be too sensitive to hear the following story. It contains vivid and explicit details." Everyone laughs, even Gabe.

I sit on the couch to cushion myself. I have never told anyone the stories that led to me getting cancer. Should I be doing this? I just told Jeff today I didn't want to talk about my past. And here I go.

"I was the third born of four boys. That was at least two too many for Mom and Dad. They were always too busy with basics to give us the necessary emotional and psychological attention. They mostly gave orders, criticisms and punishments. Usually, they argued. We got the typical white-bread upbringing with a heavy measure of brutal discipline baked in.

"My trauma began in Denver, Colorado. Mom and I had just come home from the hospital several days after my birth. I was lying in my crib looking upward at the mobile that dangled above me. I wasn't fond of the wooden mobile because it was painted stark primary colors, so I chewed on my hand. That ugly mobile gave me cancer." Everyone laughs.

"My brother Doug watched me from outside the bars of my crib. I couldn't see his nose because he was barely tall enough to see over my mattress - he was standing on something. His furrowed brow leaned against the bars and his dark eyes stared at me vengefully. Nausea overwhelmed me.

"He reached through the bars and pinched my thigh slowly until I screamed and cried. The pain was excruciating. Then he reached for my hair and yanked. He ran to the doorway with a waddle; his diaper was falling a little. He watched for Mom to come while I screamed. She didn't. He came back and pinched my arm until I screamed bloody murder. He ran back to the door."

I take a deep breath. I feel a lump forming in my throat but I continue, "Sometimes he did this for ten or fifteen minutes. Finally, Mom decided that something was wrong. She investigated. But she never caught on. Still, I was always happy to see her. I guess she assumed the red spots and bruises came from me banging around in the crib."

"My God. Was your mother a zombie? Couldn't she tell what was going on?!" an attractive matronly woman sitting on the floor in front of me asks. A tear runs down her cheek. Her tear makes me sad.

"Doug, who was eighteen months older, would pretend to like me. But when Mom left the room, or sometimes just turned her back, he hurt me. I don't think Mom could have imagined that one of her babies was so angry. She may have been in denial, I don't know. I tried to alert her. I believe everyone comes into this world telepathic. I was. I'm no different than anyone else. I knew when Doug was on the brink of hurting me. A couple of times I screamed to signal Mom when he approached. Doug leaned forward. He stared intensely into my eyes and I heard, 'If you ever let her know, you'll really suffer.' But his lips didn't move! Mom didn't hear!"

Someone gasps. I notice Jeff looking distressed.

"At that moment I realized I was living a nightmare. Doug was still telepathic enough to know some of my thoughts. He knew just when to threaten me."

Someone else gasps.

"But Mom and Dad were deaf and dumb to my way of communicating. I wasn't able to learn language."

"That's horrifying! How could you have been so aware at that age?!" the woman in front of me asks with tears streaming down her face.

"You actually remember all of that at only a few days old?!" Gabe asks annoyed, a challenge more than a question. I hear someone blowing and sniffling.

"I guess I remember because of trauma. Hasn't everyone heard enough?! You want my guts too?" I ask humorously.

"We'd like to know the gravity of it," Gabe challenges again.

"I remember the first time I fought back. It was the Easter Sunday before my second birthday. Doug was three-and-a-half years old. Mom, my two brothers, Don and Doug, and I were in our church clothes standing on the sidewalk outside our home in Oak Ridge, Tennessee. I watched the clouds my breath made in the frosty air while Dad took 8 mm moving pictures of us. Doug jabbed a knuckle in the soft of my spine without anyone seeing. I ached. Adrenaline rushed into my blood. It seemed to race through my spine and into my nervous system. I lost control. I turned on Doug. I hit and frightened him. He was afraid that Mom and Dad would realize he caused me to do it, so he froze up. I pounded on him.

" 'Stop that!' Mom yelled at me. Doug learned he could get me into trouble. Every time he furtively hurt me and I defended myself, Mom and Dad spanked me. I looked like a mad child. He looked like an angel. But he began hurting me less.

"I came to believe that I couldn't trust anyone. Not even my parents. I kept to myself as much as possible for the next two and a half years. I didn't care to talk to anyone unless I was forced to with an, 'Answer me, or I'll wallop you,' from Mom, Dad or Doug.

"The day my semi-victories with Doug ended was the day my father betrayed me. Doug had begun kindergarten. I wanted to go too. I followed him to school. He got enraged and started pushing me. I beat him up. A paper boy stopped the fight. He took me home and told my parents. Dad said to Doug, 'He's smaller than you. Don't let him get away with that. Look, hold your hands like this. Clench your fists like this. Keep your hands up like this, so you can block his fists when he tries to hit you. Like this, see? Then punch him back, like this. He'll stop hitting you.' "

I hear a gasp among a few sniffles and groans.

"Didn't you learn to fight the same way?" Jeff asks hopefully.

"Doug was stalky, a full head taller than I with much longer arms. I had a squat build. There was only one thing Doug feared from me after that. If I could talk I could prosecute him before my parents. He made sure I was too afraid to talk. This caused me to be borderline autistic and severely dyslexic.

"Schools worsened my problems. Mom is Catholic and put us in Catholic schools. The nuns in my first and second grades ridiculed me and smacked me with rulers because I couldn't read a word. I thought the whole world was full of raving maniacs. They solved their problems - so they thought - with intimidation and violence.

"At age seven, I decided that I would make Doug my friend. But his animosity was immense. He continued to hurt me. The constant stress and abuse drained and weakened me. I got sick more often as the years passed. Excuse me. I have to catch my breath. I feel as if I'm going to cry. Crying in private was the only release from my childhood traumas. Crying felt so good that I still cry, or at least tear up, from pain, joy, tenderness, and just about anything that touches me deeply."

Three women come and hug me. I start to weep. We weep together. Another woman and Jill join in the hug, weeping. Jeff joins us. Then, everyone but Gabe joins in.

I begin to laugh. Then I break down crying.

"I feel like a water pipe with no valve to turn me off. Would somebody please turn me off?" I joke. Everyone laughs. "Okay," I sniffle. "Let's try to get through this in one piece. Let's see. So, my being compassionate and understanding with Doug rarely helped our relationship. He accused me of trying to be a saint. He said I was really the devil. He called attention to my anger. I felt my anger. It felt destructive. I began to believe that I was evil.

"At age eight, I stopped trying to be his friend. I became brazen enough to try to communicate with Mom and Dad that he was hurting me. They repeatedly told me, 'You must have done something to make him hurt you.' I wanted to sass back, 'Yes, I was born!' I hadn't learned the sound patterns to express my concepts.

"Then at age ten, a light of inspiration struck. I took on Doug's criminal attitude. I immersed myself in his emotions the way an actor does. I became the frustration, the anger, the hostility. I was a better thief than he was. He shared in the loot. I fought and beat other kids. He enjoyed it. Sometimes I flipped. I waved a knife at him. Or my Knights of Columbus sword. Or a BB gun. At those moments he was frightened of me. As a result, I spent ten minutes, a day, a week, or three weeks without being harmed.

"But, I had exchanged one set of terrors for another: I could get caught. When Dad caught us he went wild on us with either belts, wooden clothes hangers, whiffle ball bat, 9-iron golf club, or wooden 2x4 paddle. (He forced Doug to make the paddle. I had to sand and finish it.) Child abuse was called discipline in those days.

"Because fighting and sharing-the-loot were social activities, I began to play with other kids. I was attracted to 'nerds' because they were rarely verbally violent, and never physically. But I still couldn't communicate well because I couldn't articulate my thoughts. I had difficulty forming sentences. The 'nerds' thought I was an imbecile. I chose to play with girls who were smart and compassionate."

Jill weeps by herself. I hold her while I continue. Jeff smiles supportively.

"Mom realized I needed help. She hired a reading tutor for me when I was in fifth grade. Kitty was a cum laude college student. I was delighted. But Kitty didn't have the understanding or patience for my problem. She laughed uncontrollably at some of my pronunciations. I was humiliated because I admired her and thought she was beautiful."

Gabe laughs. Everyone rebukes him.

"I think Gabe laughed because he identified with me," I say.

"You're too kind to him," the white-haired woman says in a witty tone.

"Sorry, Gabe. I guess cynicism breeds cynicism. Mom fired Kitty after the first session. A year later my parents shut Doug and me in the same room every Saturday. They gave each of us a book and a dictionary. (What use a dictionary is to someone who can't read, I'll never know.)

"I don't know if Doug had my problem or just hated reading. I was losing my telepathy. I was afraid of knowing Doug's thoughts. He knocked the wind from me when I did. Several times I fell unconscious thinking I wouldn't awaken. That would have been okay with me if a place called "hell" hadn't existed for me then.

"We couldn't leave the room until we had each read at least four chapters. I was resourceful enough to hoodwink Mom and Dad. I chose books they would never read, from the 'Tarzan' series. I had seen the Tarzan movies at Saturday matinees. I had learned enough sound bites to tell a little of the story by deduction and imagination. It worked and I was released from confinement after six Saturdays."

"Didn't Doug ever change, to make a long story short," Gabe jests.

"You are so rude!" a voice spews.

"I thought we had out-grown our childhood irritations, but at a family reunion only nine years ago, when Jeff was thirteen, Doug mashed water-melon in Jeff's face. Jeff couldn't breathe. Because Doug had always been a good father to his children, I realized it was an extension of his hostility for me. Doug seems to be a likable man to everybody else. To maintain compassion and equilibrium, I think of him as a dark angel who helped me face fear and disease head-on, and to reverse and heal them.

"I cheated throughout my schooling. I was always terrified of getting caught. But I didn't know any other way. There was no help to ask for as far as I knew. I had been led to believe that my inferior mind couldn't be fixed."

Jeff stirs restlessly. He looks hungry and tense. I decide to finish and take Jeff home, "Then I married at sixteen and had Jeff at seventeen. I was divorced at nineteen. So, a lifetime of toxic medical drugs, pollution in everything, especially diet, and daily traumas made me weak enough to quickly develop cancer from medication, surgery and radiation treatments. I was on my deathbed when I began to read well at age twenty-two. I literally woke one morning several weeks after my initiation into carrot juice and diets and I could read. I know it was my change of diet and not coincidence. It was as if my brain ran on high octane and my new diet supplied it. Then I began reversing all the deficiencies that my lifetime of severe stress and poor diet caused.

"Jeff and I have to leave. I will return in a couple of weeks, if you'd like. At that time I will answer specific questions about diet."

"You really have to go already?" Gabe asks sadly.

Everyone is upset that I am leaving except Jeff and me. We are exhausted. But no one else presses us to stay. I am relieved that they don't and touched that Gabe did.

I look at Jill and say, "Very few bone marrow transplants are successful without side effects. About 2%. Plus it is frightfully expensive. If you will stop radiation and chemotherapy, and eat fresh, unfrozen raw bone marrow with organic raw beef, your chances of remission and recovery from leukemia are as high as 96%."

"How did you know I was going to have a marrow transplant?!"

"The medical profession only has three ways of treating bone cancer. I can see by the side effects that you already have had two of them."

"Can my mother call you?"

"Sure. Here's my card. Take care."

She gives me a hug. "Thanks for coming. I feel better. 'Bye," Jill says.

"Good-night everybody," I say.

"Good-night, and thank you," Jeff says and we leave. Still drugged, Jeff moves slowly and almost stumbles over his own feet. I start to help him but I stop myself. He might feel embarrassed in front of everyone if I treat him as if he can't walk. He recovers his balance.

Outside, Jeff says, "You had a rough life. I'm sorry."

"Thank you."

"I need to tell you something," Jeff says hesitantly.

"What?"

"I assume you know something about what happened before the accident."

"Stacey and Ralph told me a little."

"I had to stop myself from hurting Stacey and Ralph. I drove into the trees on purpose."

18

Three days later

I stand in the kitchen hand-juicing oranges. I notice Jeff in bed stirring. He sits up.

"What are you doing awake at nine o'clock in the morning?!" I ask.

"Jus' woke up."

"Beatriz is in the bathroom. She'll be out by the time you get there."

He moves at almost normal speed to the side of the sofa bed and stands. He wavers, as if dizzy. He sits back down.

"Here." I hand him a large glass of a mixture of orange juice and certified raw cream. "Most people have extremely low blood sugar in the mornings. That's why it's so difficult to awake and do anything. Stand up too fast with too low blood sugar and you'll get dizzy. Even black out. I can hardly believe that you are so much more focused, and moving this fast. You've only been eating steak for three days."

"It's also that I haven't taken my medication in four days - since the day before we talked about it three days ago."

"You haven't?!"

"I'm a little scared."

"Well, you've had five months of fear-conditioning. Don't worry, with each day the fear will shrink and finally disappear."

"I trust you."

"Thank you. Neither of us will regret it," I say with my eyes filling.

"How can you be so sure?"

"Seventeen years experience. I've taken greater risks. And I didn't know as much as I do now. But good instincts and intuition, and common sense got my clients and me through successfully."

"Do you always eat the same things day after day?"

"I go with my cravings and desires for food. Sometimes I'm into lots of raw bland fruit, like cucumbers, tomatoes, summer squash, corn on the cob, zucchini and fresh peas, and a few vegetables like lettuce, alfalfa sprouts, parsley and young spinach with a few ounces of carrot juice. I mostly eat head lettuce because that's the kind my body has a taste for. I know people say that it isn't nutritious. They determine that by the specifics that researchers look for. They don't research unbiasedly. I trust my body. I am doing excellently for someone who has been through a lot. Trusting my body, what it wants and eating those foods raw, has been advantageous for me. But although my body mainly craves fruit, I try to limit fruit and eat plenty of fat and meat."

"The day of my accident Stacey and I broke up. I was really upset and jealous. I drank half a fifth of one-hundred-and-one proof Wild Turkey. If I hadn't of drunk that liquor I would never have been thinking like that. But I get crazy once in a while."

"Are you asking for suggestions?"

"Do you have any?"

"Probably more than you want to hear." Jeff laughs. "I recommend that you never use salt. It irritates nerves and destroys cells. When you feel anger or rage, do not eat cooked meat and, frequently, eat small amounts of cooked starch with tons of raw fat. That recipe takes approximately forty minutes after eating to take effect, so you would be wise to exert extreme self-control and do some physical activity until it does. In general, eating antibiotic-free and hormone-free fertile raw eggs, raw meat, raw cream and no-salt-added raw cheeses, soothe and calm the body."

I talk to Jeff about nutrition for awhile longer.[25]

"I don't expect you to remember much at first, so ask me to repeat anything. I'll write you a book someday." I pause a moment. Then I say, "Your conscious or unconscious decision to drive into the trees rather than kill your friends was loving - in a broad sense. I believe that your mother's, Ben's, Stacey's and Ralph's hurts will all heal. You are alive, whole, still healing and not in jail. I'm glad you are here." Jeff smiles and his eyes tear up.

"I haven't asked you about the details of your accident, not because I don't care, but because I don't want you to distort what really happened by telling abbreviated versions. Everything in your life led up to that event. It is my belief that if you can see and remember it clearly and honestly, you will make choices that will prevent that from happening again. I mean, unless you enjoy having near-death experiences."

---

[25] *See* Appendix S, page 154.

"Yeah, I don't think it's good to talk about it. You think I'll be all right?"

"Like I said, isn't your future made by your everyday choices? You have a good mind, strong will and you know how to take care of yourself. If you lack anything, wouldn't it be better to trust yourself to handle problems without drugs and self-destructive behavior?"

"I can make my life good."

"Great. I'm starving! How about you?" I ask.

"I'm starving!"

"Let's get dressed and buy some steak. What would you like."

"Sirloin and porterhouse."

"Those are my favorites!"

19

Nine days later

It is 8 a.m. I am dressed in my painting clothes. I go into the kitchen and pack my food in the cooler. I hear Jeff moving on the sofa bed.

"You goin' on a picnic at this hour?!" Jeff calls to me.

"I'm off to paint a house. If you feel like working I could use your help. Could you use ten dollars an hour?"

"Sounds good to me. But I don't know if I can do any good."

"What are you talking about? You have full use of your brain and both hands now."

"I'd really like to. It'll take me a few minutes to get ready."

"Beatriz is going to work with us, come with her. I'll meet you there."

"Awesome! I never thought I'd work again. Or at least for a long time. All right!"

Two days later

Wearing a dust mask, Jeff sands an area on the north wall that I patched. I watch him. I see how quickly he is regaining his more subtle motor responses. I amble over to him and we talk through our dust masks. "Jeff, you are doing great! But may I show you how to sand so you won't make ridges?"

"Sure."

"The hardness of the patching compound and the wall are usually different. I fill the cracks several times leaving only the slightest film higher than the surface of the wall. Then I sand lightly in circles."

"Looks easy enough. Thanks."

"I'm stopping for lunch. You can have lunch whenever you get hungry."

"I'm starvin' now!"

"Me, too," Beatriz says.

"Then let's all do lunch," I say.

We clean our hands and saunter to the porch with the cooler. I remove a jar of ground beef, butter and honey. "Would you like some?"

"No, I feel like eating some fruit right now," Jeff says.

"Help yourself," Beatriz says.

"Thanks. Dad, did you smash your thumb with a hammer?"

"No. It pusses like this every so often," I say as I look down at my thumb. At the side of my nail is an inflamed and blackened area with pus. Where it is blackened, a hole has been eaten through the nail.

"Is it painful? What is it?" Jeff asks.

"An infection that is very painful at times. When it first happened it lasted for seven weeks. Then it disappeared for three months. This makes the seventh time it has reoccurred. The blackness and eating away of my fingernail and skin usually indicates molds. After the fourth time it happened, I had a lab test the pus for molds. The results came back positive for penicillin. I hadn't had penicillin in fifteen years."[26]

---

[26] *See* Appendix T, page 156.

"Wow," Jeff says.

"Fifteen years and it's still in your body!" Beatriz says.

"If it can eat a hole through my nail, imagine what it has done to the inside of my body. Of course, the air may have rendered it more volatile than it was inside my body."

"I'll never take antibiotics again!" Beatriz says.

"Dad, how did you get into raw meat?"

"That's a jump in subject." I pause trying to remember. "I recall thirteen years ago. I had already stabilized my cancers and mitigated many of my other problems. But I wasn't satisfied. I had had a taste of good health and I wanted more.

"Everything I read was contradictory. So I decided that I had to enter the wild to learn the truths about optimal health. I hadn't realized at that point, that it was a matter of difference. Everyone's body is different. Every body reacts to food differently. Because specific foods and amounts are proper for someone, doesn't mean that those foods and amounts would be proper for others. And vice versa. That is no contradiction.

"Anyway, I traveled North America on my bicycle and lived off the land for almost three years. I occasionally lived with Native American tribes for a month at a time. A very wise native suggested that I eat raw meat.[27] I rejected the advice because I was a diehard evangelistic vegetarian.

"The experience that changed me was...unusual. After two and a half years traveling on my bicycle, I became discouraged. I had gotten too thin and was weakening more everyday."

"I thought you said you were always overweight?" Beatriz asks.

"I was overweight when I ate cooked foods. I got slender when I switched to all raw but meatless diets. And then, when I bicycled and lived outdoors the stress was so great that I deteriorated.[28] I regularly ate as much as three pounds of nuts daily, six avocados, enormous amounts of fruit and every day I awakened a bit thinner that the previous morning. But I didn't want to return to civilization with its pollution and its survival-of- the-fittest attitude. I had seen in the wild

---

27 *See* Appendix U, page 156.
28 *See* Appendix V, page 161.

that only malnourished animals lived by that rule. Otherwise, life outdoors was peaceful. I loved living outdoors. But, physically, it was too stressful on a raw meatless diet.

"Rather than go back to civilization, I decided to fast myself to death.

First, I dug in and built a ten-by-ten foot stone house in what I was told was an ancient Indian burial ground. It was in the foothills of a mountain range twenty miles northwest of Salton Sea, here in California.

"Because the house was sunken, the roof was only four and a half feet above the ground. At night, I jumped onto the flat wood roof with my sleeping bag. I loved falling asleep while watching the stars. A coyote woke me one night around midnight. She made sounds like a laughing crazy person. She stood fifty feet away. I could see her because I had night vision. Night vision is something I had developed while living outdoors.

"After several consecutive nights, I realized she had a purpose in waking me. But what it was I didn't know. Another night I sensed a coyote passing in the wash twenty feet behind me. I turned and saw him. I wondered why the laughing one woke me when they could have easily passed me while I slept. This game went on every night for two weeks. Each night I sensed another coyote, without using my eyes or ears. (I think that that was what they had intended - for me to strengthen my sixth sense.) Then I turned in the direction where I felt he or she was. And there was another coyote. Within two weeks I had sensed each one as he or she passed through the narrow canyon by me. There were eleven in the pack.

"One unusually warm night it rained lightly. I slept on the ground inside the house. My sleeping bag was unzipped and I had one leg sticking out. I was awakened by a cold nose rubbing the side of my bare leg. It was a coyote. I wasn't alarmed. The coyote dashed away and up the steep grade of the entrance. He stood looking down at me. He looked straight into my eyes. He motioned his head as if he were indicating that I should follow. I thought I must be crazy. But he did it again. I trailed behind him to the pack. They all nodded at me. I returned the gesture.

"They leapt, butted and played as they started off into the desert. I followed behind. I was weak from fasting. They waited for me to catch up. We had gone about a half mile when they caught a whiff of something up wind. The group quietly separated and made a half circle about two hundred yards wide. The one that stayed with me, looked me in the eyes. He motioned his head for me to follow. I did.

"We crept about three hundred yards up wind. Then he sped off to the side zigzagging down wind. He laughed like a crazy person. I heard the others start to howl and laugh from afar. They were approaching like an ever-shrinking half circle toward the lone coyote. He was making his way toward them.

"I ran to see what was happening. A jack rabbit was caught in the half circle. It zigzagged and leapt around. But it was trapped by the encroaching chorus of coyotes. The rabbit stopped, paralyzed. I thought I saw an apparition leave the rabbit. It seemed to no longer have a consciousness.

"A female coyote took the stiff rabbit and broke its neck. It dangled from her teeth. Another coyote bit into the skin between the rabbit's front legs and ripped open its entire torso. She brought the rabbit to me. She dropped it on my bare feet. The rabbit was hot and bleeding. I felt sick.

"All eleven of them stood staring at me. I kept getting this thought: It's what you need, take and eat it. They seemed to be sending me that thought. I flashed back to my childhood. I remembered the way my brother Doug sent me his thoughts. This was the same, but this thought had a gentle feeling about it. The coyotes were communicating with me.

"I looked down at the rabbit. It was warm and moist as if it were alive. I looked at the coyotes and said, 'I don't know, guys, I haven't eaten meat in six years.' Then the idea came to me that these coyotes were here to help me quickly end my life. A fast could take months (another oxymoron, I thought).

"I picked it up. I took a bite. I forced myself to swallow. It came right back up. The coyotes looked at each other as if it were a joke. I sat down for five minutes and psyched myself into eating it. After five bites, it tasted delicious. I ate about three and a half pounds. The coyotes shared what was left: the hind, head, skin and bones.

"They went on food-shopping and I walked back to my rock house to die. With every minute that passed, I felt lighter. I thought that the poisons were taking effect.

"I got my sleeping bag and laid down on the roof. I felt a peacefulness that I had only felt during my death experience on the heater with the fresh pizza stains on my shirt. I was sure I was about to leave my body again. I fell asleep.

"I woke the next morning after the best sleep of my life. The raw rabbit meat made me strong for three more days. And so I became a raw meat eater. I had found the missing link to my health! I killed and ate rattle snakes and birds. I traded my hard labor on farms for eggs, chickens and raw goats' milk. My muscles developed easily. Several months later, I returned to Los Angeles to spread the great news of my discovery. Everybody thought I lost my mind."

"You are! But that's one reason I like you so much, Dad. You are strange," Jeff says laughing.

"I remember you saying you liked to bowl. Would you like to go bowling?" I ask.

"I don't have enough strength in my right hand."

"At the rate you are healing, you will soon," Beatriz says.

"I don't know," Jeff says.

20

Five days later

Beatriz' friend, Wilma, and Jeff sit in the back seat. Beatriz sits shotgun. I drive us into Mar Vista Bowl's parking lot.

"I'm warning everybody right now, I haven't bowled but once in twenty years. I have never been very good at it, but I loved it," I say.

"Wilma and I aren't good bowlers either. We just enjoy it," Beatriz says.

"Before the accident, I was very good. I was in a league. But I don't know if my hand will be able to control the ball."

"That makes us all about even, doesn't it? So, the worst bowler wins. Hey, Jeff, your mother and I met at Brentwood Bowl."

"I didn't know that."

"No, I guess she wouldn't have talked about us."

We exit the car and walk to the building.

"Your accident changed you into John Wayne, I swear. You walk and talk real slow like," I say, mimicking him.

"Wish I made his kinda money, pilgrim," Jeff says.

Jeff wipes his hands and passes them over the blower. He lifts his bowling ball and moves into position. He inserts his right hand fingers into the ball. He hesitates and flexes his right wrist. He brings the ball into position. He makes his approach, slides and brings the ball forward. He drops it. It bounces hard down the lane and into the gutter. Jeff looks frustrated and disheartened.

"You expected a strike on your first bowl?" I ask.

"Crazy, huh?" He steps back and waits for the ball to return. "Dad, I think that health has a lot to do with your state of mind. If you think about good health you make it happen."

"To what extent?"

"Whatever."

"If you are saying that, because I desired good health and focused on it, found the means to achieve it and acted on it with successful results, I'll buy that as a general statement. But if you are saying that I didn't have to do anything other than think about, desire and pray for good health to find myself miraculously healthy one day, you're talking mind over matter, and I don't buy it. I mean, you can take your body for granted like any male chauvinist dominates a woman. The body will respond. But there will always be dire emotional, psychological and physical side effects."

"That's what I believe," Jeff says.

"Let's do one of those man things. You know, challenge each other - without the kill-to-win attitude," I say playfully.

"Watch out, Wilma, the boys are getting started," Beatriz says wryly.

"Who goes first?" I ask.

"You," they all say.

"All right. Jeff, tell me why were you taking that medication that was interfering with your healing if all you had to do was believe you wouldn't have seizures? And why, once you started eating the raw diet and stopped taking the Dilantin, did you begin healing after nearly four and a half months of limbo? Your state of mind was that you were afraid you would have a seizure. Why didn't you have a seizure? (Don't answer yet.) Instead, you are able to work and even bowl."

Jeff passes his hand over the blower as his ball returns.

"Jeff, I would love for what you believe to be true. I would have preferred an easier way to health. Lord knows I tried. And I'm not saying that because I couldn't do it, it can't be done. I'm just asking you to help me see it."

"It takes a certain kind of faith," Jeff says as he lifts his ball and moves into position.

"I've seen some of the greatest gurus of our time. Everyone of them had health problems. Why is that so, when they lived very cushy, protected lives? They purported to heal people yet they couldn't heal themselves. Why was that?"

"I couldn't begin to tell you," Jeff says looking back at me.

"I lived in a yoga ashram for two months, once. One of the most disciplined young men I had ever met, Sadashiva, was in charge of the Los Angeles community for Sri Vishnu Devananda. He had been celibate all of his young life. He had witnessed Vishnu Devananda levitate, that is, float up and remain suspended or bounce in mid air. But what good was that talent when Vishnu Devananda couldn't come into agreement with his body? He witnessed Devananda's cravings for pizza, canned pineapple, salt and ice cream. Every time Devananda ate any of them, he got either immobilizing stomach aches, flatulence or headaches. He ignored that Devananda's mind-over-matter concept, taught to him as spiritual fact, was not working there.

"Anyway, Sadashiva was completely sold on mind-over-matter. I was explaining to him that diet could alter a person's state of mind as easily as a person's mind could alter the physical being. He said that that was completely opposed to everything he had studied in metaphysics, short of poison. I decided to prove it to him, and myself, without telling him.

"I was the dietitian at the vegetarian ashram of which Sadashiva was in charge. I was responsible for selecting and buying food for the entire community. I chose a food combination that acts as an aphrodisiac. I intended to turn the ashram upside down by stimulating everyone's sexual desires. Sexual pleasure was the absolute no-no there.

"Except at dinner, most people ate on the fly, grabbing whatever fruit was available. I had observed that most raw-food fruitarians and vegetarians were often hungry. Only a handful assimilate enough protein to satisfy the body's needs. At the ashram we were no different. If delicious food were available, we ate often. I bought cases of oranges and avocados. Everyone ate the combination on the fly several times a day.

"Within five days, Sadashiva and the other Hatha yoga instructors, excluding me, began talking about the anatomy of their female students. As the days went on, they became randy. Some started to touch the students - not in lewd ways but unconsciously sensual.

"I stopped feeding them oranges and avocados. Within five days everyone was back to normal. I told my friend Monica about the experiment. (Monica and I had been lovers, but by this time our relationship hadn't been sexual for about a year.) She didn't know whether to believe me or not. It seemed so far-fetched. We decided to repeat the experiment and she would be witness.

"I supplied the kitchen with avocados and oranges again. Within five days they started talking about anatomy. Within eight days, the touching began. I mentioned to everyone that they were getting awfully randy (without mentioning the food) and shouldn't they be careful. They said I had a few screws loose, that they were just playing around, and nothing was going to make them lose control.

"Although I wanted to prove to them that their mind-over-matter concept was flimsy in reality, my conscience persuaded me to stop. I bought pears and apples for them to eat with the avocados instead. Everyone settled.

"Monica and I debated about the results. Among other things, she said it could have been the full moon that stimulated everyone. I agreed that that was a probability. I let a week go by.

"I supplied avocados and oranges again. By the fourth day, the conversation was wild. Touching began. I considered ending the experiment. Monica agreed that things were getting heated but she argued against my belief that food would drive these ascetics from celibacy. They continued eating avocados and oranges.

"On the sixth day, one of the instructors shared passion with a woman he had admired. On the seventh night, Sadashiva called on Monica. She thought Sadashiva was gorgeous and had mentioned her desire for him. They shared intimacy through most of the night.

"So much for mind over matter, or should I say, life in chaos. I'll take mind and matter in cooperation - life in balance."

"Avocados and oranges, I'll have to remember that," Jeff says.

"Me too," Wilma says.

"I don't know if it works on people who are not raw-fooders or vegetarians. Since then, I discovered that watermelon and avocados together stimulate me more. Add raw fish, especially raw oysters to that and I don't have to wait a day or two for it to work. But the body acclimates to almost anything. So I found that an aphrodisiac works for only so long."

"This conversation is making me lose concentration," Beatriz says, laughing.

"Me too," Jeff says as he takes his bowling stance again.

"God, wasn't everybody fat from eating all those avocados?!" Beatriz asks.

"Because the fats were raw, their bodies utilized the fat perfectly.[29] Beatriz, for you, I recommend three avocados a day with oranges and raw oysters."

"Awesome! Sizzling," Jeff remarks.

"Get some cold water for this boy, now!" Wilma says about me.

Everybody laughs. Beatriz gives me a twisted smile.

"Are you guys gonna let me bowl or what?" Jeff says.

Everybody laughs. Jeff starts his approach, hastens his step, slides and sends the ball spinning. It takes all of the pins down for a spare.

"All right!" we all say.

"Hey, hey!" Beatriz says, "Nothing like ending the first frame with a bang."

"You are going to make all of us look like the worst bowlers in the world," Wilma teasingly chides.

Jeff says, "Well, Wilma, we'll just have to feed you some avocados and--"

"Don't say it," Wilma says.

"Hey, not bad bowling - for a vegetable who's predominantly

---

[29] *See* Appendix W, page 162.

paralyzed for life. We should be filming this to show Dr. Braisley. Wouldn't he have a baby?" I say.

"You got that right," Jeff says as he approaches me and offers his right hand. We shake hands and he hugs me.

In Conclusion

Jeff called me after he had seen Dr. Braisley. He asked Dr. Braisley if he could stop taking Dilantin. The doctor became alarmed and warned Jeff of possible seizures. Jeff told him that he hadn't taken the medication in three months. Dr. Braisley stammered. Then he said, "If you haven't had a seizure by now, you don't need to take it." And Jeff stopped pretending to his mother that he was taking the medication.

Jeff went on to study electronics and computer technology, and graduated.

Ten years later

Jeff is still normal and has not had a seizure or any complication as a result of that accident.

Owanza is completely healed from her cancers, and - she insists that I mention - she has healed her sagging arms and bottom.

Jill, the teenage girl, reversed her leukemia within a year on this Primal Diet. She is married with a successful career in education. However, she hides the fact that she eats raw meat because of the narrow-mindedness within the academic community.

And, finally, my patience and tenacity were rewarded with complete recovery from the mushroom- poisoning. It took my body eleven years to recover to vibrant health.

Appendix to Volume I

Appendix A

(From page 10.)

If a mother isn't eating a healthy diet or can't breast-feed for one reason or another, feeding an infant fresh raw (not heated above 96°) cow's or goat's milk will most often resolve colic and make her baby healthy and strong. But there are some babies (and people) who can't even digest raw milk properly for several months. Two ounces of unheated honey and 4 tablespoons of unsalted raw butter blended with a half gallon of raw milk will make the milk digestible.

I remember one infant who could not digest pasteurized milk, raw milk or the raw milk/honey blend. Three years ago a young Korean couple came to Owanza and me (Owanza is a friend and nutritional colleague who was at one time my nutritional client). The distressed mother held her five-month-old infant who screamed just as Jeff had. Owanza and I could see the couple's humiliation. It seemed to me that their gestures at soothing the baby were to show us that they cared and were helpless.

In hopeful gesture, the mother tenderly placed a bottle to the baby's mouth and circled the nipple around her lips. The infant's little hands grabbed it and sucked. Within five seconds she pushed it away and screamed fiercely. The mother sighed.

"Does she cry like that often?" I asked.

"She cries all the time, almost all day," the mother said tensely.

"Doctors not able to help. Five months now," her husband said.

"May we try giving her something?" Owanza asked.

"We have tried all formulas," the mother said.

"If it works she'll stop crying," I said.

"Okay," the father said with bitter resignation.

Owanza blended one raw fertile egg with two ounces of Evian water for 30 seconds on low speed so that the egg would completely liquefy and not clog the nipple. For a moment, the high-pitched blender noise distracted the infant from crying.

Owanza poured the mixture into an empty baby bottle and handed it to the mother. The mother ran the nipple over the infant's upper lip. The baby grabbed the bottle and sucked. Within three seconds she pushed it out, screaming.

The mother looked more discouraged. The father sighed, disgusted. Then, in an instant, the baby's eyes widened. She grabbed the bottle and nursed it dry within four minutes. She pushed the nipple from her mouth and then smiled.

"She has never smiled before!" the mother said.

"Look, she happy," the father said proudly.

Appendix B

(From page 12.)

Commercially available unpasteurized raw fresh dairy products are outlawed in most states except California. Every state health department is administered by medical doctors. All doctors are taught to fear raw dairy - afraid that it is a carrier and cause of disease. Although there have been thousands of testimonials for the healthy benefits of raw dairy and there has not been one case of disease or illness as a result of certified raw dairy in California, California health officials still try regularly to outlaw raw dairy and deprive the people. Their argument rests solely on germ theory. They recently forced the raw dairy industry to put a warning label on their products. These labels scare people away from eating those healthy foods. Health conscious people who are fully aware of the benefits of raw dairy in California have had to fight hard and long over the years to maintain their right of choice. "Health" officials allow people the choice of cigarettes and alcohol which have been proved harmful, why not allow us the healthful choice of fresh raw dairy? *See* Obtaining The Foods You Want And Need, page 208.

Appendix C

(From page 20.)

Medical science removes cells from the natural environment of the body and isolates them in "controlled" environments, like test tubes. It administers chemicals to these isolated cells and observes the reactions. It treats cells as if they were machines that have no intelligence and that repeat exactly the same movements and functions. Medical science says that this is the only way experiments can be valid. But it fails to see that cells do not behave or react the same in "controlled" environments as they do in the body. Therefore, it can never predict how a person will react to a drug. And every body reacts differently.

I have employed a very different approach to experiments. I see that the body is its own ecological system. Every body part, gland, cell and particle of blood makes the body the magnificent creature that it is. Eliminate any organ, appendage, hormone or cup of blood, and the body loses a function and/or precise ability. My approach is wholistic. All of my experiments have been employed on the whole person and whole body with food as agent.

There are always side effects with drugs - sometimes seemingly minor, other times disastrous. A side effect with raw food is extremely rare.

To prove that medication prevents healing, I employed research methods formulated by Owanza. I repeated the following experiments with seven individuals. 1) I had a blood analysis performed on each person before and after his or her doctor administered a drug (seven different drugs). The analyses were specifically focused upon RNA and DNA. Blood analyses were done twelve hours after drugs were taken. Mutations were found in the RNA and DNA when compared to the RNA and DNA of the blood taken before drugs were administered. 2) I also had a urinalysis performed on each person before and after a drug had been administered, specifically focusing on bacteria. In all cases the analyses taken before drugs were administered showed a normal live bacterial count. In all cases the analyses performed ½ hour after taking drugs showed large quantities of dead bacteria.

The next step was to show a correlation between greater bacterial levels and healing. Bacteria, like bears and flies, go in and out of hibernation. When conditions are right they wake from hibernation. Are bears and flies contagious? Bacteria consume particular damaged, decaying and dead cells when weather, other environmental conditions and bodily cycles are right, and when an individual's body is ready to detoxify. To prove that higher bacterial levels advance healing, I observed ten subjects, each with three open wounds. On each person, I treated one wound with alcohol. I treated another with the subject's urine only. (Urine contains most of the same constituents as blood, except that it contains very few red blood cells. The practice of using urine as both a cleansing and healing agent has been employed for thousands of years in Ayurvedic medicine.) The third wound on each person was left untreated to heal on its own. The wounds treated with urine healed about three times faster than the ones treated with alcohol. The wounds that were untreated healed a little quicker than those treated with alcohol. Conclusion: Alcohol destroys bacteria and retards healing. A high bacterial level inspires healing.

In another experiment, I observed several groups of people who had stomach ulcers. One group took either Maalox or antibiotics. Another group drank his or her own urine. A third group drank urine and ate a raw diet. The ulcers in those who ate raw foods and drank urine healed two times faster than those who only drank urine. The ulcers in those treated with medication grew larger.

I asked those who were taking medication to discontinue medication. After one week I observed that their stomach secretions had higher bacterial levels. Concurrently, I observed that the ulcers had diminished in size and/or were less inflamed. Conclusion: Drugs kill bacteria and retard healing. Bacteria inspires healing.

To explore the phenomenon that infection also inspires healing, I observed a person who was suffering from polio. When the person was treated with the standard drugs, I noticed that there was a drop in body temperature and a loss of bacteria and virus in the blood. The urinalysis showed very few poliomyelitis virus in the urine and blood. However there was no improvement in the condition or symptoms. I asked the person to discontinue drug therapy. After three days without drugs, the person drank five raw smoothies a day and drank Perrier water when thirsty. (Each smoothie consisted of 2 raw eggs blended with a whole green – unripe - banana.) No other food was eaten. After this nine-day procedure there was about 50% improvement in the condition and symptoms. I reexamined the blood and urine. I found a lot of poliomyelitis virus and bacteria. In ten weeks this person healed completely without paralysis. Conclusion: Drugs destroyed bacteria, prevented cells from manufacturing virus, and interfered with healing processes. When the subject stopped medication and began to eat the right nutrients, bacteria and virus increased and healing began and continued until complete. Bacteria and virus are necessary for proper cleansing and healing.

To prove that medication stores in the tissues, Owanza suggested that I examine people who had a long history of drug treatment. I found hard dry areas on their skin. I had small tissue samples cut from these hard dry spots and had them analyzed for chemicals. Every tissue sample was found to contain small amounts of medical chemicals, specifically those containing alkaloids.

In another test I conducted, I had small tissue samples taken from the throats of people who had long histories of taking drugs such as Emperin, codeine, aspirin, Fiorinal, and other drugs which effect the mucous membranes. I had the tissue samples analyzed. All of the analyses showed trace amounts of drugs.

In another experiment, I worked with subjects who had long histories of taking antibiotics. I asked them to discontinue taking medication for at least two weeks. Then blood and urine samples were taken and specifically analyzed for drugs. These samples showed only trace amounts of drugs, or no drugs at all. I suggested that the subjects follow a diet for six weeks. First thing in the morning each of them ate ½ cup raw fatty beef with one tablespoon of unheated honey. When the stomach growled, indicating hunger, each of them ate 2 fresh oranges and a tablespoon of unheated honey. Again, after the stomach growled, each of them ate another ½ cup raw fatty beef with one tablespoon of unheated honey. They continued to eat the beef and oranges, alternately, throughout each day until they went to sleep for the night. They always waited until their stomachs growled before eating the beef or the oranges.[30] They drank as much unfiltered, unadulterated spring water as desired, but no sooner than 30 minutes after eating meat. They ate no other foods. After this six week diet, blood and urine samples were taken again and analyzed for drugs. Analyses showed large quantities of drugs in both blood and urine. Conclusion: Drugs store in the body. Certain foods cleanse the body of drugs.

Appendix D

(From page 27.)

I am reluctant to mention the harm that vaccines produce because most everyone is adamantly brainwashed that vaccines produce immunity. However, I would be negligent to ignore how vaccines actually affect health.

Allopathic medicine is based on the "germ theory", that microbes and viruses, cause disease. Medical science bases the use of vaccines on the theory that the body forms antibodies to "fight" natural viruses. They believe that these antibodies live on after the virus is contained, thereby creating immunity.

First we must consider the facts known to evaluate medicine's viral theory. Science has proved that virus are not alive, that they are predominantly protein but that they contain organic DNA. Science has proved that virus increase only in the presence of live cells, and that they cause certain cells, and/or parts of cells to dissolve. What is believed and taken as fact but not proved, is that viruses are non-discriminatingly destructive "things" that self-replicate. That is like saying that laundry soap, because it is found in homes inhabited by

---

[30] When doing this detoxification diet, which helps the body eliminate stored drugs without much harm to the body, it is important to eat only when the stomach is completely empty. That is because some drugs will be dumped into the stomach and be arrested there. Eating during the dump/arrest phase, or mixing the beef and oranges in digestion - by eating either before the other has completely been digested - causes indigestion, increases nausea, and sometimes causes vomiting. (Vomiting is beneficial and the quickest and easiest way for the body to eliminate drugs after they have dumped into the stomach.)

humans, self-replicates. Those assumption and conclusion are shallow and ludicrous. Medical science operates from fear, and it attacks the body. All medical procedures for treating disease are written by pharmaceutical-related individuals and groups. That is a severe conflict of interest. Self-produced health or medication-dependent profit, which do you think that they want?

A rational and logical conclusion would be that virus are solvents (cleansers) manufactured by individual cells to dissolve degenerative tissue (disease) caused by accumulated waste and industrial toxins, including medicines. Virus contain DNA because cells have used substances within themselves to synthesize virus; DNA is a part of that. When the cleansing and healing processes cease, cells stop producing large amounts of virus.

Normally, healthier bodies symbiotically utilize bacteria and parasites to cleanse themselves of cellular degenerative tissue and organic waste. They are the bodies preferred janitors. Bacteria and parasites consume the degenerative tissue and organic waste and reduce it to a tiny fraction of the original mass eaten. They can consume 100 times their weight and reduce it to 1-percent excretion. When eating a healthy raw diet, our bodies easily secrete and/or excrete the 1-percent excretions from bacteria and parasites.

However, when bodies become too toxic with industrial toxins, including medicines, the bacteria and parasites are poisoned to death. Under such toxic conditions, the only cleansing method that the body can utilize is virus. So, cells synthesize viruses. I reiterate, viruses are solvents that dissolve degenerative tissue and organic waste. They are beneficial in preventing disease; they do not cause disease. The symptoms that accompany viral, bacterial or parasitical detoxifications are a necessary process but can be mitigated with the consumption of plenty of raw eggs and raw dairy fats.

The key is: We should trust, nurture and understand the body and Nature, not fear them.

Inoculating people to prevent viral infections is ridiculous and dangerous. After many years of experimentation, Louis Pasteur realized that the idea of vaccination was doomed. He confessed on his deathbed to his assistants that a poor (toxic) environment within the body creates disease. Microbes do not cause disease.

Regarding the immediate trauma that vaccines cause in many people, the eminent scientist and physician, Dr. William F. Koch, M.D., Ph.D. said:

> The injection of any serum, vaccine or even penicillin has shown a very marked increase in the incidence of polio - at least 400%. Statistics are so conclusive no one can deny it.

The long term effects of vaccines are just as harmful. Vaccines are made of disease, mercury, aluminum, formaldehyde and other poisonous chemicals. Pharmaceutical houses manufacture diseases in animal tissue. The diseases are sterilized to make vaccines. Sterilization alters the RNA, DNA, structure and actions of diseases and viruses. When a sterilized disease or virus enters the body, the body tries to analyze it and create antibodies to regulate the disease or virus. The body cannot find the logical reason for the unnatural disease or virus. Nor can it find the key to the time that the bacteria or virus will be active. Therefore the body creates mutant antibodies that do not go dormant for up to decades.

These mutant antibodies remain active long after the disease or virus becomes inactive. The mutant antibodies eat sub-particles from the inside of amino acids (proteins) in the blood.[31] That renders proteins unstable. The amount of proteins damaged and lost to mutant antibodies depends on the number of vaccines. Because amino acids are the primary building blocks of cells, the consequence is cellular malnutrition. In all animals, the malnutrition causes gradual genetic mutations, resulting in weaknesses, diseases, malfunctions and deformities.

The life span of mutant antibodies varies, from at least 1 year (penicillin) up to 50 years (polio).[32] Each vaccine multiplies the number

---

[31] The nature of the sub-particles eaten from proteins is explained in THE PERSECUTION AND TRIAL OF GASTON NAESSENS by Christopher Bird, H.J. Kramer, Inc., P.O. Box 1082, Tiburon, CA 94920.

[32] The body reacts to antibiotics (like penicillin, tetracycline, etc.) the same as it does to vaccines - that is, mutant antibodies are created.

of mutant antibodies, which increases cellular malnutrition and results in greater weaknesses, diseases, malfunctions and deformities.

Table 1 shows the reported incidents of polio in the year 1958, before the compulsory polio vaccine law, and the year 1959, when the law was adopted. Only four states and one city kept records. The statistics show that the polio vaccine actually created the disease that it was purported to have prevented.

Table 1: Number of Polio Cases Reported in 5 areas, Before and After Polio Vaccine became Compulsory

	1958	1959	% Increase
Compulsory Vaccination?	NO	YES	
Connecticut	45	123	273%
Los Angeles, CA	89	190	213%
North Carolina	78	313	401%
Ohio*	17	52	306%
Tennessee	119	386	324%

*Ohio had an escape clause and many people declined inoculation. Therefore there were fewer incidents of Polio.

Eighty-two percent of all of the people who had polio in 1959 (listed above) had been vaccinated with one or more polio vaccines. Twenty percent had at least three polio vaccinations. Polio vaccines create polio.

Vaccines have other immediate side effects. There is temporary or permanent paralysis (Guillain-Barre) associated with any type of vaccine, including flu shots. Almost everyone receiving a vaccine of any sort suffers some of the following side effects: blindness, brain damage, convulsions, death, dizziness, other serious diseases, fever, headaches, hepatitis, impotence, irritability, muscular pain and soreness, nausea, skin eruptions and disease, sore throat, stiffness and vomiting.

Former Secretary of War, Henry L. Stimsom, reported that at a military boot camp in only a six-month period, there were 63 deaths and 25,585 cases of hepatitis "as a direct result of the yellow fever vaccine."

Yet, doctors and pharmaceutical houses say vaccines are miraculous - choosing to ignore the harmful effects. Is it because vaccines generate several billions of dollars a year? Isn't it frightening that our children are the main target?

I experimented with vaccines in animals (rats, cats, and rabbits) and found that the mutations compounded with each succeeding inoculated generation. In the second generation, with all three types of animals, mutations started as slight deformations of an ear, or eye, or jowl; or a shortened limb; or scoliosis. Glandular malfunctions were prominent. In some animals, temperaments became unruly. In the sixth and seventh generations' mutations were severe: loss of glands, organs, limbs, features, motor and neural functions; brutal suicidal and homicidal tendencies; and impotence resulting in extinction.

In my experience, of all the pharmaceuticals that are accepted as miracles, vaccines are the most dangerous because the side effects are most often subtle, or attributed to another problem, or ignored. These side effects become obvious after the third and fourth generations. That is when the mutations start to become exaggerated and pitiful. With humans this will probably be apparent by the year 2015.

There are many books on the dangers of vaccines. Read them. I've listed the ones I've read - both well written and not - in the reference section. *See* Bibliography, page 340.

While I was experimenting with raw moldy foods as possible remedies for particular health problems, Owanza, who was assisting me, discovered that eating moldy berries affected the mutant antibodies caused by vaccines. She placed raspberries, blackberries and strawberries in separate glass containers with lids that were not tight. She allowed them to sit at room temperature until a healthy mold had formed. Then she placed them, still in glass containers with loose lids, in refrigeration for ten weeks. After these ten weeks, Owanza strained the moldy berries through a porous sieve, separately. The mold-juices were ready for my subjects.

Blood analyses were done on eleven people with long histories of vaccinations, with specific focus on amino acids. All subjects had minor complaints, ranging from headaches to joint pains. For one time only, each person drank ½ cup of one kind of mold-juice - of the particular berry that normally appealed to their taste. Their diets were not altered. Blood analyses were done 30 days after drinking mold-juice. Analyses showed an average of 30% increase in stable amino acids over previous analyses. There was only one side effect as a result of drinking the mold-juice - everybody became lethargic for a period of 30 days. After that period, everyone's level of energy and health increased sharply above what it had been before drinking the mold-juice. Health complaints either diminished or disappeared.

Between 13 and 18 months after they drank the mold-juice, three of the people planned to get vaccinations for travel reasons. Blood analyses were done before inoculations and again a month after inoculations. The post-inoculation analyses showed a 30% drop in stable amino acids.

Twenty-four months after taking the mold-juice all eleven had blood analyses. In eight of them the stable proteins in their blood remained high. In the three who had recent vaccinations, stable proteins were still down and the health complaints that they had prior to drinking mold-juice returned.

Appendix E

(From page 39.)

I would have substituted raw plain kefir (a liquid yogurt) in place of the butter, to replenish her intestinal flora destroyed by the antibiotics, but plain raw kefir wasn't on the market at the time. I didn't give her yogurt because yogurt is made with milk heated to at least 112° to make it congeal quickly. Even low heat above 100° Fahrenheit makes the nutrients in milk inferior. By the time Monica came home I had made a raw kefir using kefir grains and raw milk.

Appendix F

(From page 40.)

The formulas I fed Monica were: (1) the tomato mixture; (2) plain raw kefir blended with unheated honey and whatever fruit appealed to her at the time, and (3) an orange and banana blended with a primary yeast that had been grown on raw milk and dried below 95° Fahrenheit.

With what I know now, I would have used raw chicken and fish marinated in fresh lemon, or lime or pineapple instead of formula 3. Eating raw chicken and fish better ensures that nerves heal properly and promptly.

Appendix G

(From page 52.)

To ensure that my high adrenaline level didn't overtake, irritate or exhaust me, I ate some starch. I had a taste for raw pistachio nuts with raw butter, raw egg and unheated honey rather than cooked starches. I knew this combination would cause my blood sugar to drop, so I put some non-steamed dates (most dates are steamed) on the counter, to be ready. I'm glad most people's blood balance isn't as delicate as mine.

Appendix H

(From page 53.)

I know that when I eat raw fat with fruit 1) my blood sugar level doesn't get too high because the fat time-releases the fruit sugar into my blood for better equilibrium and therefore I don't have the sugar top and drop, 2) I don't have to eat constantly to keep sugar in my blood, and 3) I get two to three times more energy than when I eat fruit alone. I eat rich delicious foods that balance me without side effects like getting too fat, or wired and then exhausted from caffeine, or the sugar highs and lows (mentioned above). The benefits of eating raw fat and fruit together would apply to most people most of the time.

Appendix I

(From page 64.)

I remember my childhood and think how wonderful it would have been if aloofness were my only complaint about my father. Dad probably recalls his childhood and thinks how much easier my childhood was compared to his. But Dad wasn't sick or injured six months out of every year as I was. Although, I do remember a story he told me.

When Dad was three years old, he was walking in the barnyard and a Clydesdale horse kicked him in the face and put him in a coma. Everybody thought Dad would die. Nearly every year as a child thereafter Dad got severe migraines with an infection under his cheekbone. The doctor literally hammered a horseshoe nail through Dad's skin and cheekbone to drain the infection. No anesthetic was used. Dad's migraines continued through the years.

I believe Dad's trauma never healed because his nerves didn't properly heal. He didn't eat raw meat. And he ate a lot of salt, which causes high blood pressure in the brain (the main reason for headaches[33]). His high salt intake along with his tremendous adrenaline flow made Dad extremely irritable, sometimes violent and regularly suffered migraines.

I believe that almost all violent and antisocial behavior has biochemical and biological roots because I have witnessed that it can be turned on, off or mitigated by what a person eats. And I have seen that if we don't become aware and take care, our relationships and lives fall victim to our biochemical imbalances.

---

[33] *See* Appendix J, page 140.

Appendix J

(From Appendix I, page 139.)

I worked with people who had long histories of headaches. Ninety percent of these people ate a lot of salt. When they stopped consuming all types of condiment salts (which are radical, that is, harmful), including sea salt, they stopped having frequent headaches.

Periodically their headaches returned. Whenever the headaches returned, I had their blood and urine analyzed. Each analysis showed sodium molecules clumping - just as if they had recently consumed condiment salts. They assured me they hadn't. Also, all of the analyses showed high levels of dead cells, especially liver and brain cells. The conclusion I drew was that radical salts had stored in the body and killed the surrounding cells by dehydrating them. I realized that the salt and dead cells in the blood and urine indicated that the body was cleansing salt and dead cells. And that salts store throughout the body, especially in the brain and sometimes liver and brain.

See also Appendix M, regarding salt, page 143.

Appendix K

(From page 67.)

All nutrients - proteins, starches, sugars, vitamins, minerals, enzymes and millions of unknowns - interact. Each requires all of the other nutrients in varying amounts to be properly utilized. All supplements lack most of the balancing nutrients, especially bioactive enzymes. If all are not present, the body leaches nutrients from its own supply (if it can afford to). Supplements create a balance/depletion see-saw effect.

I experimented with supplements for two years. I started this research while I was the nutritionist at a health food store. Of the 1,200 supplements we carried, I observed that only nine had any significant benefits. Those nine supplements were all prepared at temperatures below 82° Fahrenheit and were not chemically treated or extracted.

Over those two years, I observed that the remaining 1,191 supplements created toxicity throughout people's bodies, especially their glandular systems.

For example, many people who regularly consumed iron supplements had iron deposits somewhere in their systems. The worst deposits appeared as rust spots in Iridology. Almost all mega-dose-Vitamin C-takers suffered irritability, psychological problems and frequent hunger - sometimes compulsive - for ice cream, chocolate and/or other rich foods. This is because supplemental Vitamin C is spiky, like glass, irritating blood and nerve cells. It depletes fat from the blood and makes the blood highly acidic.

People often reported an increase in energy from taking supplements but I observed that the increase in energy was most often a toxic effect. The toxicity forced certain hormones to rush into the system, similar to caffeine or nicotine rushes that ultimately have damaging effects on the entire body.

Unless supplements are prepared correctly, the side effects outweigh the benefits. By the time I left supplement research, 6 of the 9 beneficial supplements had been destroyed: wheat germ oil, 2 brands of cod liver oil, shark oil and 2 brands of primary yeast powders. The pharmaceutical houses and the American Medical Association created a myth that synthetic, natural and organic were all the same; so why pay more? The media circulated the myth. So preparation and temperature quality controls became moot points. Manufacturers altered their processing to compete in the cheaper markets. The public are deprived and consequently suffer.

Appendix L

(From page 70.)

Most often, depression is caused by too much carbohydrate sugar and sugar byproducts in the blood, lymph and nerves. Carbohydrates made into blood sugar result, unfavorably, in high sugar byproducts, causing the blood, lymph and nerve serums to be sticky, causing reduced bodily functions and hypoglycemia.

Naturally, when too much carbohydrate sugar enters the blood, the pancreas produces insulin. Insulin helps regulate blood sugar levels by binding with sugars and turning them into glycogen which can be stored in the body and used later. When mutant sugars enter the blood, the pancreas overproduces insulin even if the blood sugar is low.

Refined sugars are mutations, including flash pasteurized products. They enter the blood too fast. When refined sugars are eaten, the body first tries to turn them into a more natural sugar. However, most of the sugar just passes into the blood as mutations. They over-stimulate the liver and pancreas. Eventually, bile and hormones, like insulin, bind with the sugars and leave the blood low in sugar (hypoglycemia). Over a period of time, this can lead to the eventual exhaustion of the pancreas (diabetes). Although it would take considerably longer, the same can result from eating too much raw fresh fruit and fruit juices.

The best way to resolve the blood-sugar problems that cause depression is to eat a lot of raw meat. When the body forms blood sugars from meat, the blood sugar is called pyruvate. The body's use of pyruvate results, favorably, in low sugar byproducts allowing clean body serums, including in the nerves.

For some people, simply changing to a raw diet, that includes lots of raw meat, relieves depression. For a few, adding only raw fats to their diet is the simple answer because without proper fat, proteins cannot be assimilated for many purposes. Eating raw meat with raw fat, and reducing fruit intake to once daily in the afternoon only, feeds the liver and pancreas, regenerates and rebuilds them and, over a period of many years, repairs them to where they cease to automatically over-dump sugar into the blood and over-produce insulin.

Another cause of chronic depression is too-low of bacterial levels throughout the body. When high levels of bacteria are present, proper detoxification occurs. Bacteria are janitors who consume organic cellular waste, keeping the body clean. When the body is low in bacterial levels, the body becomes overloaded with organic waste and toxins, causing cellular depression that is experienced throughout the body and mind, and expressed emotionally.

The low-bacterial cause of depression can be alleviated by eating stinky bacterially decomposing meat, as several cultures do, such as the Eskimo. The Eskimo call that meat "high" meat. Eating an ounce of high meat usually relieves depression in 10-20 minutes and may last for weeks. I demonstrated that there is no danger from eating meat with enormous amounts of bacteria on Ripley's Believe It Or Not (it first aired internationally on July 17, 2002). The recipe to make high meat is in my recipe book, The Recipe For Living Free of Disease.

A less favorable way to keep the blood sugar level balanced is to eat one cooked starch (like French bread, rice cakes, pasta, air-popped corn, baked or steamed potato) with lots of raw fat (like avocado, unsalted raw butter, no-salt-added raw cheese, raw cream, raw eggs, stone-pressed olive oil or fresh coconut) with a little fresh fruit. For people with severely overactive pancreases, that combination - in small amounts - may have to be consumed two to four times daily. However, the cooked starch always results in accumulations of sugar byproducts and toxins.

How the last recommendation works is that the cooked starch easily binds with excess insulin. Then the raw fat binds with the starch-insulin mass and escorts it to the bowels.[34] The fresh fruit raises the blood sugar level to normal. Depression is gone or mitigated within forty minutes. However, many sugar byproducts and other toxins from the cooked starch accumulate in the body and could eventually cause disease.

Appendix M

(Part of the conversation cut from page 74.)

"Should she continue drinking a lot of distilled water?" Ray asked as we stood in the vitamin and supplement aisle.

"Distilled water makes all problems worse in the long run. It's hungriest water that starts leaching nutrients from the digestive tract and blood, then from the rest of the body. All water disturbs the balance of the digestive juices and intestinal flora. Sometimes, that causes people to lose a little weight and they falsely think it's healthy.

"Balanced minerals in natural unadulterated waters, if drunk moderately, help dissolve and bind with toxins in the body. Then blood fat or protein, if available, binds with the mineral/toxin mass and are

---

[34] If the fats reach temperatures above 104 degrees Fahrenheit, they have a greater tendency to store in the body and solidify instead of dumping into the bowels. Therefore, eating fats warmed above 104 degrees Fahrenheit is <u>not</u> suggested for optimal health.

eliminated from the body. Balanced minerals in natural unadulterated waters help dissolve and neutralize toxins, cleanse and soothe.

"The only naturally distilled water I would ever recommend would be fresh unpolluted rain water with its high bacteria content. It may cause diarrhea for a few days, but that's always a healthy cleansing process. To balance the effects of diarrhea, I suggest any or all of the following: raw plain kefir, a little banana, no-salt-added raw cheeses, and a Nut Formula [page 194]. Oh, and your wife should not eat salt in or on anything."

"She craves salt! What's wrong with salt?" Ray asks alarmed.

"It causes sodium molecules to clump in the blood. That reverses ion magnetism and pulls the guts (so to speak) from cells. The affected cells can no longer eat anything and they shrivel and die. Four little bitty grains of salt - including sea salt - destroy approximately two million red blood cells. It takes at least three hours to replace the blood cells and about 24 hours to cleanse the dead cells. During those processes important nutrients are leached from the blood and body. As a result, salt speeds aging.

"The craving for salt is symptomatic of a mineral deficiency. To satisfy her craving for salt, I suggest that your wife eat any or all of these foods: fresh raw tomatoes, no-salt-added raw cheeses, fresh celery juice and raw fish. (Eating raw shell fish, like oysters and clams, several times a month is particularly effective in quickly correcting a mineral deficiency.) These foods will supply a concentrated balance of minerals that the body can utilize easily and pleasurably."

Appendix N

(Part of the conversation cut from page 76.)

"Where did you get the beef?" Mary asks me, worried.

"At the shopping center."

"Isn't raw meat toxic from all the antibiotics and injections animals get nowadays?"

"Yes, but most toxins store in glands, some organs and bone marrow because of the concentration of fats in glands, bone marrow, and some organs. I don't recommend eating glandular tissue and certain organs (that is, pancreas, thyroid, adrenals, testes, ovaries, liver, kidney, brain, etc.) and bone marrow unless they are from organically grown animals raised without injections and without deworming medication. Fresh muscle meat - steaks and ground - are okay even if you buy them at regular markets as long as they don't add coloring and you don't cook them. If toxins are in the meat, cooking the meat releases the toxins from the fat and some or all will accumulate in the body, eventually causing disease. Organically grown is always more nutritious and preferable. But if organic isn't available, regular is healthier than none."

Appendix O

(Part of the conversation cut from page 84.)

"I'm allergic to everything but grapefruit juice that I squeeze myself. Literally, I can't eat anything. Not even whole grapefruit. If I do, I break out in hives that itch so intensely that I feel like I want to tear off my skin," Owanza said.

"I see two problems. You do not form enough healthy resilient mucus. And you are not lubricating and protecting your cells. There are two basic reasons for that. Either you do not eat enough fat and proteins, and/or you are not digesting, assimilating and utilizing fat and proteins properly. Eating raw protein and raw fatty foods will relieve the hives in time. Probably within two hours," I joke.

"Oh no, you're a raw-fooder? I did raw-food fruitarianism for years and I never felt balanced. I had to eat cooked pastas, and I got better. So you see, raw food doesn't work for me," Owanza said and her eyes filled with tears.

"Did you always eat a raw fatty food with fruit?"

"No."

"A strict fruitarian diet often robs the body of fat, protein and minerals. If you had eaten avocado, raw eggs, no-salt-added raw cheese, raw cream or fresh coconut cream, the fruit would have digested and utilized the fat you ate. Instead, the fruit leaches the fat from your blood and body. Therefore, it was impossible for you to get balanced."

"Avocados caused acne with me, and they sat on my stomach."

"What did you usually eat with avocados?"

"Nuts, salads, in sandwiches."

"Some people lack the digestive enzymes to digest avocados. Eating any raw fruit that appeals to you with avocado will help you digest avocado properly. Raw fruits include sweet, acid and subacid fruits, tomatoes, cucumbers, fresh corn on the cob--"

"I'm not a skinny person, I'll get fat!" she said.

"You look trim to me."

"But I have this sagging flesh and cellulite on my arms and bottom."

"If you feel puffy or bloated, it's mainly water retention. Fat has to be soluble to be absorbed and utilized properly. Cells absorb fat to lubricate, protect themselves, gain energy and clean waste. When vegetable oils are cooked they most often do not stay soluble at body temperature. They harden and the body can't dispose of them. The body stores them - sometimes as cellulite and/or plaque.

"When hardened fat stores in a cell, the cell will do one of two things. It will try to liquefy the hardened fat, or try to soothe as much as possible its non-lubricated, vulnerable self. The end result in both cases is water retention. Eating raw fats will eventually alleviate the need for water and water retention.

"Would you rather have two to three extra inches of raw healthy fat to lubricate, protect and soothe you, or would you rather suffer your case of hives and heightened fear of life?"

"I pride myself on not being vain, but I guess that's a delusion," she said.

"Only about 28% of those whom have done a high-fat raw diet of unsalted butter, no-salt-added cheeses, cream, avocados, fresh coconut cream, eggs and meat gain more than an inch or three and retain it for awhile.

"I use size rather than weight because body weight on a raw food diet with raw meat is considerably heavier. On the "normal" weight chart, a person of my frame and height is supposed to weigh around 147 pounds. I actually weigh 169 pounds but look like I weigh no more than I should. So I go by inches."

"I'm vegetarian. I can't eat eggs and meat," Owanza said firmly.

"How long have you been vegetarian?"

"Fourteen years. I can't kill, it's against my religion. It's also unhealthy to eat meat," she said.

"You have done the balanced-protein-type vegetarian diet?"

"I've followed the chart and rules to the tee."

"If vegetarianism hasn't made you healthy in fourteen years, do you think that you're plagued with these problems for some spiritual or psychological reasons?" I asked.

"Maybe, I don't know."

"Could it be simply that a vegetarian diet is not appropriate for your body?"

"I don't think so," she said, offended.

"Generally, herbivores have several stomachs and a digestive tract more than twice the length of ours. They have sixty thousand times more digestive juices to disassemble vegetable cellulose. Most humans can't digest the proteins and fats from legumes, grains and vegetation enough to satisfy the body's needs.

"According to the archaeologist, Dr. Stuart Struever, in charge of the excavations of past Native American civilizations at the Koster site in Illinois, evidence showed that the more Native Americans became a cultivating society and lived less on meat, the more diseases they got. So maybe eating raw meat is necessary for most humans to live without disease.

"My approach is very existential when it comes to health. It has been my experience that health is the basic gift of all life - as the sun shines on everybody. Food, what one does to it and what one eats, determines health. Unless someone has a genetic digestive or assimilative problem. (Often congenital problems can be healed, but it takes longer.)

"Since your problems have developed over time, I will assume you are not eating what is proper for your body. And since you have rejected what I have suggested, I can't help you."

"Please. I have a thirteen-year-old son and a husband. What will happen to them? I can't eat anything. I know I'm going to die. I have been diagnosed as having thirty very small malignant tumors in my spine, sixteen in my liver, six in my uterus, and innumerable nonmalignant ones in my brain. They said I had maybe three months to live. I have one week remaining," Owanza pleaded, weeping.

"What do the doctors want to do?" I asked.

"Radiation and chemotherapy. But I've seen several people suffer terribly from those therapies and die miserable deaths. More miserable than I am dying. None of them lived very many years after those treatments. Medical treatment is not an option. I haven't told my family that I have cancer. I don't want to be forced into radiation and chemotherapy," she said.

"You don't have to convince me. I'm against all medical treatment for cancer from personal experience. Okay, I'll try to help you without meat, but you have to eat what I tell you, how much and when. Because I'm not a medical doctor, you will have to sign a release. Is that agreeable with you?"

"Yes."

"My research and experience has brought me to view cancer as a condition where the body no longer eliminates dead cells, for various reasons. So the malfunctioning body develops tumors, or catacombs, so to speak, and contains the dead cells within them.

"Cancer cells are only the caretakers of the catacombs. They are not the problem that created the inability to eliminate dead cells. Does a rooster crowing at sunrise cause the sun to rise? Calling cancer cells responsible for tumors is like calling roosters responsible for sunrise.

"Killing all the roosters and all other creatures near and around will not stop the sun from rising, no more than killing cancer cells with countless other cells will stop cancer. If clouds pass during rooster killings, one may believe that the killing has stopped the sun from rising, just as, occasionally, a body stops mutating normal cells into cancer cells during and after radiation or chemotherapy.

"Cancer, then, is basically a fat deficiency. A deficiency in utilizable cholesterol that normally binds with or dissolves, carries away and eliminates dead cells. Certain properly digested, assimilated and utilized fats, like those in stone-pressed olive oil, dissolve dead cells. Then other fats, like those in raw eggs, act like sacrificial garbage collectors, binding with dead cells or the dissolved waste and dump themselves and the toxins wherever the body is able to eliminate them from the body.

"A fat deficiency forms when a person stops eating fat; or a person doesn't eat the particular fat his or her body digests, assimilates or utilizes properly; or the body is unable to digest, utilize or assimilate fat at all. Therefore the body becomes as much a vessel for death as for life.

"Eating anything cooked depletes the body of enzymes, vitamins, minerals and innumerable unknowns that could be used to properly digest, assimilate and utilize fat and proteins. Antibiotics destroy digestive ability. They kill more of the beneficial intestinal bacteria than so called "bad" bacteria. Cooked or processed sweet foods, like sugar cane and beets from which table sugar and molasses are derived, work like acids and destroy digestive abilities. Coffee, teas and chocolate, even if caffeine free, create acidic conditions and neutralize digestive juices. This disables the body's digestive abilities in varying degrees. All of these, and many more problems, gradually and completely deplete the body of its ability to digest fat and therefore create a condition where the body is susceptible to countless health problems (cancer merely being one).

"Eating many raw fatty foods daily with the foods that supply enzymes for fat digestion, utilization and assimilation (that is whatever bland, sweet or acidic raw fruits, or unheated honey, you have a taste for) shrinks the odds of getting cancer in our society to 10%. We could reduce that to 0% if we were not exposed to medication, pollution and chemical additives.

"Fifty percent of your diet will be raw fat. Every meal will have to include either the unsalted raw butter, no-salt-added raw cheeses, raw cream, avocado or fresh whole coconut. If you live beyond the week, will you at least consider eating raw eggs?"

"It's against my religion to kill anything. I won't even kill a cockroach," Owanza said.

"I think killing cockroaches is inappropriate too, unless you're a bird or other creature who eats them. Everything is alive, even vegetables. You kill vegetables when you uproot or cut them. You dismember them when you tear off their leaves. If you bite into a fruit and leave it, it rots very quickly. Eggs are as immobile and as faceless as fruit and vegetables. I'm not asking you to make a decision now, but think about it."

"Why didn't you mention beef? Was Owanza of the blood type[35] that doesn't do well with red meat, even if raw?" Beatriz asks.

"No. At that time I didn't believe raw beef was healthy. A friend and I had had a very bad experience with raw liver and sweet breads - that weren't organically grown. She vomited and I had terrible hallucinations. It wasn't until after my poisonous mushroom experience that I discovered that animals store most of their toxins in glands and bones. That's when I realized that it was okay to eat muscle meat of non-organically grown beef, but not the glands. It was almost a year after the poison mushroom before I ate raw red meat."

Appendix P

(From Appendix O, page 145.)

There are three basic blood types when determining what meat someone should eat regularly. These types are: 1) People who naturally have acidic blood easily produce red blood cells. They do not naturally produce enough white blood cells. Generally, this type should eat mostly white raw meat (fish, fowl, rabbit) to be balanced. If they eat red meat more than occasionally they will have a tendency to be irritable, impatient, overanxious and overaggressive. 2) People who naturally have alkaline blood easily produce white blood cells. They do not naturally produce enough red blood cells. Generally, this type should eat mostly red raw meat (beef, lamb, venison) to be balanced. If they eat white meat more than occasionally they will have a tendency to be lethargic and tired (anemic) 3) People who naturally have a balanced blood pH produce a balance of red and white blood cells. Generally, this type should eat both red and white raw meat to remain balanced. Few of this type can do fairly well as vegetarians.

Type 1 usually has a ruddier complexion, holds a tan easily, and/or has a high adrenaline level (that is, they have a lot of physical energy). Type 2 usually has a light complexion, his or her tan fades moderately to quickly, and/or he or she is more emotionally and mentally oriented

---

[35] *See* Appendix P, above.

than physically oriented. Type 3 normally has a balanced complexion, tanning cycle, and a near-even balance of physical, emotional and mental energies.

A person can change from one of these blood types to either of the other types many times throughout his or her lifetime.

Appendix Q

(Part of the conversation cut from page 96.)

"Byron, a nutritional client and friend, got a call from the Health Department one day last year. They told him that a woman with whom he had had an intense sexual relationship for three months was in second stage syphilis. He called me immediately, horrified:

> "Byron," I said, "in order for syphilis to flourish in your body, you would have to have acute toxicity in your nervous system. You have been on a raw diet for years, so you're clean enough of toxins. Go down to the clinic and have the test, but I suggest you do not take medication. It is meant to poison the virus but viruses are not alive and cannot be poisoned. The medication poisons millions of healthy cells and causes the body to stop manufacturing detoxifying virus."
>
> "But Aajonus, this is syphilis," Byron shouted.
>
> "Go get the test done and then you will know."
>
> About a half hour later, Byron called again. He was at the clinic. "Everyone here is panicked because I refused the medication. They say that no one is immune to syphilis and that it could already be in my brain because the woman is in advanced second stage. Aajonus, I'm going to take the medication. What should I do to counteract the side effects?"
>
> "The medication is a poison. Just buy billions of cell caskets and kiss your energy and sexuality good-bye, because they will diminish for years to come - pardon the pun."
>
> "Aajonus, don't kid around, this is serious."
>
> "Something has to make you rational again. Take a look at who's promoting the fear and who's profiting. Trust me, you do not have syphilis. You have sex more than anyone I know. That exercise in

conjunction with your raw diet keeps you clean and healthy. Use your common sense. Panic persuades people to do all sorts of things that are not beneficial. Who in their right mind is going to drink poison because someone tells them to? One or two more days isn't going to melt your brain, Byron."

"Aajonus! This is syphilis."

"I have said all I can. It is your body, your life and you have to live it. It is your choice."

"Okay. Thanks. 'Bye.' "

Five minutes later, Byron called again, "Aajonus, they say I have to take the medication. This is syphilis."

"Would you tell me it's syphilis one more time, just to make sure I remember?"

"Will you stop joking around?! We're talking about my brain and nervous system."

"Byron, right now we're talking panic and fear. I told you the choice is yours. They cannot make you take the medication. It has dangerous side effects."

He handed the phone to the man at the clinic, and the man said, "Excuse me, how can you be human and put this man's life at more risk? Don't you care about him, or is he just a client you take money from? I mean, get rational, sir, this is serious. This is syphilis."

"Now, now, be nice, and calm down. How long will it take to get the results?" I asked.

"As early as tomorrow, if we rush it through. But he has to begin the medication now."

"Would you read the specific law stating that he has to take medication, and the procedures to enforce it."

"It could take weeks to go through the procedures," he said.

"Exactly, so until a judge would rule that he would have to take it, he does not have to take it. And for a judge to order that, a syphilis-positive blood result would be required. Am I right?"

"You have no idea the danger you are putting your client in."

"Let me ask you this, does the medication have side effects?"

"Of course."

"If Byron's test comes back negative for syphilis, would you be putting him in danger with medication?"

"This is crazy. This is syphilis. Your ignorance is really sad."

"I have been exposed to the medical profession my entire life, so ignorant regarding it, I am not. I have also been experimenting with raw food diets for 15½ years, so ignorant about that I am not. Have you ever experienced anyone on a raw diet like Byron's who tested positive?" I asked.

"I'm not aware of anyone exposed to syphilis who was on a raw diet. Have you worked with syphilis like I have?"

"I admit ignorance to your experience, but not about syphilis. Since you are absolutely certain, would you be willing to pay one thousand dollars in damages if Byron does not have syphilis as a disease or as a carrier?"

"You are crazier than I thought," he said and hung up.

"Byron did not take the medication and the test results were negative. They demanded he take the test again. He did. It was also negative."

Appendix R

(Part of the conversation cut from page 102.)

"If a medicine gets a 20% effectual rate, it's considered worthy. The pharmaceutical houses then conduct isolated tests on individuals most likely to react favorably and the effectual rate increases, and consequently the results are biased. Although they know a drug is going to be effectual on very few people, the manufacturers sell it to the masses and doctors as if it would help most people. Drugs don't work on most people and not without side effects, and most people develop a tolerance for them, so people stop taking them. To keep the hopeful masses buying, pharmaceutical houses create new drugs regularly. And advertise heavily," I say.

"But drugs have to go through so much testing before they're approved," Jeff says.

"The people who approve the drugs have not witnessed anything.

They read the test results as viewed by researchers who are being financed or influenced by a pharmaceutical house and/or the medical establishment or researchers who would like their names associated with medical progress whether exaggerated, fabricated or real. It has been my experience that drugs are ineffectual 91% of the time. It seems to me that people are being sold the old snake-oil-panacea pitch with every drug."

Appendix S

(Part of the conversation cut from page 115.)

"Back to your question about eating the same thing day after day. I eat meat almost every day, but which meat I eat changes. Once, for sixteen months, I craved only raw organic chicken. I couldn't eat any other meat, except fish several times a month. Another time, for six months, the only meat I could eat was lamb. One year I craved meat two to three times daily, eating as much as four pounds a day. Another year I could only eat about one third of a pound once daily. Other times I had to eat parsley and fish with beef because beef alone made me too acidic and I got sores around my mouth. I just stay in touch with my body's taste and needs."

"Do you think raw foods would work for everybody?" Jeff asks.

"I don't know if the few hundred people I've counseled who have actually done it are enough proof that my approach could help everyone, but it's the most effective diet for developing and maintaining health that I know. Everyone's body is different and everyone will eat differently, but basically we were raw-food eaters for millions of years before cooking became convenient and changed our sense of taste.

"I've seen that most people are ill because they don't digest cooked or processed foods well enough. Not many of us have mutated to handle cooked foods to create or even maintain health without disease.

"But everybody has to follow their own instincts, that is, whatever they have a taste for. Generally, I suggest that whatever it is one craves, he or she should eat it raw. Most often I've found that foods artificially heated above 104° Fahrenheit are inferior for creating and maintaining optimal health. Very few people who have eaten a cooked-and-processed-food diet lived without any health complication throughout a long lifetime.

"If people are satisfied with their health, then my view isn't for them. If they are not, as I was not, I suggest they cultivate a taste for raw food.

"If, for example, you like sauces, discover what is in them, buy the raw ingredients and mix or blend and eat them raw. Pay attention to whether you digest them well. If you have problems or discomfort, simplify the ingredients. Experiment until both your taste buds and digestive system are satisfied. Sometimes quickly, but most often gradually, you will achieve better health.

"A few rules of thumb, but not absolutes. If you are feeling shaky, it most often indicates too low of a blood protein level. Eat whatever raw meat appeals to you (no-salt-added raw cheeses - a fat that is high in concentrated minerals - will also help this symptom but not as effectively). If you are feeling depressed, it's most often low blood sugar. Eat some fresh fruit with raw fat and a cooked starch. If you are feeling hyperactive, anxious, impatient, or irritable, it indicates one of two things: either you are overproducing adrenaline and/or other stimulants, or your blood fat level is so low the body's own acids irritate the nerves. Eat cooked starch with lots of raw fat and/or raw meat. If you are feeling headachy, nauseous or just have no appetite, it most often indicates that your blood is over acidic and/or toxic. Eat some no-salt-added raw cheese and drink some fresh-squeezed lemon or lime juice with some unheated honey and naturally carbonated water. Sometimes a salad or fresh raw vegetable juice is also helpful. If you can't sleep or can't get to sleep easily, one of two things will help. Eat two to three raw eggs blended with fruit at least twenty minutes before bedtime, and/or eat raw fish in the evening.

"Caution, anything in a can or bottle is at least pasteurized and is relatively a lifeless food, unless labeled raw, unheated or unpasteurized. Concentrates are adulterated and cause ill health.

"Again, get in touch with your body's signals and trust them. Sometimes nothing seems to work fast enough. Patience. Your body didn't grow in a day. Finally, if you get a cold, flu or allergy, eat the following: blend two to three raw eggs, one to three tablespoons of unheated honey and one to two tablespoons of unsalted raw butter with either an orange or a banana. That mix is a panacea that speeds detoxification. It cleanses and binds with the toxins that cause symptoms. It helps you feel better through the detoxification."

Appendix T

(Part of the conversation cut from page 117.)

"That pus test inspired me to investigate athletes foot, other fungus, some yeast infections, and the like. I have most often found that antibiotics were the cause. (However, I have found that drinking coffee is the worst cause of yeast infections.)

"Because all antibiotics create unnatural antibodies inside the human system, the body has to get rid of them. If it doesn't, they disrupt normal functions, consume vast amounts of blood nutrients and destroy tissue.

"I found that most penicillin stores in joints, especially of the hands and feet. When people get a fungus and the skin itches and peels away, it's most often the body throwing off antibiotics or some other medication that molds, or causes molds, within the body.

"Women who take antibiotics while pregnant or nursing are putting their offspring at very high risk of anemia, leukemia, malformation of cartilage, weak joints and other bone problems."

"Does that include Candida?" Beatriz asks.

"Not as much. I've found a large correlation between alcohol, and drugs in the aspirin family causing Candida."

Appendix U

(From page 118.)

"I was on a vision quest at Pine Ridge Indian Reservation, South Dakota, in the summer of 1975. As my Oglala Sioux friend, Spotted

Deer, had instructed me, I was alone, meditating, praying and fasting for four days and nights. I was expecting a vision that would answer my health dilemma. It was sunset and the third day of my quest on a butte. I hadn't seen a vision. I wondered if Spotted Deer had been pulling my leg.

"Actually, I didn't care because the days had all been beautiful. Clouds formed shapes that inspired me to think of prehistoric, Medieval and futuristic times. I was enjoying just being alive.

"I heard something climbing toward me. An ageless wise man came into view. He had the most beautiful smooth vibrant deep red skin. It seemed to glow. He wore supple deer skin tribal clothing as I had seen in pictures. He didn't pant from climbing the butte as I had. He was clear of the normal thickened leathery skin that I'd seen on other Native Americans.

"I got excited. Surely this healthy man could tell me his secrets and to heck with visions. I stood and he bowed his head. I returned the gesture.

"I'm Circling Feet. That's what I'm called here because I've been living off a bicycle for two years. 'Circling Feet,' makes me think of myself as the Road Runner cartoon," I said.

He laughed. "I am Elk-of-the-Black Moon," he said and we shook hands, wrists to hands, while he put his other hand over my diaphragm. "You have been cut by Wasichu[36] medicine."

"You can see my scar through this shirt?" He smiled without answering. "I've been here days waiting for a vision about my health. What's your secret?" I asked.

He sat in my vision-quest square made of a thin bed of sage with its fragrance turning heavier, flatter, stale, but still pleasant. I sat down beside him. We faced east where the sky was turning dark and the clouds were multicolored with a mauve hue.

"If you listen to all that your body tells you, as you most often do, you will have the health you want," he said.

"Are you saying, this is all there is, I'm as well as I'll get?"

"Maybe yes, maybe no. You could add something to your diet," he said.

---

[36] A term referring to Caucasians.

"What?"

"When you were a child, what did you often take more of than your mother told you you could?"

"Cookies, candy and sodas."

"For your lunch?" he said laughing.

"You're very psychic. Luncheon meat."

"Does your body ever have a taste for it now?"

"I've been a fruitarian/vegetarian for five years now."

"Do you ever have a taste for meat?"

"I stopped eating meat some time after medical treatments for cancer. Meat always made me nauseous and increased my skin problems and made me irritable. It seemed to just sit in my intestines."

"Do you remember how eating cooked peas instantly made your body want to throw up?"

"Yes. All cooked vegetables made me want to vomit. Why do you suppose that was?" I asked.

"Cooking altered them into chemicals that were toxic to your body. Your body was telling you not to eat them cooked."

"My parents forced me to eat them anyway."

"That is the first and most harmful assault against all of Nature. Like in your holy book, there." He lifted my Bible beside me and opened it to Genesis. "Eve's apple is any bad food that creates havoc in the body and mind. Bad food makes life difficult and distorts perception, like bad fuel makes a machine run poorly, become faulty, wear and die too soon. Life becomes imbalanced and painful. Fear and ugliness dominate the mind. Then life is seen as dangerous and we live defensively, attacking the outside when it all begins inside. That is the banishment from the Garden of Eden. Paradise was the state and feeling of health and balanced happiness. You like and digest raw peas well, right?" he said.

"They're delicious. I do well with almost all raw foods."

"Three hundred years ago, my people didn't use fire on food. Only for pottery, some tooling and warmth. Then Wasichu came and drove us from our cultivated lands. All tribes of all Indians everywhere became hungry. We began fighting and killing so much then - even members of other tribes - for land to live on.

"To stay healthy we had to eat mostly meat, as my ancestors did thousands of years ago, and as the plains Indians did. But our food supply was always in jeopardy. Wasichu grew like mold on rotting fruit. They pushed further and further westward behind us. They slaughtered us, our buffalo, deer and all animals for greed and sport and again we were no longer able to get fresh meat daily. We had to cure it into jerky to survive.

"When we ate it fresh and raw, Wasichu said that it was a savage ritual. They said we would evoke their devil and infect them with disease. They ordered us to cook our meat or they would kill us. Consequently, we got sick.

"Everything we did, Wasichu used against us as an excuse to kill us and take over all our land and resources. This weakened us more. Wrinkled us like grapes to raisins. Our bones and teeth began to rot rapidly. We became crazy like Wasichu - sick in heart and mind. Many of us drank to forget our pain and fought like the worst of them. Wasichu were used to eating cooked foods and living with the ill consequences. We weren't," Elk-of-the-Black Moon said.

"I'm sorry. I think Native Americans were and still are treated horribly. Like Hitler treated Jews. As you said, white men proliferate and live without respect for balance. They have child after child simply because they want to. It doesn't seem to matter whether they can care for and raise them healthfully and happily. I don't feel like I'm one of them," I said, lowering my head in shame.

"On your mother's side, you have Sioux blood," he said.

"Yes, my mother said she's one-eighth Native American Indian. Do you think you could teach me to be as psychic as you?"

"Let me teach you this: raw meat will make you strong."

"Spotted Deer put you up to this, didn't he?" I said laughing.

"I live alone out here," he said, insinuating he didn't know Spotted Deer. "The next time you have a taste for meat, eat some raw."

"I can't kill animals. I mean, even though I didn't actually kill them, eating meat is the same as killing," I said.

"To uproot vegetables, or bite into fruit is also killing. But when someone only kills to eat, it is according to the goodness of Nature. It is a natural agreement between all species. Death is quick in the hunt. Suffering is a lifetime in disease. You choose."

"No. I believe the reason people are so hateful and aggressive is because they kill and eat meat," I said.

"As I said, the cause, or 'sin' as you might call it, is any fruit of evil. Cooking food is one of them. My people lived very peacefully for thousands of years eating raw meat under strenuous environmental conditions without severe diseases. Only those of us who accidentally or purposely ate foods that were not good for them became diseased. Everything in your society is confusing. Science and business try to formulate everything and everyone. Soon your scientists will name fat and red meat 'evil' and say they cause much disease."

"That would be a shame. Fat is the main nutrient that has kept me alive. They research people who eat cooked fat, so they are right about that, but they're wrong regarding people who eat only raw fat. Meats are all poison. They turn into uric acid in the body," I said.

"As you are for plenty of raw fat and against cooked fat, the same is true for meat. When I was a boy, my friends and I would greet food-hunting parties with our knives drawn. We would cut and spread the hides and cut handfuls of buffalo fat and eat them like Wasichus eat cookies, candy and cake. And then we ate the meat with some leaves to make our breath fresh or sweet. We never got sick from either. It made us strong against disease and gave us rich skin. Now, you haven't answered my question: Do you get a taste for meat?" he asked.

"No."

"Well, if you do, have it raw and you will become much stronger over a period of many years."

"I love animals. I can't kill them," I said. A wind twister whipped around us and Elk-of-the-Black Moon stood up.

"I will continue my journey. May you find peace in Wakan-Tanka. Your God and Wakan-Tanka are the same by different names."

"I know. God bless you, too. Thanks for stopping," I said as I made the peace sign. He smiled and disappeared into the dusk, opposite from the direction he had come. I had no vision on my four-day quest.

I told Spotted Deer about Elk-of-the-Black Moon and he said,

"You spoke with Black Elk?![37]"

"Black Elk has been dead for years. He died of very old age. This man's name is Elk-of-the-Black Moon," I said.

"No Wasichu knows him by that name. I don't believe this."

Appendix V

(from page 118.)

Living outdoors in the wild was more stressful on my body than living in the city. I had to deal with hunger, constant sunrays or wind, drastic temperature changes from day to night (up to 50° Fahrenheit in deserts), and insect bites. A few times I awakened in humid swamp areas with at least a hundred mosquitoes sucking my blood at once - my mosquito net had opened. But I never got lice or parasites. I did not eat meat at that time, so living in the wild aged me faster than normal. I weathered. I developed deep lines in my face.

Psychologically, living outdoors in the wild was less stressful than living in the city. There was no pollution or rat race to maintain. I loved that.

Since that three-years period, I have lived outdoors for a month or two at a time. The addition of raw meat to my diet has changed my outdoor experiences considerably. (It also reversed my aging process.) When mosquitoes light on me, most often they leave without sucking my blood. I tolerate the cold and hunger more easily, and sunrays and wind no longer wizen me.

---

[37] Black Elk was a revered Oglala Sioux holy/medicine man who lived from 1863-1950.

Appendix W

(From page 125`)

Most cooked vegetable fats harden so much that most bodies can't get rid of them, especially vegetable and seed oils. Rarely can a body utilize cooked fat properly, especially after the body reaches its mid-twenties. After several years of eating my Primal Diet, if the body stores excessive raw fats, usually we can lose them with exercise. However, I prefer that people maintain excess weight. The reason is, sometimes our bodies go through a major detoxification, like a cold, flu, pneumonia, or whatever, and we may crave lots of fats and store them in our bodies. This makes detoxification much easier, reducing and mitigating symptoms. By the time detoxifications are over, all or most of the stored fat is gone without leaving us weak and exhausted. Excess fat is very important for optimal health in our toxic bodies and environment.

VOLUME TWO

of

WE WANT TO LIVE!

Expanded and Revised in 2005

Healthfully

(the facts)

UNDERSTANDING THE PRIMAL DIET ™

I've learned that if I eat donuts today I look and feel like donuts tomorrow, and maybe for the rest of my life. -- Jill, School teacher

This volume was written for better understanding of how food and nature affects us. The remedies are based on results, not conclusions that were based on speculation and assumptions that were based on theory and disseminated mainly for profit. The efficacy of all of the dietary wisdom given herein was born from 35 years of nutritional experimentation, trial and error. It does not depend upon our chemical understanding and explanations.

This material is for educational purposes (*read* Warning/Disclaimer, page 6).

INTRODUCTION

The Raw Truth

by Rob Strauds

As a researcher and practitioner of the healing arts I have devoted a great deal of time and energy to the study and application of what is variously referred to as "alternative", "holistic" or "natural" healing, which embody most of the "modalities" currently in use. After many years I concluded that while the "alternative" approaches to illness and health are generally more organic in principle than conventional drug-based allopathic medicine, many of them still treat symptoms rather than whole organisms. They often merely substitute herbs, supplements and other substances for drugs. It became apparent to me that neither medical science nor alternative medicine was going to resolve the issues of degenerative illness, radiant health, and longevity, in the laboratory. The number of variables and the vast complexity of biological and subtle energy processes and reactions in the miraculous human "body-mind" seem to defy any attempt by man or machine to ultimately "figure it out" at the biochemical level. Intelligent and talented men and women have devoted decades of their lives to researching tiny fragments of human biochemistry and still their conclusions are often contradictory, incompatible with one another, wrong, or limited in their healing applications. Although there have been remarkable advances in medical science, the foundational understandings necessary to resolve degenerative disease and produce radiant health and significant longevity are still not evident.

In the field of natural healing in the Twentieth century, the work of pioneers such as Bernard Jensen, Paul Bragg, Paavo Airola, and others, has led to a greater understanding of the single most fundamental principle of health and healing. These landmark health practitioners embraced <u>food</u> for detoxification, regeneration and rejuvenation. The human body is, after all, a "food body", and although there are emotional, psychological and spiritual components to health, any system that does not incorporate food as a primary healing therapy is seriously negligent.

My investigation, therefore, led me to the confusing and contradictory world of diet and nutrition: vegetarianism, dairy-free veganism, macrobiotics, Chinese dietary therapy, raw foods, etc. In the course of studying and experimenting with each approach, a significant factor seemed to emerge (based on successful results): the health of living organisms is dependent on the use of live, organic food in raw form, rich in enzymes and other nutrients that have not been destroyed or reduced by heat or other processing. Consequently, I pursued the work of Ann Wigmore, Victor Kulvinskas and other advocates of vegetarian raw-foodism.

As time passed I observed that the completely raw vegetarian diet was not for everyone. While some benefited, many tended to become weakened by it. Some could not easily digest raw vegetables, even with enzyme supplementation, making it difficult or impossible for them to eat salads. In one instance I observed a rapid decline in the health of a cancer patient (who had been improving somewhat on a modified macrobiotic diet) when he switched to an all-raw diet. Doubts surfaced. The questions kept arising: Is there a fundamental dietary approach to prevention, healing, and longevity? If so, on what basis would that diet vary from one individual to another?

I decided to approach the matter in a different way; to start from the desired result and work backwards. This took two forms, 1) to seek and research the work of health practitioners who were consistently (75-90%) reversing deep-seated pathology (cancer, AIDS, chronic fatigue syndrome, etc.) and evaluate and compare their methods, 2) to study the diets and lifestyles of cultural groups that enjoyed radiant health and significant longevity and look for commonalities. In phase one, I found that such practitioners were hard to come by, for several reasons: a) they often work alone rather than in the context of a larger organization or clinic, b) they are generally not mainstream or even well known, and c) they generally maintain low profiles because of the political and economic dangers of curing diseases in a society controlled and policed by medical and scientific prejudices.

I began to hear about the work of Aajonus Vonderplanitz, a practitioner who had apparently facilitated 232 cancer remissions (of 240 cases) as well as many recoveries from heart disease, chronic fatigue and other serious illnesses. Even more remarkable was the fact that these healings were effected almost exclusively through diet. I contacted him immediately and ordered the manuscript *The Primal Diet; We Want To Live*. The book was a revelation. The first reading left me astonished.

After months of enjoying significant health improvements from the diet, I found myself involved in a week-long face-to-face apprenticeship with its creator. I was pleasantly surprised at my first encounter. His general appearance was that of a man ten years younger; his skin and hair possessed the healthful glow that develops from the inside rather than from the mere use of topical cosmetic products; his musculature exhibited a tone that results from regular work-outs, despite the fact he had not done any significant exercise in seventeen years. The most amazing characteristic was the clarity of his eyes. Iridologists will tell you how very rare it is to find a human being alive in today's toxic world, whose irises show little or no signs of disease or toxicity. An examination of his irises revealed a complete circle of solid blue filaments radiating outward from the pupils. There were none of the yellow, green, brown, white or dark discolorations and telltale shapes that appear in most eyes and reveal states of less than optimal health. The man was a living testimony to the validity of his work.

His dietary approach postulates two fundamental principles: 1) food of any kind is best eaten in its live, raw condition, rich in enzymes and other nutrients, and 2) a diet resplendent in raw fats and raw meats taken from natural sources is essential to excellent health. The latter may be hard for us to grasp since we live in a fat-phobic, meat-phobic, and bacteria-phobic society, where fats, meats and bacteria are blamed for just about everything short of the depletion of the ozone layer. When we speak of raw fat and raw meat, we must think of them as new food groups, utterly different in their biochemistry from the fats and meats we have been taught to avoid in cooked form. The diet primarily encompasses: a) raw animal meats (beef, fish, poultry, organic eggs), b) raw dairy products (unsalted raw butter, raw milk, raw cream, unsalted raw cheeses, raw kefir), c) raw whole fruits and vegetables (especially vegetable juices), d) unheated honey.

Traditional Precedents

The idea of consuming raw meats and raw dairy products in raw diets has many historical precedents. Much of this history was brought to light by two pioneering doctors who researched the subject extensively in the first half of the Twentieth century. Francis Pottenger, Jr., M.D., was a physician and researcher who demonstrated that raw foods contain unique nutrients vital to health. His research included a now-classic series of controlled experiments that involved more than nine hundred cats for more than ten years. Pottenger proved that raw foods (including raw milk and raw meat) were required to maintain these animals in excellent health. He applied elements of this knowledge to the care of his patients with tuberculosis and other chronic diseases, with excellent and well-documented results. Unfortunately, while his work was initially well received by the medical profession, it has been ignored in the ensuing years.

Weston Price, D.D.S., was a contemporary of Pottenger who, during his years in practice, began noticing in the children of his patients problems which their parents had not experienced. Besides having more decay, in many children the teeth did not fit properly into the dental arch, causing them to be crowded and crooked. He noticed also that the condition of deformed teeth reflected the overall state of compromised health. Considering possible reasons, the idea occurred to him that perhaps there was some deficiency in modern diets. While others in his profession looked for causative factors in dental decay, Price searched among primitive people for one or more nutritional factors protecting them. His travels took him to the corners of the earth. He and his wife lived with and studied Swiss people in high Alpine valleys; Gaels on islands of the Outer Hebrides; Eskimos in Alaska; Indians in the far northern, western and central parts of Canada and western United States and Florida; Melanesians and Polynesians in the South Pacific; Africans in eastern and central Africa; Aborigines in Australia; Malay tribes on islands north of Australia; Maori in New Zealand; and descendants of ancient civilizations in Peru.

Fortunately, Price traveled and conducted his research during the 1930's when the cultures he observed were still primarily indigenous, and groups of people still lived entirely on local foods that they mostly ate raw. He found cultures without tooth decay and children without misshapen dental arches or crowded teeth. He interviewed an American medical doctor living among Eskimos and northern Native-Americans who reported that in thirty-five years of observation, he had never seen a single case of cancer among natives subsisting on their traditional foods. When natives eating "civilized" man's processed foods developed tuberculosis and other diseases, this doctor sent them back to their native villages and foods. They usually recovered.

In the course of his travels, Price specifically searched for groups that maintained immunity to dental and chronic disease on diets consisting entirely of vegetable matter. He did not find any. Every healthy native culture he studied ate many animal foods raw; tradition often dictated which foods. The milk, cheese and butter of Swiss villagers and African herdsmen were seldom heated. Animal glands and organs, in every traditional culture, were often eaten raw. Eskimos of Arctic regions, where no plants were available much of the year, ate a lot of raw meat and fish. This tradition prevented scurvy; the vitamin C in meat and fish is destroyed by cooking. Islanders in the South Pacific and coastal Australian Aborigines ate most food raw, including shellfish. As Price's studies progressed, it emerged ever more clearly that healthy, free-ranging animal life of the land and sea provided humans everywhere with essential nutrients apparently unobtainable in adequate quantities from plants alone.

It is useful and inspiring to study the diets of these indigenous people in order to break through the conditioning and fixed ideas that dictate what we should and shouldn't eat. An obvious example is the objection to eggs as a food that contains cholesterol that is dangerous to the heart and arteries, particularly in individuals who already have high cholesterol levels. The fact is, however, that harmful cholesterol accumulations result from cooked fats; accumulations decrease when raw fats, including raw whole eggs, are eaten. To quote Edward Howell in his classic work, *Enzyme Nutrition*:

> ...when fats, either animal or vegetable, are eaten along with their associated enzymes, no harmful effect on the arteries or heart results. All fatty foods contain lipase in their natural state. Cooking or processing removes it.

While similar to traditional diets, most of the principles and formulas contained in *We Want To Live* constitute a unique discovery, one which opens an entirely new healing paradigm. The work of Aajonus Vonderplanitz, as presented in these two volumes, is truly a pioneering effort which should become a significant breakthrough in the health-care revolution that looms on the horizon.

If we don't take responsibility and care for our individual health, how can we have more than limited abilities, limited happiness and limited control over our lives?

Understanding Food That Nourishes Us With Radiant Health

QUESTIONS AND ANSWERS

WHY DOES LIVE FOOD ASSIST HEALING?

We are born with a given supply of nutrients in our bodies to facilitate all bodily functions. Enzymes, vitamins, minerals, sugars, fats and proteins are just some of the known nutrients. As we grow, we require greater quantities of all nutrients. We eat to supply this need so that we develop fully, healthfully. Many nutrients are expended during bodily processes. Those nutrients must be replaced. We eat to supply them and maintain or achieve the most efficient bodily functions and optimal health.

Enzymes are catalysts for every metabolic process from thinking, to smiling, to healing, to cleansing, to cellular regeneration. Vitamins, minerals, sugars, fats, proteins and all other nutrients cannot be digested, assimilated or utilized properly without a myriad of active enzymes.

Raw foods contain a myriad of active enzymes and have plentiful supplies of vitamins and other nutrients. Eating raw foods ensures optimal digestion and functioning, and replaces expended nutrients, promoting excellent health.

HOW DO COOKED AND PROCESSED FOODS CREATE DISEASE?

I have found that all sickness is rooted in malnutrition, pollution and the accumulation of toxins. This includes allergy-related conditions and genetic diseases. Malnutrition results from a person not getting the nutrients (or combination and balance of nutrients) that his or her body needs. Disease most often results from a combination of malnutrition and accumulated toxins, or an instant poisoning, such as results from many vaccines and other industrial substances. Under this heading, the toxins that result from cooking food will be our focus.

Cooking and processing foods destroy nutrients by altering their shape, size and chemistry. This causes biochemical confusion, and toxicity in the body (the accumulation of harmful substances, residues, and debris). Immersing fully charged batteries into boiling acid would cause batteries to lose charge, be destroyed and become debris. That is analogous to the destruction of nutrients by cooking.

Because nutrients have been destroyed in cooked and processed foods, eating cooked and processed foods forces the body to leach enzymes from its own supply to digest, assimilate and utilize whatever is eaten, breathed and absorbed. Enzymes are not the only nutrients that are leached. Our bodies leach cells, vitamins, minerals, proteins, and hormones from our constitutions, gradually weakening us. Leaching increases work that the body and enzymes must do. Consequently, increasingly, work does not get done. Gradually, inert and volatile toxins accumulate. Cells weaken. Cellular functions decline, causing bodily deterioration and disease. We call this aging.

Therefore, cooked diets lack what the body needs to more easily build, protect and cleanse itself. Many people over age 20 easily succumb to gravity and lose muscle tone because they eat cooked and processed foods. Most people have at least one ailment because they eat cooked and processed foods.

If instinct and intuition were not muddled with traditional dietary habits, and if healthy foods were available, we would eat only for good health and the body would never get to the state of gross toxicity that is disease. Disease would be a concept rather than a fact. However, while we lack intuitional and instinctual connectedness, symptoms of illness are as necessary to achieving good health as ears are to good hearing. A body that does not manifest symptoms would behave like a little girl who had no feeling of hot or cold. Sadly, she burned off her backside from her waist to her knees when she sat for five minutes on a hot radiator.

Symptoms are the body's way of telling us that something needs to change. In all cases it is a change in diet that is needed. But in some cases, other changes may be necessary in conjunction with a dietary change. Simply avoiding certain foods and environmental pollutants, such as smoke, poisonous fumes and radiation, sometimes corrects an ailment with time. In others cases, besides a change in diet, physical or psychological changes may be needed. For instance, leaving a cynical mind-set and becoming more open-minded, accepting and creative. Or sometimes what is needed is to leave an unhappy or inappropriate or non-improvable relationship.

Sabotaging symptoms with drugs puts a person in greater danger of disease, suffering and early death. Correcting the causes of illness is the cure. Adopting a healthy diet and environment naturally lessen and eventually eliminates symptoms, indicating that health gradually improves.

WHY ARE SOME PEOPLE HEALTHY EVEN THOUGH THEY EAT COOKED AND PROCESSED FOODS?

The body, as a whole and on a cellular level, always strives toward good health. The changes in shape, size and chemistry of nutrients from cooking forces the body to invent and manufacture unusual forms of enzymes to facilitate all metabolic processes. We will call those ENZYME-MUTATIONS. Some individuals have a full spectrum of enzyme-mutations, and are better able than others to digest, assimilate, and utilize the mutilated nutrients in cooked and processed foods, as well as discard the enormous waste. Consequently, those people are healthier than people who do not have a full spectrum of enzyme-mutations. Each body handles nutrients and toxicity differently.

There are so few people who do very well on cooked foods that we are genetically an unstable species. As a whole, mankind has not come close to altering himself to live on cooked and processed foods without disease. Diseases are changing form and increasing. They are not being eradicated.

Genetic illness is the same malnutrition carried on for generations; that is, dietary habits are learned and followed from generation to generation. When a deficiency is continued in a particular family, the genetic plan for proper functioning of one or more body parts or systems is misplaced, but usually not lost, at birth or during the lifetime. Most genetic illness can be corrected in time if the right nutrients are eaten.

The onslaught of pollution has created a need for more nutrients and enzyme-mutations to neutralize, constrain, and eliminate more toxins. We have an even greater need to eat fresh raw foods, especially raw fat, today than we have had in the past.

WHY ARE SOME PEOPLE MORE ILL-AFFECTED BY COOKED AND PROCESSED FOODS?

Some ailments are a direct result of a lack of enzyme-mutations for handling certain cooked foods. This causes the toxic resins and residues from those cooked and processed foods to accumulate. These ailments are basically allergies to those cooked and processed foods. Therefore, some people are more sensitive to and ill-affected by cooked foods than others.

Fat resins, especially from vegetable oils, and protein residues from cooked or processed green foods first collect in intestinal cells. Secondly, they collect as gummy resins in the glands (as in prostatitis leading to prostate cancer). Thirdly, they collect as gummy resins in the brain (as in Alzheimer's disease). Finally, the gummy resins frequently crystallize, hardening cells and creating disease such as hardening of the heart, arteriosclerosis and multiple sclerosis.

The resins and residues from cooked or processed red fruits and vegetables most often collect in the lymph and skin cells, causing acne, sickly looking tongues, hard and brittle bones, and deep lesions in the skin when the weather turns very cold. Most children with chronic illness within their lungs and nasal passages, like colds, sore throats, tonsillitis, and swollen adenoids, lack enzyme-mutations for eating cooked or processed red or orange fruits and vegetables. By simply eliminating cooked red and orange fruits and vegetables from their diets, and by eating raw red and orange foods, most often those symptoms normalize so that those children will have only occasional colds, flu, and/or sore throats.

People who lack the enzyme-mutations for digesting, assimilating and utilizing cooked or processed yellow foods most often look pasty around the nose and eyes, and have very slow digestion, especially after eating a cooked or processed yellow or orange food.

People who lack enzyme-mutations for eating all three food groups - cooked or processed green, red (including orange) and yellow (including orange) foods - have a predisposition toward HIV positive.

IF I LACK ENZYME-MUTATIONS, WHAT FOODS SHOULD I AVOID?

If a person lacks enzyme-mutations to digest, assimilate or utilize cooked or processed green foods, she or he should avoid eating or drinking cooked or processed green foods such as ordinary olive oils, cooked leafy vegetables (including steamed), artichoke, celery, green beans (string beans), green peppers, broccoli, any pastas made from green foods such as spinach, cooked vegetable juices (canned or bottled), teas (including herbal unless sun-steeped) and food coloring.

If a person lacks enzyme-mutations to digest, assimilate or utilize cooked or processed red fruits and vegetables, she or he should avoid eating or drinking cooked or processed red or orange fruits and vegetables, like store-bought strawberry preserves and jams, cherry, cranberry, tomato, vegetable and orange juices and drinks, tomato sauces, catsup, carrots, peppers (including cayenne and paprika), red and brown beans and food coloring. Other cooked foods to avoid that have red in their pigment are coffee, chocolate, boysenberries, grapes and blueberries. Therefore cooked or processed apple, strawberry, cherry, boysenberry, grape and blueberry jams, juices, syrups and pies should be avoided.

If a person lacks enzyme-mutations to digest, assimilate or utilize cooked or processed yellow foods, she or he should avoid eating or drinking cooked or processed yellow or orange foods, like ordinary corn oils, cooked corn (including steamed or popped), carrots, yellow squashes and onions, corn bread, banana bread, pasteurized or frozen juices (including pineapple, lemon and orange) and food coloring.

COULD I BENEFIT FROM EATING VITAL FOODS?

Sick and healthy people have benefited from eating vital foods. If you are a person who is in perfect health, does not have disease, is balanced emotionally, physically, mentally, and sensually, is happy, has great patience and stamina without intoxicants such as coffee and chocolate, and ages without deterioration, you have mutated to eat cooked foods completely. You are an evolutionary wonder! You can eat cooked and processed foods. Please give this book to someone who needs it.

If you are like me and most people who have some kind of health problem, including genetic, you have not mutated well enough to handle a cooked diet without sickness or disease. We can struggle to try to change millions of years of dietary evolution in our short lifetimes, or we can experiment and probably discover that this raw Primal Diet is healthier.

WHAT SHOULD I EXPECT IF I CHANGE TO EATING A VITAL-FOOD DIET?

People who have completely changed to a raw diet have had different experiences. In thousands of cases, every person experienced improved health. Coincidentally, some people entered a detoxification period at the same time they began this Primal Diet. However, the detoxification was not directly caused by the change of diet. Their bodies were detoxifying accumulated toxins that were in their bodies from the mass quantities of toxins from cooked, processed and chemically grown food prior to the diet change. I have never seen a bad physiological reaction directly caused by a complete change to the Primal Diet.

Squeamishness toward eating raw meat, especially raw chicken (even though antibiotic-free and hormone-free), was a psychological block in some instances that was overcome by those people eating a few bites of raw meat several days weekly until their bodies developed a craving for it. Another psychological block I encountered was that people, especially women, who were thin-conscious and fat-phobic, and who gained weight and size in the initial stages of a raw diet, got upset. Sometimes those people chose to discontinue the raw diet so that they would stay slim, even though a cooked diet made them anxious and irritable and gave them one or more serious health problems. I tried to reassure them that their tissues were being hydrated, cleansed and strengthened, and that the increased size is temporary, lasting no more than 30 months (except in women who had cesarean surgery or disease, in which cases size retention averages 74 months). If you are a person who is thin-conscious and has one or more health problems, you must ask yourself, "Would I rather gain and retain 10-20 pounds and put on a few i0nches while my body cleanses and improves my physical, mental an2d emotional health, or would I rather continue with my present state of heath and progression toward more disease?" *See* Weight and density, page 339.

Some bodies are so starving for nutrients that some people eat twice as much on a raw diet as they do on a cooked diet. However, most people's hunger is easily satisfied on the Primal Diet. Eating excessively usually lasts only 1-2 months. Eating more is healthy, especially if you are underweight. Even if you do not crave food, it is good to eat more if you are underweight.

Some bodies crave so much sleep that some people sleep more during the first month or two on a raw diet. Sleeping more is healthy because it promotes healing. Most healing occurs during sleep. Yet some people sleep less than before they began the raw diet because they don't spend so much energy on digestion and toxicity. Occasionally a person will feel sluggish because her or his body has to slow or rest certain functions to cleanse and rebuild.

In my thirty-one years of experience, everyone gained general vitality within a month and maintained it, except during some detoxifications. Digestion significantly increased. Bad breath was either eliminated or reduced significantly in most people but increased in some for awhile. Usually, bowel movements were easy, except in people with a history of constipation. For them, it took 1-2 years to produce relaxed, smooth bowel movements. However, some people did not have bowel movements for 2-5 days when they began the diet because their bodies utilized almost everything they ate without discarding much. After many months on a raw diet, a perpetually increasing calmness of body and clarity of mind usually were beneficial results.

Specifics About Particular Foods

Note: To the categories of carbohydrate, fat, and protein, I add the category starch because certain starches, like nuts, seeds, grain and potato, contain substances (such as gluten) that can bond with toxins (including excess hormones) and neutralize them. See Cooked Starch, page 183, and Nut Formula, page 194.

ALCOHOL: For some people, raw organic wine is beneficial. It helps break down and remove some hardened fat from the blood and body. However, any kind of alcohol robs the liver of fat. This weakens the liver and causes it to become lethargic. Eating 2 raw eggs within 10 hours of consuming raw wine restores fat to the deprived liver. Most often it is healthier to eat raw unripe pineapple, raw lemons, or raw oranges to dissolve hardened fat rather than to drink alcohol. Raw natural alcohol in slightly fermented raw fruit facilitates the making of internal natural body soaps to cleanse the body of internal toxins. All hard liquors - bourbon, whiskey, cognac, etc. – and wine are damaging to glands, brain and nervous system.

ALKALIZING FOOD neutralizes acidity and volatile toxins, refreshing an acidic and toxic body. Except for wheat grass juice, all edible raw fresh vegetable juices, raw fruits and raw fresh fruit puree are alkalizing. Raw fresh tomatoes, raw fresh figs, raw fresh pineapple, raw fresh lemons and raw fresh parsley are the most alkalizing. Alkalizing foods do not need to be eaten together or eaten exclusively except during particular ailments. But if they are included - when you desire them or have a toxic problem - in a balanced raw diet, physical, emotional, and mental life will be easier. Although tomatoes, apples, citrus fruit and raw unpasteurized apple cider vinegar are considered acidic, they alkalize the blood and body. *See* pages 201 and 213-216 about acidic and volatile toxic conditions.

See Salad dressings for dressings that alkalize, page 199.

APPLE CIDER VINEGAR, RAW, UNPASTEURIZED AND UNFILTERED is a must for all home remedy kits. This quality of vinegar promotes healing in a wide variety of ailments. *See* Remedies, pages 212-339.

BLACK PEPPER: *See* Pepper, page 196.

BUTTER/HONEY MIXTURE is made of equal portions of unsalted raw butter and unheated honey. Where raw butter is not available, the following 3 alternatives may be substituted in the remedies that suggest the butter/honey mixture: 1) raw avocado mashed with an equal portion of unheated honey; 2) fresh coconut cream (juiced from the meat of fresh whole coconut) mixed with an equal portion of unheated honey, or 3) a stone-pressed or cold-pressed-below-96° Fahrenheit oil mixed in equal portions with unheated honey. Those alternatives produce similar effects, but in some cases, take a little longer.

Here is a recipe that makes the honey/butter combination more desirable for some people: Place 1 cup of room temperature unsalted raw butter in a tightly sealed jar and immerse the jar in hot water that is not hot enough to burn your hand. While the butter is melting, blend ½ cup of shelled raw walnuts (or other soft nut) until it is powder. When the butter is melted, add 4-6 tablespoons of unheated honey and the powdered nuts and blend. This mixture can be refrigerated and kept up to 3 months. It can be eaten with any food or just eaten off a spoon or finger (if mothers and fathers allow), or spread on toast (after toast has cooled a little) or other bread, or it can be included in smoothies and milk shakes.

CANNED FOOD is cooked food. Therefore, canned foods are all nutrient-deficient and difficult to digest and utilize. Most canned and bottled food, like fruit and tomato purees and sauces, were rotten. Then they were very processed and chemicalized to hide the rotten taste. If food is moist in the can, it is contaminated with metal from moisture leaching metals from the can. Metal-leaching causes low-grade, gradual toxic mineral/metal-poisoning that complicates and promotes numerous diseases. The metal from all canned food is toxic in the human body. Aluminum never occurs naturally in the human body and is toxic. Cooking food in aluminum foil and eating canned food, including beverages stored in aluminum, cause many complications in the body. In thousands of hair analyses performed for measuring mineral content of the body, each person had high levels of aluminum. Most of the hair mineral analyses also showed unnaturally high levels of lead, iron, cadmium and other toxic metals. Cooking and storing food in metal vessels also cause gradual toxic metal-poisoning that helps disease blossom.

CARBONATED BEVERAGES AND WATERS: If a label reads "carbonation added" or "carbonated" it means that the carbonation is synthetic. Synthetic carbonation causes radicals and free radicals, resulting in mineral and oxygen deficiencies, sometimes resulting in headaches. If a label reads "naturally carbonated", or "natural carbonation added" or "naturally sparkling", the carbonation is natural from the well and highly charged with healthful electrolytes. *See* page 72.

In combination with unheated honey, naturally carbonated waters relieve most headaches. Naturally carbonated waters help relax adrenal glands. Therefore, if you are an individual with low energy, it would probably be better to drink naturally sparkling water only when needed in a remedy.

CAYENNE PEPPER: *See* Pepper, page 196.

CHEESES, RAW, NO-SALT-ADDED, are made from raw milk and there is no salt added to the milk. Similar to clay, cheese supplies concentrations of minerals that bind with radicals and poisons that the body dumped into the stomach and intestines. Also, cheese draws the poisons from the blood, nervous and lymphatic systems as they pass through the stomach and intestines. Unsalted raw cheeses act like a sponge to absorb those toxins, relieving nausea. Since cheeses lack most bioactive enzymes, causing dehydration, eating raw fat with cheese, such as unsalted raw butter or coconut cream, helps prevent constipation.

CHOCOLATE is mainly made of fat and approximately 20% sugar. People crave chocolate because they need fat accompanied with sugars to digest the fat, especially during stressful times. However, because the fat and sugar in chocolate are cooked and processed, they have a tendency to store in the body without being properly utilized, especially during stressful times, and should not be eaten. Chocolate also contains the toxic nerve irritants caffeine and theobromine.

CHOCOLATE SUBSTITUTES can be made by combining 4 parts raw fat to 1 part unheated honey. For instance, place ½ cup unsalted raw butter in a small canning jar and place it, with the lid tight, into a bowl of hot water to melt (water should be no hotter than your hand can stand without burning when immersed for 4 seconds). After the butter is mostly melted, add 2-3 tablespoons unheated honey and 1-2 tablespoons raw carob powder. Mix until it has an even consistency. To harden it, you may refrigerate it. Or eat it warm by itself or on something you desire, like bananas topped with crushed raw nuts.

To make another chocolate substitute, juice the meat of fresh coconut, rendering a coconut cream, and use the coconut cream in place of the butter in the recipes above.

For anyone who likes peanut butter and chocolate together, the following recipe may be substituted: 1 cup unsalted raw butter, ½ cup raw peanuts or other soft nut (blend alone until nuts become flour), 4 tablespoons unheated honey, 1 whole raw egg, and 2 heaping tablespoons raw carob powder. Butter should be room temperature (soft). Blend all ingredients together until dark and rich-looking. That mixture may be refrigerated or eaten soft.

Unlike chocolate, those mixtures have no ill side effects and they promote good health. You may eat as much of those chocolate substitutes as are appealing to you, and they will usually satisfy your cravings for chocolate.

CLAY, POWDERED, SUN-DRIED, binds with toxins both inside the body and topically. I suggest clay in several remedies, even if the clay is labeled not for consumption, provided that it is pure without additives. It may be purchased in most health food stores in the cosmetic department, or the best that I found was at www.terramin.com. Do not use clay from volcanic activity, such as most bentonite clays. Those clays are full of molten heavy metals, including mercury.

Prepare the clay by mixing it with good drinking water in a glass or pottery container until it is a thin plaster-like mixture. Cover and let it stand for 5 days in a dark cupboard. When premixed and aged, clay is 3 times more effective.

COFFEE SUBSTITUTE AND COFFEE DETOXIFIER: The first and best choice is always raw fresh green vegetable juices, containing at least 80% celery juice. I suggest drinking 8-16 ounces first thing in the morning. That juice provides many nutrients that alkalize excessive and toxic acids in the stomach and blood, healthfully waking the body for the day. The second choice would be to heat 5 ounces of good mineral water until it is <u>not</u> hotter than an immersed finger can tolerate for 4 seconds. Stir in 2-5 tablespoons unheated honey and fresh juice of ½ lemon or 1 lime (optional: 1 tablespoon raw unpasteurized apple cider vinegar). This mixture also supplies most of the enzymes necessary to get the blood and digestive system energized. A coffee substitute for people with sluggish thyroids could be the same as above but with an added 1/8 teaspoon organically grown vanilla extract (*see* Vanilla extract, page 201). Coffee is a catalyst for many diseases.

CONCENTRATES have been extensively processed and heated to at least pasteurization temperature. Concentrates do not promote health; they mostly damage health.

COOKED FOOD is any food heated above 104° Fahrenheit, whether by baking, barbecuing, boiling, broiling, frying, irradiating, microwaving, pasteurizing, steaming, stewing or toasting. The destruction of enzymes is not significantly observable until cooking temperature reaches 118° Fahrenheit. However, I have consistently noticed subtle to substantial declines in digestibility when food is heated at 106° Fahrenheit for more than 2 minutes. I found that sick people digest food best when food is not heated over 104° Fahrenheit.

Pasteurized food is food heated between 140°-160° Fahrenheit. Nowadays, almost every bottled food is heated to at least pasteurization temperature to kill what is alive in it, lengthening shelf life but decreasing nutrients for human life.

Irradiated food is food that has been exposed to radiation, more commonly to toxic radioactive material. *See* Irradiated food, page 190.

Dehydrating food, even at low temperatures, causes nutrient loss, especially of enzymes and mineral/nutrient couplings. Even natural weather conditions above 104° Fahrenheit continuously for one or two days can destroy nutrients by dehydration.

Utilizing refrigeration or cold cellars preserves many enzymes as well as prolongs shelf life.

COOKED STARCH: Eating cooked grain or potato starch is important for some people with excess hormones or toxicity. The reason for eating a little cooked starch is that cooking releases starch and gluten that some individuals cannot obtain from any other source. However, most people can obtain raw starch from eating nuts in combination with raw fat and unheated honey. See Nut Formula, page 194. Released starch or gluten can bind with excess neurological hormones and toxicity if the starch or gluten is refined, that is, without the bran and germ.

Eating refined starch goes against the established concept that more fiber is better, but people rarely utilize starch and gluten in whole grain products because the starch and gluten often attach to bran and germ and cannot be absorbed. (Also, cooked fiber robs the blood and intestines of available fats. That often causes dryness, irritability and/or lethargy.) If starch and gluten are not properly utilized, they will not arrest excess hormones, toxic hormonal byproducts, including psychological, and other related toxins. Therefore, refined flours that are unbleached and not fortified or enriched are better for that purpose than whole grain flours. Normally, the human body requires no vegetable or grain fibers on the Primal Diet.

As when eating any cooked food, eating too much cooked starch causes the accumulation of acrylamides and advanced glycation end products, creating obesity and/or cellulite, and diseases. Generally, an individual should not eat as much cooked starch as she or he may crave. Eating small quantities of it when necessary reduces anxiety, depression, anger, symptoms of detoxification, etc. Plenty of raw fats must be eaten with every cooked starch to help prevent more toxicity, cellulite- and acrylamide-storage, and constipation. If constipation ensues, not enough raw fat was eaten with cooked starch. An equal amount of raw fat to cooked starch is healthier.

Most people, most of the time, don't need to eat cooked starch because they obtain and utilize the starch that is present in raw meat, raw nuts and raw seeds (*see* Nut Formula, page 194), and raw vegetable juices. However, people who need cooked grain and/or potato starch may require it regularly for as long as two years. After one to two years on a raw diet, cooked starch should be eaten sparingly or not at all. Cooked starch may be cooked at normal recipe temperatures. When putting unsalted raw butter, raw oils, self-made raw sauces and raw jams, and any other raw food on hot cooked starch, make sure that the starch has cooled to the point that it won't burn the raw food. This temperature test can be done by sticking a finger deep into the hot food after steam no longer rises from it - if it is too hot for your finger, it will burn the raw food and diminish nutritive value. Wait until it cools just enough that it doesn't burn.

Where I have recommended cooked starch, I am referring to baked, boiled or steamed potatoes, plain grain pastas, air-popped corn, and breads (for instance, French, Italian or sourdough) that are made with only unbleached flour that is not fortified, yeast and water. (A little salt in the baking is acceptable because gluten will not easily release salt into the body; however, breads made without salt are best for health).

Most often it is better not to eat cooked potato skins. Cooking potato skins often creates toxic resins and concentrated residue. People lacking enzyme-mutations for eating cooked red fruits and vegetables should not eat yams or red or purple potatoes. Air-popped corn and rice cakes are good for some people and indigestible, or unassimilable, or non-utilizable for others. If anyone has an ailment that relates to a lack of enzyme-mutations for eating cooked yellow food, he or she usually cannot eat yellow popcorn, yellow potatoes or cooked whole grains easily or properly.

When cooking, it is healthier to cook ingredients in oven-safe glass or pottery. (*See* Canned food, about metal poisoning, page 179.)

EGGS: Should always be from chickens that are not fed antibiotics or hormones. Fertile eggs are eggs that have been laid by chickens that have fraternized with roosters. Eggs should be at least "free range" if not fertile. "Free range" means that the chickens run on the ground and are not cooped in tiny cages. Chickens that are permitted to roam in pastures are healthier. When consuming large quantities of eggs, there is a need for vegetable iron. Therefore, it is necessary to eat deep leafy green (for example, spinach or parsley) or purple (for example, red cabbage) vegetables or 4 ounces of their juice once weekly.

It is believed that large quantities of whole raw eggs should not be eaten because avidin (an amino acid) in egg white binds with biotin (part of the Vitamin B complex) in the body, causing side-effects. The avidin/biotin bond is beneficial because it helps to dissolve biocarbons and helps muscles retain carbohydrates. Whole raw eggs contain a wonderful natural balance of nutrients, including bioavailable lutein (an antioxidant) that is an important carotenoid for eye and skin health.

Empirical experience proved to me that the body properly alters any chemically-identified enzyme-inhibitor in eggs, allowing raw eggs to be eaten in their entirety at once. I have eaten up to 24 whole raw eggs daily for 28 years with no ill effect. Thousands of people have eaten up to 33 whole raw eggs daily for up to 25 years with none of the symptoms associated with biotin deficiency. People need to stop making conclusions based solely on laboratory analysis.

In my experiments with animals, including humans, who ate only the yolk and not the white (along with other foods on a raw diet), metabolism was considerably increased, usually with<u>out</u> increasing energy. The side effects were that often hunger increased to a frenzy and dispositions tended to be irritable. It has been my experience in every case and condition that eating the whole raw egg was more nourishing, and better for metabolic and emotional balance.

The cautions listed by many sources regarding raw eggs are from rhetoric and not experience. I suggest that you forget all of their precautions regarding freshness and salmonella. For centuries, the Chinese have been consuming eggs that were as old as 25 years to increase health and stamina. Many of my patients purposely "spoil" eggs to increase bacteria and digestibility, which almost instantly relieves poor digestion, constipation, and chronic depression for days.

FAT FOR GREAT HEALTH: Because fat cleanses, fuels, lubricates and protects the body, it is needed more than any other single nutrient - that is, more than protein, sugar and starch. Fat is a necessary catalyst for utilizing minerals and protein. That is why a diet resplendent in raw fat is so important to excellent health. People who eat diets low in fat often develop immune deficiencies sometime in their lives.

The body can, to some extent, turn sugars, starches and proteins into fats, but not nearly enough and it is a long and exhausting process for the body. When fats are eaten raw, they can and will clean, fuel, lubricate and protect the body properly. And raw fat ensures cellular reproduction when raw meats are eaten.

If fats are heated above 104° Fahrenheit they are rarely digested, assimilated or utilized properly. (*See* Appendix O, pages 145-150, and Appendix W, page 162.) The following raw fats are easiest to digest, assimilate, and utilize: unsalted raw butter, raw eggs, raw cream, the fat in and on raw meats (all flesh food), no-salt-added raw cheeses, fresh coconut, avocados, stone-pressed olive oil, and other non-vegetable cold-pressed-below-96° Fahrenheit oils.

Most often the body utilizes the fat in raw eggs and avocado to bind with toxins, carrying the toxins to the bowels and from the system. In the case of cellulite and other cooked fat that has bound to toxins and stored in the body, raw fruits and raw fruit puree (including raw unpasteurized apple cider vinegar), and raw vegetables and raw vegetable juices gradually break down and releases those old storages of cooked fat. Eating raw eggs or avocados provides fat to bind with the released cooked fat and toxins and escorts them from the body. Without the raw fat to escort toxins to the bowels, toxins often restore in the body. Avocado is especially helpful for cleansing and strengthening the liver.

The fat in raw cream and full-fat raw milk soothes and lubricates nerves and muscles, including heart, gently cleanses and lubricates the liver, restores moisture to the thyroid and heals intestinal lesions from dryness. Often drinking too much raw dairy cream causes bloating and slows digestion. Dairy cream is the fat that is most complicated for the liver to digest. Raw eggs and raw butter are easiest for the liver to digest. The fat in unsalted raw butter strengthens organs and glands, heals eyes, cleanses arteries and vascular system, dissolving plaque made from hardened and/or crystallized cooked fats (mainly vegetable fats), chelates and escorts byproducts and waste from the body and lubricates bones, cartilage and teeth. It is utilized for all body-fat needs:

cleansing, dissolving, lubricating, fueling, protecting, rejuvenating and helping to reproduce cells.

The body uses the fat, protein and minerals in no-salt-added raw cheeses to absorb toxins, including free radicals like aluminum and mercury that exist in the stomach and intestines. No-salt-added raw cheeses act like a sponge in those areas of the body, allowing minerals in fresh raw food to be utilized intercellularly for all purposes, such as relaxing and strengthening nerves, and reversing bone diseases.

The fat in raw meat is the most valuable for healing, soothing and lubricating tissue faster than all other fats. Meat fat and coconut cream have all of the healing properties of all other fats and oils. *See* Oils, page 194. Raw coconut cream eaten with cucumber gradually dissolves hardening of the nerves (e.g., in early Alzheimer's), and eaten with banana, gradually dissolves glandular, organ and dermal hardening (e.g., sclerosis, and cirrhosis of liver).

FIBER: is not normally necessary on this Primal Diet. *See* Cooked starch, page 183.

FISH that are grown in fish farms where they are fed processed foods - for instance, alfalfa pellets and fish meal - grow very malnourished and anemic. Those fish are not healthy to eat. *See* Index: Meat.

FISH OILS, including Norwegian cod liver oils, are all purified with solvents (chemicals) and contain toxins. As of April 2005, the only way to get pure raw fish oil is to eat raw fish. All advertising that claims pure fish oils are false claims. Before we begin to give credence to any pure and raw claim for oil, we must receive in writing on the producer's letterhead that at no time does the oil come in contact with any chemical, including but not limited to chlorine and alcohol, or any heat greater than 96° Fahrenheit from ocean or lake to commercial container (usually bottle). Distributors cannot make any verifiable claims because they do not know the details of producing oils, only the producer of any oil knows the process. Any oil that is encapsulated, has been subjected to high temperatures when sealing each capsule, and absorb chemicals from the capsules. Capsules are all chemically and thermally constructed.

FOOD-COMBINING: Each person must pay attention to her or his digestibility. Eat whatever combinations appeal to you, unless you have digestive problems after eating. However, most problems come from eating red animal meat within 1 hour of eating sweet ripe fruit, and sometimes too much tomato. Papaya and pineapple are exceptions; most people can eat them with any meat.

FROZEN FOOD: Freezing, like cooking, destroys nutrients. The colder foods get, the more nutrients are destroyed. Therefore it is always healthier to eat foods that have never been frozen.

The nutrients in meat are especially harmed by freezing. The protein in raw meat that has been frozen is only 25% utilizable in the human body, whereas in fresh raw meat, the protein is nearly 100% utilizable. Freezing meat causes the Escherichia coli bacterium (E. coli) in meat to flourish quickly. When only frozen meat was fed to carnivores, they developed mange and other skin disorders, and sometimes scurvy. When the same meat unfrozen was fed to carnivores, they remained healthy and happy. *See* Refrigeration, page 197.

Some fats, like raw cream and butter, seem to maintain well when frozen for short periods. *See* Ice cream, page 189.

FRUITS are produced by vegetation. Vegetation is the plant; that is, the leaves, stalks and roots that constitute the plant, like spinach, parsley, celery, rhubarb, carrots, onions and garlic. The following foods are often thought to be vegetables but are fruit (bland fruit): tomatoes, peppers, broccoli tops, cauliflower tops, corn on the cob, mushrooms, cucumbers and other squash.

Fruits are mainly used for cleansing (including detoxification), hydrating the body, and supplying sugars for fuel and enzymes for digestion, utilization and assimilation. Fruits that are not bland fruit are best eaten unripe and very firm. When unripe, they contain less sugar and more enzymes. Fruit eaten highly sweet and ripe causes much over-emotionality.

GARLIC is believed to be a blood cleanser. It contains nutrients that transmute toxic substances into less volatile forms. However, many people are ill-affected by eating it too regularly, interfering with blood pressure (increasing or decreasing) and overstimulating adrenal and sexual glandular activities. Eat garlic if you crave it, not simply because it can be a stimulant and cleanser. *See* Halitosis, page 267, to mitigate garlic breath. *See* Body odor, page 233, to mitigate garlic body odor.

GELATIN and gelatin products are made from very processed and cooked pulverized bone and cartilage. Eating it creates mineral imbalances in many people that often ill affect every part of the body. Eating gelatin is often partially responsible for bone overgrowths and deformities.

HONEY, UNHEATED, that is, honey that does not reach temperatures beyond 93° Fahrenheit; *See* pages 12-13. Bees fan honey inside hives to prevent honey from reaching over 92.8° Fahrenheit. If the honey reaches higher temperatures, bees abandon part or the entire hive. They will not eat the heated honey unless they are starving. If they have to eat heated honey, they become agitated. Eating plenty of unheated honey helps replace missing enzymes for nearly all purposes throughout the entire body, but especially for protein digestion. When the bees collect nectar, they swallow it and predigest it, synthesizing an insulin-like substance that prevents excessive sugar problems. For most diabetics, unheated honey replaces absent insulin and eliminates the water retention caused by missing insulin and enzymes. Unheated honey is a major promoter of youth when the diet includes raw meat.

HONEY/BUTTER MIXTURE: *See* Butter/honey mixture, page 179.

ICE CREAM, RAW: Self-made raw ice cream is fine if eaten within 24 hours after making it, but it is most digestible if eaten shortly after it is made. Ice cream can be made by using raw cream, unheated honey, raw fresh fruit(s) and raw eggs (optional) in an ice cream maker. After 24 hours, raw ice cream may become too difficult to digest, causing fat build-up around the waist and abdominal areas. Here is a raw ice cream recipe that tastes like French vanilla (makes about 2 quarts): 1 pint raw milk, 1 pint raw cream, 1 papaya, 1 or 2 raw eggs and 4 ounces of unheated honey. Blend milk, peeled and seeded papaya, eggs and honey together. Then stir in cream and pour into ice cream maker.

A fat-burning, energy-producing raw ice cream is: 1½ pints raw cream, ¼-½ raw fresh pineapple, 1 or 2 raw eggs and 3-4 tablespoons of unheated honey. Slice pineapple into little chunks. Blend 1 cup of pineapple chunks with eggs and honey. Stir remaining pineapple chunks and cream into the blended mixture. Pour into ice cream maker.

A toxin-absorbing raw ice cream recipe that tastes a lot like gingerbread eaten with ice cream and makes about 2 quarts is: 1 pint raw milk, 1 pint raw cream, 2 raw eggs, two-inch section of fresh ginger root, 4 ounces unheated honey and 1-3 ounces raw carob powder. Slice ginger root (peeled or not) into thin circular slices. Blend milk, eggs, honey, ginger and carob powder together. Then stir in cream and pour into ice cream maker.

Delicious frozen ice on a stick can be made by blending fresh fruit(s) - with a little unheated honey if desired - into a puree. Pour into molds and freeze. *See* Frozen foods, page 188.

IRRADIATED FOOD is food that has been exposed to radioactive materials for the purpose of lengthening shelf-life. The radiation destroys enzymes that would cause normal fermentation and molding. It also alters many other nutrients and causes many toxic byproducts. Eating irradiated food increases your chances of developing cancer.

Many potatoes and packaged spices have been irradiated. Fruit and meat are increasingly being irradiated and are supposed to be labeled as irradiated. The label is a deceiving encircled rose. The FDA does not require manufacturers to label foods that have been irradiated when they are blended with other foods, such as sauces and seasonings. Manufacturers and suppliers are fighting to change the law so that they do not have to label irradiated food. They do not seem concerned that they are slowly poisoning us into painful disease and/or early death.

KEFIR, PLAIN RAW is similar to yogurt, that is, milk that has been predigested by bacillus (*see* Yogurt, page 203). Kefir is healthier when not thickened with gelatin (*see* Gelatin, page 189). The difference between kefir and yogurt is that plain raw kefir is thinner than yogurt and can easily be made without heat above a cow's body temperature (about 100° Fahrenheit). Yogurts are heated to at least 112° Fahrenheit to further thicken them.

The fat, lactose and protein in raw plain kefir have been predigested by the bacillus cultures for easy digestion, assimilation, and utilization. Kefir improves general digestion because the milk is mostly predigested. Blending or mixing in some unheated honey increases digestibility. Along with unheated honey, raw unripe fruit may be blended with kefir if desired, but not if you suffer from pain. If you blend or mix fruit with kefir, you should not drink it within an hour of eating beef, lamb, venison, and other red meat.

Flavored kefir is flavored with concentrates, and concentrates destroy much of the nutritive value of raw kefir, even if the concentrates are made from fruit only (*see* Concentrates, page 182). Raw plain kefir may be flavored by blending fresh raw fruit and unheated honey with it, as mentioned above. Kiwi fruit is the only fruit I would not recommend blending with kefir because the taste of the combination is repulsive to many people.

LIVE OR VITAL FOOD: When I use the words "live" or "vital" in conjunction with food, I use them as synonyms for raw, meaning that the food is not heated above 104° Fahrenheit. When I use "live" referring to raw fruit, I mean that the fruit should not be cooked or dried. For instance, live pineapple denotes that the pineapple should be fresh. When fresh is not available, sun-dried fruits that have not been sulfured may be substituted but they lack bioactive enzymes and have high sugar levels that may cause over-emotionality.

MEAT, RAW: Wherever I have used the words "meat" and "meats", I have not referred only to beef. I have referred to any flesh food, whether fish, fowl (like chicken) or animal. I don't recommend eating the skins of meat; they are all too difficult to eat and digest. I do not recommend eating any glands or bone marrow from fish, fowl or animals unless they are organically grown, because most toxins store in the glands and bones. To help a person decide which meats are right for her or him, *see* Appendix P, page 150. *See* Index: Meat.

MILK, RAW, AND RAW DAIRY PRODUCTS: For someone who gets stomach or intestinal discomfort, gas, or flatulence from drinking raw milk, try adding and blending up to 1 tablespoon of unheated honey per 8 ounces of raw milk to correct the enzyme deficiency that causes digestive problems. Pre-blending ½ gallon (64 ounces) raw milk with ¼-½ cups unheated honey and ½ cup raw cream makes it convenient when you want a glass. Drinking cold milk from the refrigerator often causes lactate and milk-protein to pass into the blood without digestion, causing allergic reactions. It is best to warm milk, or let it stand in a dark warm cupboard several hours before drinking it. I let mine stand for at least 24 hours prior to drinking to allow the natural bacteria in milk to predigest it for me.

A very small percentage of people will have intolerance to raw warm milk or raw milk that has unheated honey added to it. Those rare individuals should not drink milk at all. However, some of those rare individuals may be able to drink raw cream, and eat no-salt-added raw cheeses and unsalted raw butter without difficulty because those milk products contain very little lactate.

In the remedy section I have suggested full-fat raw milk. This means that the milk should be approximately 10% cream (the way it came from cows when I was a child). Raw cream facilitates proper digestion and utilization of the minerals and protein in raw milk. Dairies usually skim the milk, reducing the cream content to 2-4%. Milk containing 2-4% cream is usually labeled "skimmed milk." Milk containing 4-7% cream is labeled "whole milk" - which of course it is not. Add enough raw cream to the raw milk so that the cream content is 15%. For example, add ½ cup of raw cream to 6 cups of raw milk.

The only "raw" cottage cheese that is available (at the time of this writing) is not really raw. It is heated to about 120° Fahrenheit. Many of my clients, especially women, developed thyroid sluggishness and swelling throughout the thyroid area (neck) from eating that cottage cheese. Like other cooked foods that are not starches, I don't recommend that people eat that misnamed "raw" cottage cheese.

MILK, PASTEURIZED, HOMOGENIZED AND GENETICALLY ENGINEERED: Like all other cooked and processed foods, pasteurized and homogenized milks are nutritionally deficient foods. Pasteurized and homogenized milks create dry and coarse hair, skin, glands, and brittle bones that can easily break. Pasteurized and homogenized milks have been linked to causing osteoporosis and diabetes (*see* the book The Recipe For Living Without Disease, Chapter 31).

A hormone has been genetically engineered that forces cows to produce more milk. This also makes the cows anxious. Genetic hormones are passed on to the consumer through the cows' milk, and may have side effects besides creating anxiety. For instance, in young laboratory animals, one or both breasts overdeveloped. In adult humans, the hormones in milk may cause over-production of milk while nursing, spontaneous lactation when not nursing, or difficulty in ceasing lactation. It was found that, for children and adults, it was carcinogenic when that milk was drunk pasteurized. Other side effects have been swollen and overdeveloped thyroids, causing thick necks, especially in females. (Were any women on the engineering team that developed hormonally stimulated milk?) I observed that infants who nursed from mothers who drank those milks developed rashes, colic and frequent odorous bowel movements including diarrhea. Within days after mothers ceased nursing and fed their babies healthy raw cow's milk, the rashes, colic and irregular bowel movements stopped.

MOLASSES is the thick resinous matter that is left at the bottom of the caldrons when cooking sugar cane to make table sugar. It is given a "healthier-than-sugar" blurb simply because it contains so many minerals, like iron. Those minerals are mostly indigestible, unassimilable and unutilizable. They are most often toxic. Since molasses is extremely high in toxic resins it clutters the entire body, causing kidney stones. It's another by-product marketed only for profit.

NUTS AND SEEDS, RAW AND UNSALTED: Even if raw, nuts and seeds are indigestible in the human system because they contain phytic acid that prevents proper protein digestion and absorption. Most people can digest only 1 cup per week if they eat them in combination with raw fat and unheated honey. That combination neutralizes phytic acid. If you crave nuts but feel blah after eating them raw and unsalted, I suggest that you eat the Nut Formula. Nuts and seeds help heal the vascular system and brain lesions. Seeds fortify the immune system. It is better to eat nuts and seeds only in combination with the other foods contained in the Nut Formula recipe. It is better to eat nuts and seeds rarely for the first 7-9 months on a predominately raw diet, unless you crave them or need them to help prevent depression.

Most "Raw" cashews are not raw. They are blasted with a laser that pops the shells open and cooks the nuts. I discovered this only after years of trying to analyze why cashews were so indigestible. If you crave cashews, raw macadamia nuts are a good substitute, but raw macadamias must be dried at temperatures below 104° Fahrenheit. Diabetics should not eat seeds unless they crave them because seeds thicken the blood. Insulin-deficient blood is usually too thick.

NUT FORMULA 2 to 4 ounces raw pecans or walnuts, pine or hazel nuts, sunflower or pumpkin seeds, or peanuts, 4 to 8 tablespoons unsalted raw butter, 1-2 raw eggs, 1½-2 tablespoons unheated honey. Blenderize nuts in an 8- or 12-ounces jar on high speed until they are flour. Add remaining ingredients and stir. Blenderize on medium speed for 20-25 seconds, until smooth. ALTERNATIVE: Substitute coconut cream for butter.

Many people need starches to bind with toxins (including excess hormones) that stress the body. We may obtain that starch by eating a Nut Formula once or twice weekly. Some people may need to eat a little cooked starch with plenty of raw fat if they cannot digest the Nut Formula. That may be determined by eating the Nut Formula when we are extra-stressed. If we become more self-controlled within 12 hours after eating the Nut Formula, we do not need to eat cooked starch.

OILS must be stone-pressed or cold-pressed below 96° Fahrenheit. Write or call the producers or distributors of cold-pressed oils. Discover the maximum temperature each oil reaches all times during processing and bottling. Many producers and distributors label their oils cold-pressed but temperatures will be as high as 250° Fahrenheit depending on the speed and friction produced by the machinery. Cooked vegetable oils, such as margarine and safflower, are primary causes of many ailments, including hardening of the heart and arteries, multiple sclerosis and some cancers. Hydrogenated oils have the molecular structure of plastic. Would you knowingly eat plastic for nourishment? The tribes that eat cooked animal fats do not have hardening of arteries or heart disease.

I have been using a little unheated-above-96° Fahrenheit fermented coconut oil for awhile now. Its virtues have been impressive, especially for the skin. I mention those virtues throughout the remedy section. I do not know if the virtues would increase if the coconut oil were fermented, for the 12-19 hours of fermentation, below 96° Fahrenheit. I do know that the virtues diminish if heated above 96° Fahrenheit. Eaten a little at a time, the body uses coconut oil to help unclog organs and glands, strengthen liver and heart, and heal vascular lesions. The natural fermentation process helps digestibility of the coconut oil.

The olive oils that I have been using have been either stone-pressed or cold-pressed bellow 80° Fahrenheit. I do not know if the virtues that I have stated throughout the remedy section would diminish if the olive oils were cold-pressed above 80° Fahrenheit yet below 96° Fahrenheit. I do know that the virtues diminish if heated above 96° Fahrenheit. The body uses olive oil to cleanse blood and vitalize lungs, soften and then dissolve scar tissue. Eating citrus fruit or tomato with or immediately after olive oil helps digest olive oil.

The cold-pressed flax seed oil that I have been using has been pressed below 96° Fahrenheit. I do not know if its virtues would increase if it were pressed at temperatures below 96° Fahrenheit. I do know that the virtues diminish if heated above 96° Fahrenheit. The body uses flax oil to help prevent cancer cells from forming, heal nerve tissue, soften liver and kidneys, reverse cirrhosis, and substantially strengthen the heart. It is better drunk not more than 1 tablespoon at a time, in the morning, in a few ounces of fresh raw citrus juice.

Unheated-above-96° Fahrenheit fermented coconut oil may be used in place of olive or flax oils but not as replacement for coconut cream. Coconut oil is more of a cleanser, except on the skin where it is a health-stabilizer. Internally, coconut cream is more a health-stabilizer.

ORGANICALLY GROWN food is always preferable. That means, foods that are grown without any chemicals including fertilizers and sprays. Regarding animals, "organically grown" means that animals are grown on organically grown feed, and not fed or injected with chemicals or hormones. However, this label is abused. If you have doubts, call the manufacturers/farmers that produce the food. There are many poultry producers who claim to sell organic chicken. They feed their chickens mainly soy (50-85% of the diet). Poultry would be poisoned by eating raw soy. So feed manufacturers heat and chemically process soy for poultry feed. Even though the soy may have been organically grown, the chemically treated and processed soy is no longer organic. Then, farmers who feed their fowl soy as a protein supplement are not raising their poultry organically grown but will sell it as organically grown, such as Rosie Organic chickens. When a product is chemically treated and processed, it is no longer organic. Animals that eat such a feed are not organically grown. Governments allow producers to lie to us and harm us. So we have to do the best we can by choosing the best we can, until we change the laws and get farmers to grow crops and animals truly organically grown.

PAPAYA helps to increase taste, health of the spine, and general digestion.

PEPPER, dried and ground, when eaten too much or too often, irritates the digestive tract and glands. Processed black and cayenne peppers are partially responsible for many kidney problems and "high" hernias. Those peppers may be eaten in moderation for flavoring. Fresh raw hot peppers, like jalapeño, banana and chile, promote good circulation, and prevent and expel parasites when very very hot.

PRESERVATIVES AND PESTICIDES, airborne, or in or on foods, create volatile substances inside the body that are dangerous to the life of cells, often causing faulty development and functions, faulty production and utilization of body serums, cellular mutations and overall impaired cell and body constitutions. Some people have severe reactions (allergies) to preservatives and pesticides, especially children: sores, eczema, psoriasis, nose bleeds, severe irritability, headaches, numbness, dizziness, panic, nausea, fatigue, anxiety and hyperactivity. *See* Edema, page 260; and Overweight, page 296.

RAW BROWN SUGAR is a misnomer. It is nothing other than table sugar with about 5% molasses added back to it. *See* Molasses, page 193.

REFRIGERATION AND STORAGE: Refrigeration that is too cold dulls taste. Setting the refrigerator temperature no lower than 48° Fahrenheit ensures more taste. As room temperatures fluctuate through seasons, so will refrigerator temperatures. Adjusting refrigeration temperature every two months ensures more flavorful refrigerated foods.

Meats are best kept in the coldest area of the refrigerator but not frozen. Raw meat wrapped, sliced or cubed and placed in large wide-mouth glass jars, usually keeps 10 days (the average is 7 days) without developing a strong odor. The lid should be tight. I found that raw poultry stays fresh 5-7 days without developing a strong odor when the bone and skin are removed and the meat is stored in glass jars with the lid tight. However, I have not experienced any problem with eating any meat when the smell was offensive. Remember that I had my vagus nerve severed in surgery when I was 20. I am supposed to be in danger of death from bacterial and parasitical invasion from raw meat. I have been eating raw meat full of bacteria and parasites for 29 years without ever experiencing food-poisoning. I explain in my book The Recipe For Living Without Disease, more about bacteria and parasites in raw meat and the fact that they are healthful, rather than dangerous.

Raw meats stored below 38° Fahrenheit lose too many enzymes and flavor is subdued, often becoming almost tasteless. Storing raw meat below 32° Fahrenheit destroys enzymes, vitamins and protein, and causes E. coli to mutate.

Eggs should not be refrigerated. Refrigeration destroys or damages too many enzymes and protein in eggs. Therefore, when refrigerated, eggs are less nutritive, and harder to digest, assimilate, and utilize. Egg may be nonrefrigerated for at least 4 weeks. More about eggs is discussed in my book The Recipe For Living Without Disease.

Most fruits may be refrigerated to preserve their unripe state with more enzymes and less sugar. However, refrigeration quickly advances ripe bananas to the rotting stage, causing intestinal fermentation when eaten. Any fruit that turns brown or becomes mushy in refrigeration should not be eaten. Often, pears that have been frozen in commercial storage turn brown and mushy rather quickly after they thaw. When thawed, they rot from the core outward causing intestinal fermentation when eaten. If fruit is frozen, it should be eaten very soon after it thaws. Covering fruits with glass bowls or domes, or placing them in glass containers with lids and storing in refrigeration slows spoilage, keeps flavors alive longer, and prevents insects from feasting on them.

Raw butter can be left at room temperature and enjoyed soft for as long as two weeks, that is, unless room temperature exceeds 80° Fahrenheit. Even if room temperature reaches 90° Fahrenheit, raw butter remains flavorful for two days or more unrefrigerated. Do not expose butter to direct sunlight. Exposing butter to sunlight for an hour or more causes it to sour. I prefer to refrigerate my raw butter until the day before I use it. Then I put 1½ cups in a 2-cups wide-mouthed glass jar and leave the butter at room temperature so that I may enjoy my butter soft and flavorful. Many people on this type of raw diet eat 3-8 ounces of butter daily and keep a daily schedule preparing raw butter for the next day or two. Raw dairy never spoils, it simply becomes varieties of cheeses, including butter that becomes a blue cheese.

Raw cheeses last several weeks unrefrigerated in air-tight containers. Like butter, no-salt-added raw cheeses are more flavorful at room temperature. Some of my clients enjoy their no-salt-added raw cheeses left unrefrigerated for weeks. Some times a pungent white mold forms on cheeses. The mold is beneficial for some people, that is, if strong cheeses are appealing. However, for some people, moldy cheeses cause listlessness that may last weeks.

Raw milk is best consumed soon after it has been taken from an animal. However, since most of us do not live on farms, raw milk keeps better in refrigeration. Raw milk mixed with unheated honey and raw cream added, and stored in a dark cupboard without refrigeration lasts without souring for 3-4 days unless room temperature constantly exceeds 80° Fahrenheit. If it separates, shake to remix it.

Oils that are properly cold-pressed or stone-pressed, that is, pressed below 96° Fahrenheit, should be kept from light. Placing each bottle of oil inside a brown paper bag, pressing the bag around the bottle, putting a rubber band at the neck, and putting the oil in the darkest, coolest cupboard prevents the bottle of oil from turning bitter and/or flat. Olive oil should not be refrigerated. Because flax oil is so vulnerable to oxidation and light, it should be refrigerated. If and when there is ever truly cold-pressed, non-solvent-extracted wheat germ oil available, it should be refrigerated. Cold-pressed peanut oil, if we can ever get it again, is better nonrefrigerated. It should be placed in a dark bag and kept in a dark cupboard, as for all pressed oils, except flax and coconut oils.

Holding your breath for ten seconds and exhaling into containers of fruits, vegetables and oils, then sealing them, facilitates preservation.

ROYAL JELLY is food prepared just for the queen bee and brood of a hive. Eaten with raw meat and raw fat, it increases regeneration of tissue and youth. Royal Jelly should be stored in refrigeration.

SALAD DRESSINGS: An alkalizing salad dressing is 5 tablespoons each of raw unpasteurized apple cider vinegar (or raw wine/vinegar) and unheated honey. Optional ingredients are: red onion, fresh chile, fresh herbs, raw plain kefir (when available), raw cream (when available) and raw fertile egg. Unless combined with an equal portion of raw vinegar, avoid oils on salads because the nutrients in the salad foods will be bound by the oils and unable to alkalize the blood and body. However, it is okay to eat raw oil, like unsalted raw butter or stone-pressed olive oil, on cooked starch such as pasta or bread, during the same meal with a salad - the starch keeps the oil free from coating and penetrating the salad foods. *See* Wine/Vinegar Dressing, page 202.

SALADS, VEGETABLE: *See* Vegetables, page 201.

SALT: *See* Appendixes M, page 143, I, page 139, and J, page 139. Table salt is a catalyst in the development of all diseases in most people. Mineral salts are plant-food, not food for humans. If they were food for humans, we could live on dirt. The vegetable kingdom makes wonderful use of mineral salts, in balanced ratios, to grow healthfully and strong. After they make the salts into bio-actively available substances, we can juice their leaves, stalks and roots to obtain concentrations of those salts. In our bodies, mineral salts that are not naturally present in food, imbalance our systems, causing many diseases, including cellular dehydration, edema, and bone diseases and malformations.

SAUCES: Store-bought, prepared sauces are all cooked. Raw sauces may be made by using your favorite ingredients fresh and raw, and blended together. For example, here is a tomato sauce: Press 4 tablespoons unsalted raw butter against the inside walls of an 8-ounces canning jar and put a lid on it tightly. Place the jar into water that is as hot as your fingers can stand without burning them. While the butter melts for 5-10 minutes, slice one medium tomato that is room temperature and then blend it with the melted butter and fresh raw herbs, fresh raw pepper, fresh raw onion and fresh raw garlic if you like. Pour that mixture over raw meat, or not-too-hot pasta or bread, and top with grated no-salt-added raw cheese. In the book, The Recipe For Living Without Disease, there are 82 sauces that can each be made 3-5 different ways.

SMOOTHIES: When I mention smoothie, I mean a drink made with raw eggs blended with a raw fresh fruit or raw fresh fruit puree and unheated honey. Honey is optional, but in some cases it helps digestion. If you have a taste for a smoothie without the honey, you should have it without honey. *See* Eggs, page 184.

SUGARS: Table sugars and sugar sweeteners (refined sugars, sucrose) are all made from processing sugar cane or sugar beets at temperatures around 320° Fahrenheit. They interfere with and damage digestion, glandular and nerve health and functions.

Fructose is the sugar from fruit (as opposed to sucrose which is the sugar from vegetables). Sweeteners made of fructose are also processed and cause as many similar complications as sucrose. Fructose is the lesser of two evils. Unheated honeys, raw fruit and raw juices are the only sweeteners that promote better health.

SUGAR SUBSTITUTES are inorganic chemicals. They are debris that create toxins and damage health. Unheated honey and raw fruits are the only sweeteners that promote better health.

TURKEY builds strong lymph and membranes. Turkeys produce an enzyme during molting season which can make some people sick when eaten raw. Some people should avoid eating raw turkey from early Spring through Summer. If you have a taste for turkey during molting season, most likely you are not ill-effected by this enzyme and it may be important for you to eat raw turkey during molting season.

VANILLA EXTRACT should be organically grown and should contain its natural alcohol. Its nutritional properties stimulate the thyroid when a thyroid is inactive, or when it is needed to balance a sluggish glandular system. Vanilla extracts that have had the alcohol removed are less effective. Some people become hyperactive and develop insomnia if they consume vanilla extract too often or too late in the day. *See* Coffee Substitute, page 182.

VEGETABLES: Whole vegetables should only be eaten when craved; *see* page 147, about digestibility of vegetables. However, when eating vegetables - leafy, root and stalk foods - most often they should be eaten without oil dressings. Drinking very fresh raw gel of aloe vera, or juice of yam, in combination with other vegetable juices such as carrot and parsley, most often increases healing and decreases suffering.

VEGETABLE JUICES help alkalize overly acidic blood. They are also a means of supplementing our vitamin, enzyme and mineral deficiencies. Vegetable juices should mainly be celery with a little parsley. See the book The Recipe For Living Without Disease. Children under 15 should only have vegetable juices occasionally, if necessary for a particular ailment or following a cold or flu, and regularly maybe once every 10-22 days. If a child is raised on raw food, there maybe no need for her or him to drink vegetable juices.

VINEGAR: *See* Apple Cider Vinegar, Raw, Unpasteurized and Unfiltered, page 179.

VOLATILE TOXINS are substances entering the body or substances altered to a state within the body that create harmfully acidic and sometimes allergic reactions. They can negatively alter RNA and DNA, enzymes, hormones, cells and tissue, affecting the entire body. They can be the result of: low-grade mineral poisoning caused by eating canned food, preservatives, pesticides and medication; exposing oneself to chemicals, pesticides and other pollution; from an excess of hormones produced by the body itself because of those substances listed above; or from a diet that is not proper for an individual.

WATER dries the body. Drink water rarely. Analogy: continually applying water to skin dries and cracks the skin. Oiling the skin protects and preserves the skin. It is the same inside our bodies.

Eating tomatoes quenches thirst best. Dry lips and mouth are not dehydration. The brain discards many toxins, especially metals, through the gums and tongue, absorbing and spending all available fats in and surrounding oral tissues. That leaves the mouth and lips very dry, but it is not dehydration but fat deficiency. Placing 1 tablespoon of unsalted raw butter with a dab of unheated honey on the tongue and keeping them in the mouth for 5-10 minutes reverses dry mouth and lips. Drinking fresh raw milk, cream and kefir, fresh raw vegetable juices, unheated honey, and eating fresh unripe fruit provides H_20 rich in electrolytes, enzymes, minerals, vitamins and fats that prevent drying. A wonderful thirst-quenching drink is a blended mixture of 2 cups peeled cucumber, 3-6 tablespoons coconut cream and 1 tablespoon unheated honey. Of that mixture, drink 2-3 ounces at a time throughout the day. *See* Appendix M, page 143.

WINE/VINEGAR DRESSING, RAW, for salads, can be made and refrigerated up to one week only. One suggested recipe is: Blend 1/3 cup of raw unpasteurized apple cider vinegar, 1/3 cup raw organic wine, all or a portion of 1 fresh hot pepper (red, yellow banana, red or orange or black jalapeño and chilies), ½-4 tablespoons unheated honey, and a slice of purple onion. Use as much fresh hot pepper as desired but the dressing should have a little bite from the pepper. For some people, the sweetness of the honey in the dressing is not appealing; those people should have it with less honey or without honey. For some people the opposite is true; those people should add more honey. (This is the dressing that is imperative for those people who lack enzyme-mutations and need to remove the accumulated toxic residues and resins from years of eating cooked green and cooked red foods.)

For another salad dressing, decrease the amounts of wine and vinegar to ¼ cup each and add ¼ cup raw plain kefir (when available).

WHIPPING CREAM: when raw cream is available, it can be whipped and enjoyed. Whip raw cream until it starts to thicken, and then add 1-4 tablespoons unheated honey per 1 cup of cream. Continue whipping until it is as firm as you like it. Eat it with whatever meets your fancy - fruit, salads, popcorn (?!) or other cooked starch or raw meat.

YOGURT is similar to kefir. However, yogurt is always made with heated milk and will not thicken unless the milk is heated to at least 115° Fahrenheit. Most store-bought yogurt is made from pasteurized milk and is an inferior food. Raw kefir is considerably superior.

Conversations About the Primal Diet

I conclude this section by sharing parts/composites of the email exchanges between Sheri, who is a mother of 5 and has been on the diet for about 4 years, and an acquaintance Cari, a woman who was a dissenter of my Primal Diet, and finally me.

> Sheri,
> Didn't you feel this strongly about a vegan diet too? This diet says no water, this diet says no starch, this diet says no salt, this diet says eat eat eat. That will burn out your organs. I just am saying that faith is blind and you will have to see for yourself as I did. My husband's grandma lived until she was 16 years old in Poland on raw goat's milk. She came here and has been living without and now is 92 years old. She drinks coffee everyday and eats lunch meat everyday. I haven't heard of a 92 year old raw foodist. Also my sister-in-law's husband's grandma from Germany who ate her weight in chocolate lived to be 102. Do you want to be that old?
> Aajonus makes it seem that this diet will give you the vitality to jump rope when you are 95. I haven't seen the people who he claims cured themselves. I haven't even read articles about any of it. I haven't seen him share with the world his findings. Nothing is published anywhere. His first book I read 10 times. I wasn't convinced by his appearance that 20 years of eating like this was promoting youth and wellness.
> take care
> Cari

Hello, Cari,
Again. I have already considered the objections you posed. I have read, studied and applied principles of nutrition and its relation to our physical, mental and emotional health for many years, and also have put these principles to the test to see what really works. My husband may be smart in many ways, but he is not in great health and even has some fairly serious pre-cancerous symptoms. He may have a strong genetic health which has allowed him to be abusive to his body thus far, but he will need to consider making changes in his own diet, if he wishes to continue into old age in good health.

I look to Dr. Pottenger's studies and see such a mirror image of what happened to his cats and what is happening to humans today regarding the lack of health we are all experiencing. I attribute many factors, not just diet to the cause of it all. But because we have been assaulted by vaccines, medications, processed foods, and pollutants of every sort, we must take what seems to be extreme measures to reverse it. We did not have the healthy start that our parents and grandparents had with breast milk, or raw milk and wholesome foods, and free of vaccines and other chemical pollution. I am most certain that raw food reverses disease because I have witnessed it.

I have personally witnessed over and over again, the negative affect on physical and mental health when eating junk food and YES even cooked food. I conclude that it is because our organs and glands are so toxic, that even a little cooked food will give us some symptoms. I am sorry, but you are not going to convince me. As I have said, I have been there, done that, thought that already.

I also do not think that because I have not made all the right choices in the past regarding diet, makes me wrong today. As humans we must progress a little at a time. Change is a gradual thing. I learned very much from being a raw vegan, and even though it was nutritionally deficient, it still showed me that raw foods heal and make one feel better.

By the way, Aajonus is not using me or anyone to promote his business. Those of us who have benefited from his knowledge and the diet, wish to share that with others. Aajonus is one of the few people I know who is not given to pride and greed. He lets the diet speak for itself. And speak it does, if you give it a chance.

I have 4 children and one on the way, and can see a great difference between my last born when I had been on the diet for more than 2 years, and the rest of my children. I have also spoken to another mother who has been on the diet for 2 of her pregnancies and there is no doubt that this diet positively affects our children emotionally, physically and intellectually.

I appreciate your thoughts, but again, you will not convince me as I have already considered these same objections in the past, and cannot find any validity to them. We have been doing the Primal Diet now for 3½ years, and I have only seen continued improvement in my children and myself. My youngest is exceptionally smart and advanced, and that I attribute to being on this diet during pregnancy as well as her now consuming the raw meat and dairy. I have much empirical experience/evidence at this point to prove the diet, and I will confidently continue.

Sincerely Yours,
Sheri

Sheri,
There are plenty of smart people who eat cooked foods. Did Sir Isaac Newton eat raw meat? What about all the people who design machines to do the work of 200 men. They definitely pass me up as far as brains go. Doctors don't necessarily have brains. Being smart isn't a product of this diet. It's the time you take to teach your children in ways that they can absorb all the knowledge given to them. Look at your hubby, he eats cooked food and is able to work out of your beautiful house and make enough money to raise 4 children and have a comfortable life. To me that is smart!

Dr. Howell died, he looked his age. As far as Pottenger, he studied cats. Animals have far greater enzymes and acids to digest raw food because that is how God designed them. Yes they should eat raw. People are different. Another thing Aajonus said is you don't need a lot of sleep just 4-5 hours.

I am not here to judge, I just feel in my heart that Aajonus isn't telling all and is using you for his BUISNESS because that is all it is.

I am sorry to upset you, I am grateful I met you and for the farm foods.

take care
Cari

Hello Aajonus,
I think that whenever we are persecuted for this diet, it gives us some consolation if you read and comment on the exchange, only if you have time, of course.
Hope you are well.
Yours,
Sheri

Hi, Sheri,
If anyone claims to have read my first book 10 times, we must ask, "Why did that person misquote me on water, starch, sleep and salt?"

About water: I recommended that we minimize the drinking of water because very little water can be absorbed by our cells and dries the skin and membranes of cells. I suggested drinking more milk and vegetable juices, and eating tomatoes and cucumbers. All of those foods and all raw foods contain H_2O that can be cellularly utilized. I said in my first book that some people should drink a lot of water for awhile.

About starch: I said in my first book that starches are very necessary, even to the point that I recommended that a few people go against the main principle of eating raw food. I suggested that they would benefit from eating simple, cooked starches sometimes, like unsalted bread, etc. But, because I later observed the collection of toxins even when those people ate plenty of raw fat with the cooked starch, in my second book and in the revision, I advise that necessary extra starch be derived from eating the Nut Formula as much as possible. Note that all meat contains starch. That is what herbivores eat when they eat seeds of grasses, especially their preferred seeds, those that have fallen to the ground and dried.

About salt: It is a fact that people need sodium but not necessarily salt. When people drink salt water, they get sick. Eating salt is helpful in cultures that eat only a little meat and lots of starch because those people are prone to tapeworms and excessive pinworms. Salt dehydrates intestinal parasites. Some salt is helpful to people who eat cooked food and cannot utilize enough sodium to counter all the toxicity that results from eating cooked foods. I said that people who have adrenal exhaustion should eat a little salt. I said that most people who eat a raw diet should not eat salt, including sea salt.

About sleep: I stated in my books that sleep is very important because 90% of healing happens for most people in the sleep state. After my 32 years of eating raw food, I said that I need only 4-5 hours of sleep daily, unless I am in an intense healing state. Sometimes I have needed 6-12 hours of sleep per day. Most people need 7-10 hours of sleep. I did not say that everybody needs only 4-5 hours sleep.

About greed: I could have compromised many times and made fortunes. I wrote a diet for a woman named Judy. It was for a certain period of her life, for her to temporarily lose weight. Judy wrote a book of the diet called The Beverly Hills Diet and made a fortune. That diet is harmful to the nervous system if followed for more than a few days or weeks. It often made people very testy and/or irritable. Many people who followed that diet damaged their nervous systems, family relationships and friendships. I refused to do that harm to people for money. In 1971, on moral principle, I refused to be the Winston man in commercials, rejecting $7.5 million over the next seven years.

You are a very intelligent woman who has experimented and found that the Primal Diet promotes healthy emotional behavior for yourself, as well as for members of your immediate family and many of your acquaintances. You are blessed with a particular sensibility. I suggest that you trust your reality. It may be a waste of time to try to educate people about the science of nutrition if they are new to the diet and their thinking is clouded because they believe that they know everything from only a few months, or even a few years of eating some of the Primal Diet. Also, some people have learning and comprehensive disorders along with frustration, fear and impatience. They are unable to see the nutritional puzzle clearly, even though they think they see it clearly. I do not know what can be done for them but it seems like a waste of energy to allow it to frustrate us.

Healthfully and lovingly,
aajonus

Obtaining The Foods We Want And Need

Some foods necessary for optimal health, and for the remedies that follow, are not available in all states in the USA. Fresh raw dairy is commercially available only in a few states. In some states, fresh raw dairy is sold only at the farm. Some farmers have to label their raw milk "For animal consumption" or "For pets only". I will consume raw milk from cows fed raw feed and that do not receive hormones or antibiotics. I prefer organically fed, but it is not always available.

The rulings that fresh raw dairy cannot be available commercially to the people in most states is prejudicial. Health freedom is denied. You may regain this right if enough people from each state petition their state government. The process, reports and documents to change legislation to permit raw dairy to be sold are on the internet at www.RawMilk.org. Find a dairy farm that feeds their cows organically and produces raw dairy products. Or buy and start organic raw dairy farms as individuals, or as cooperatives.

For any other foods that may not be available in your locale, the need and demand create the product. Tell your local stores what you want. If they can't get it or refuse to, write to me at: Optimal Ways of Living, P.0. Box 176, Santa Monica, CA. 90404-0176. Enclose the order form at the back of this book and a check or money order for $15 (cost of service, materials, handling and shipping) made payable to Optimal Ways of Living. You will be sent a list of the brand names and addresses for Primal Diet-quality products. If you know of any raw dairy products, unheated honey and stone-pressed oils (or cold-pressed below 96 degree Fahrenheit) in your part of the country, please send me the brand names, the kind of food, and the producer's address and phone number so that I may verify rawness and quality, then pass this information on to those who search for genuinely raw products.

Brief Preparation Guide

For recipes, instructions and suggested meal plans, buy the book, The Recipe For Living Without Disease. It contains 150 recipes, including raw cheesecakes, raw pies, raw meat recipes, and 82 raw meat sauces that can be made 3-5 different ways each. That means there are approximately 400 sauces to help you enjoy raw meat.

BLENDING MADE EASY: Buy a blender, such as Osterizer. The base of the blender, where the blades fit, should be the size of a regular, small-mouthed, glass Ball canning jar (the 2½ inch diameter mouth, not the 3¼ inch diameter mouth). The rubber sealing ring, stainless steel blade, and the threaded plastic bottom of the blender screw onto the mouth of a regular, small-mouthed canning jar (in that order, that is, one side of the rubber sealing ring should be against the mouth of the jar and the other side against the base of the steel blade). Note: As of April 2005, the rubber sealing rings for the Osterizer are too thin and small, so that a proper seal is not made with the jar, causing food to leak from the jar while blending - very messy. Therefore, buy a rubber washer that is made for another blender. Buy one that is at least $^{3}/_{16}$ inch (½ mm) thick and slightly larger than the circumference of the blade-plate.

Then buy or collect regular, small-mouthed canning and jelly jars in an assortment of sizes: 4, 8, 12, 16 and 32 ounces. Select the size of jar that is appropriate for the job, such as a 4-ounces jar to make a sauce for 1-2 people. Before blending food, make certain that the blades do not strike or cut into the glass jars during blending. If one blade strikes the glass, bend it upward so that it does not strike the glass again. Usually, one blade strikes the glass on only 4-ounces-sized jars. Place ingredients into the jar. Place the rubber sealing ring on the rim of the jar. Then place the steel blades inside the jar. The metal base of the blades will rest on top of the rubber sealing ring. Make sure that the sealing ring does not fall into the jar. If any part of it does, it will become twisted around the blade, causing profuse leakage and possibly damaging the sealing ring. Finally, screw the plastic base over the base of the blades and onto the jar. Turn the jar upside down and place it on the blender and blend. If you hear an unusually low frequency or high vibrational sound when you turn on the blender, turn it off immediately, unscrew the threaded bottom, remove the blade and untwist the rubber sealing ring from around the blade. Realign the ring properly (if torn, use another sealing ring - have several sealing rings on hand because that occasionally happens). Absolutely do not blend any substance harder than shelled raw almonds in a glass jar because the jar might break and the glass could injure someone.

DISSOLVE HONEY easily and quickly into any liquid or food to puree by blending it in the appropriate sized canning jar. Always put honey in the jar last and blend immediately, especially if other ingredients are cold from refrigeration; otherwise the honey will turn hard and stick to the sides of the jar. *See* Blending made easy, above.

DRINK FOR MOISTURIZING AND LUBRICATING DRY AND/-OR HARDENED INTERNAL AND EXTERNAL TISSUE (e.g., dry skin and hair, arthritis, sclerosis, and cirrhosis of the liver): Blend 1-2 raw eggs, 3-6 tablespoons unsalted raw butter (or other raw fat, but butter is best), 1-1½ tablespoons fresh raw lemon juice and 2-6 teaspoons unheated honey. That drink has a lemon-meringue taste that appeals to most people, and works quickest to relieve dryness, stiffness and hardening.

JUICING A COCONUT: Choose a coconut by inspecting its shell. If you find any cracks or dark watermarks, small or large, or black spots, it is probably soured. Inspect the three small dark circles grouped together at the top, called eyes. If one of the eyes is open or shrunken, it is soured. If the coconut is without any of the above, the odds of having a good coconut are 9 of 10.

Juicing coconuts can seem like a chore but the healthful rewards are worth the effort. You will need leather gloves that are not heavily dyed, an ice pick, hammer, curved-ended oyster knife, and a juicer that separates cream from pulp, such as a GreenStar 1000 juicer.

Poke the coconut eyes until you find the eye that is soft. Do not puncture it, yet. Puncture one of the hard circles with the ice pick and hammer. Then puncture the soft circle with the ice pick. Pour the coconut milk into a glass. Taste the milk. If it is sour, the coconut may be partially or completely soured. If the coconut milk (often referred to

as coconut water) is good, drink it when thirsty.
Don gloves. To loosen the meat from the shell, firmly tap coconut all around for 2 minutes but not hard enough to crack it yet. Now, crack the coconut shell at the end opposite from the three eyes. Hammer the coconut into many pieces. If you find some of the meat yellow or discolored, it is partially soured. Pry the meat from the shell with the oyster knife. If black spots appear on the brown skin, it is molded where the spots appear. Separate the non-soured meat from the soured meat. If it is completely soured or moldy, begin again with another coconut. Slice good coconut pieces into strips that are approximately ¼-inch thick by ½-inch width and any length. Or (easier!) drop the chunks of coconut into a food-processor and grind.
Place the coconut meat slices or ground coconut into a juicer that separates cream from pulp, such as a GreenStar or Champion juicer. The result is coconut cream that will thicken as hard as butter in refrigeration. Use the pulp to fertilize a garden or lawn, or sun dry it to make a coconut confection for recipes. Do not mix the coconut milk with the coconut cream unless you intend to drink it within 24 hours, or it will sour. It is best to store coconut cream in many 4- or 8-ounces glass jars. Blend ½ teaspoon lime juice with each 8 ounces coconut cream. Storing in that manner in refrigeration will preserve it for up to 7 weeks. Note: Since making coconut cream requires time and tools, it is recommended that you juice 5-10 coconuts at a time. Each coconut renders 6-8 ounces of pure cream from the preferred metal twin-gear juicer (such as Green Star) not including the coconut milk.

PÂTÉ is made by cutting meat into cubes, then putting them into a food processor and chopping them until they are paste.

POULTICES are made by blending, chopping, crushing, grating, mashing or mincing raw food, and then wrapping it in a clean white cloth (cotton, cheesecloth, muslin or silk). That is then applied to an affected external area of the body. Put a strip of cloth around the poultice to hold it in place, not too tightly. When the poultice dries in several hours, replace it with fresh ingredients. The cloth should always be thoroughly rinsed before adding or replacing ingredients, and the final rinse should be with good mineral water.

Nature should not be feared; She is healing, vital and loyal. Our bodies should not be feared; they are part of Nature and are always in the process of healing. While eating our way to better health, it should be remembered that healing often takes time, endurance and requires patience. I wish you a richly healthy life.

VITAL FOOD REMEDIES

I have recommended that my clients acquaint themselves with all of the ailments listed throughout this section because most people have many of these ailments, but not to the extent that they can be diagnosed. I have suggested that they highlight all of the sentences that have applied to them sometime in their lives. Highlighting makes it easier to locate applicable symptoms, explanations and remedies.

Symptoms were usually alleviated and ailments usually mitigated in people who ate the foods that I had specifically recommended for their ailments. Where more than one food or combination was recommended, I suggested that they eat all that was recommended but not all at one meal. When someone desired more food than was specifically recommended, I suggested that they supplement the recommended food with food that constitutes a balanced raw diet. *See* the book The Recipe For Living Without Disease. They chose the foods that they desired, then prepared and ate them raw. Consequently, the speed of healing increased. But people who did not continue to eat raw food on a regular basis did not heal properly. Because optimal healing needs proper nutrients and takes time, their ailments gradually returned. Ailments that did not heal usually advanced. Detoxification and healing - to the point that people no longer felt hindered by advanced ailments - took weeks, months or years, depending on severity. Symptoms of ailments that quickly mitigated usually returned, indicating that more thorough cleansing and healing was required for better body functions. When symptoms lingered because the body continued a process of cleansing and healing, or when symptoms mitigated quickly and then returned for more cleansing and healing, people sometimes became disconcerted and discouraged. Doubts rooted. However, everyone who held fast to eating the raw diet experienced proper cleansing and healing, mitigating the severity of their ailment(s), often to the point that eventually they forgot they had had the ailment. People who trusted in Nature's raw-food precedence, and to a degree in their instincts and intuition, with endurance, patience and time, most often achieved significantly better health.

Throughout Volume 1, I gave examples of the many healthy rewards I obtained using courage and patience when going through a major detoxification and eating a raw diet. I will give you another, here. Immediately prior to the first printing of this book in 1996, a violent rash erupted on my nose, around the inside of my left eye and the top center of my forehead at my hairline. On the second day, the rash looked as if it were developing into karposi, accompanied with chronic headaches. I did not have AIDS but was concerned. I used my salve for burns, ate raw chicken every 4 hours, ate 8-12 raw eggs daily and drank raw milk constantly to keep pain to a minimum. By the fourth day, small blisters formed. I released the pus on several but it was not enough for a laboratory test. On the fifth day, a chunk of my skin fell off near my burned eyeball. I became alarmed.

I quieted myself and took the skin to a lab and requested that they test for chemical and medical toxins as well as cancer. The laboratory reported listed components used in aerospace/dental epoxy, and basil-cell melanoma. Since my nose was the primary focus of tissue, the lab technician asked me if I had splintered my nose. He told me that some plastic surgeons use epoxy in such cases because they can't pin a shattered nose together. I told him that when I was fifteen, my nose was shattered by a hard ball going about 60 mph thrown by an adult. My nose shattered into seven pieces. It took two major surgeries to correct it over seven years. The first surgeon told me that the surgery took 6 hours. He did not tell me why, or that he had glued my bone together using aerospace/dental epoxy.

The technician explained that, during an operation such as the one I'd undergone, the surgeon would have normally cut and pulled the skin covering my nose, and would have clamped it to my forehead. Then, he would have had to allow each spot-glued piece of bone to dry before gluing the next fragment. He would have had to let the epoxy dry completely, because if wet epoxy were to have come into contact with tissue softer than bone, the epoxy would have burned and melted it.

Almost 30 years after that surgery, my body decided to detoxify the epoxy. The epoxy-detoxification process took six weeks. If I had panicked and gone to a dermatologist, I would have been given antibiotics, steroid ointments, radiation and chemotherapy, adding more toxins to my body, and scarring my face as well. Now my face, skull and brain have the opportunity to live and function healthier, better and more efficiently. Already, my sense of smell is keener, and food tastes better. I'm hoping that the scars and damage to my left cornea, nose and forehead where the dissolved epoxy, causing cancer, burned my eye and burned massive holes in my skin will heal. One year after that cancer in 1997, my left cornea contained 8 layers of scars and vision loss to 20/180. Almost 8 years later, an eye exam revealed only 1 layer of scar remained and my vision improved to 20/40. I have observed consistently that the body always gains more than it loses during a detoxification. I trusted it that time, too, and I am not disappointed.

Because eating raw food provides the nutrients for the body to properly cleanse (detoxify) as well as heal and rebuild, natural cleanses (such as colds, flu, and temporary aches and pains) should be welcomed. They may occur 1-4 times a year. Cleanses (detoxification) have been shorter in duration and less debilitating than cleanses that occurred before my Primal Diet. Almost everyone on the balanced raw Primal Diet felt more energy and vitality during and immediately after a natural cleansing than they had experienced when on cooked diets.

Note that sometimes different ailments resulted from similar overall problems in different people. For instance, a frequently high adrenaline level in one person caused acute hardening of the arteries, while in another person it caused Candida, and in another person it caused cataracts.

Some elderly people who had a lifetime of accumulated cooked-food residues or chemicals (for instance, years of medication, or exposure to household or industrial chemicals and gases) spent the remainder of their lives in painful detoxification. Consequently, I learned that it is sometimes more important to feel better while getting a little healthier. Therefore, now I suggest to my elderly clients who find themselves going through an uncomfortable detoxification that lasts more than three months, that they bathe as suggested under Detoxification. *See* Detoxification, Stopping It, page 255.

The less beneficial alternative for stopping painful persistent detoxification for the elderly is to eat a cooked meal once weekly. A cooked meal discourages continual detoxification of old stored toxins. One cooked meal each week of baked, broiled or boiled chicken, not fried, usually stops and prevents extreme detoxification of old toxins stored in the body.

Volatile toxic conditions are ailments where highly reactive toxins have accumulated, whether in the blood, nerve-serum, lymph, connective tissues, muscles, bones, glands or organs. It is a state in which live cells in the affected area(s) or system(s) are vulnerable to severe irritation and cellular destruction (as in my example above). Excess hormonal production (for instance, adrenaline and insulin) along with pollution, or not eating enough raw fat and meat, or not drinking raw fresh vegetable juices, frequently causes volatile toxic conditions. Drugs (medicinal and recreational), coffee, chocolate, processed peppers and sugars, pesticides, preservatives and sodas all irritate and overstimulate adrenals and pancreas, creating volatile toxic conditions. Symptoms of excessive adrenaline are: hyperactivity and/or irritability and very dry skin or hair. Eating the foods suggested for alkalizing the blood balances the blood within 2-10 days (*see* Alkalizing Food, page 178). Symptoms of excessive insulin are hypoglycemia, irritability and edema. Completely refraining from eating ripe fruit and high-carbohydrate vegetable juices helps relieve that condition. Completely neutralizing all of those conditions has taken up to 10 years.

Drinking 1-2 cups of naturally sparkling mineral water daily helps restore the electrolyte balance and oxygen level in the blood and reduces adrenaline production.

Eating 3 ounces of unheated honey daily and 1-4 cups of raw fresh green vegetable juices at least five days weekly for the rest of one's life, gradually replaces enzymes lost or leached from years of eating cooked food.

For optimal health, research and experience have conclusively proved to me that all food, except raw oils, should not be heated above 104° Fahrenheit. Raw oils should not be heated above 96° Fahrenheit.

The following remedies have worked an average of 85% in all cases. However, by man's laws, they are not prescriptive.

When beginning the Primal Diet, a person who has not eaten many fresh foods such as raw fruits, raw juices and raw salads, may do better eating more raw fruits, an occasional salad and lots of unheated honey. Also, there are people who have diseases for which the body requires more fruit until the disease is reversed. However, after those people have eaten the Primal Diet for 1-2 years, I have observed that better health and mitigated symptoms have been achieved quicker by limiting fruit intake to once daily in the afternoon. A person who exercises may need more fruit, but usually in combination with a raw fat.

ABORTION: Scraping of the uterus (D&C) may cause scarring; *See* Stretch Marks, Scars And Wrinkles, page 338, about removing scar tissue. *See* Hemorrhage, page 210, to stop an excessive bleed. *See* Family Planning for more natural abortive methods, page 333.

ABSCESS is a localized infection (detoxification) accompanied by pus externally or internally. An abscess is helpful because it is a process of dissolving and discarding volatile toxins from tissues.

Externally, packing the abscess with a little clay that has been pre-mixed with good mineral water into a thin paste, and then applying a bandage over it absorbs and neutralizes volatile toxins. Clay is best premixed as instructed under Clay. The abscess will, most often, come to a head in a couple of days and burst on its own when as much toxicity as the body plans to remove is brought to the surface. *See* Clay, page 181.

In the case of an abscessed tooth, eating at least 15 medium-sized tomatoes per day neutralizes the condition. Eating no-salt-added raw cheese with tomatoes helps to reduce abscessed tooth pain and promotes healing. With an abscessed tooth, blending the tomatoes into puree makes them drinkable. The cheese may be blended with tomatoes. Also, *see* Pain Formula, Chapter 15 in the book The Recipe For Living Without Disease.

ACNE often comes from not having the enzyme-mutations for utilizing cooked red and orange fruits and vegetables. The fat from cooked red fruits and vegetables cannot be broken down, assimilated, or utilized properly, forming resins and residues. Therefore, the body binds the resins and residues with numerous white cells (antibodies) and fat molecules. Then the body tries to discard the mass through the skin. Because of the chemistry or size of the mass, or the sharpness of residues (often like glass) the toxins burn, split, or lacerate cellular walls of the skin as they pass though the pores, creating lesions. This causes cellular sores that weep, forming pus (acne) and causing scars. Avoiding cooked red- and orange-pigmented fruits and vegetables (including all bottled or canned tomato sauces) usually eliminates acne. *See* If I Lack Enzyme-Mutations, What Foods Should I Avoid?, page 174.

Topically: Applying a mixture of 1 tablespoon good mineral water, ½ teaspoon powdered sun-dried clay and a drop of stone-pressed olive oil soothes and usually prevents scars. Or apply some Primal Facial Body Care Cream (from my recipe book). Or simply applying a dab of unheated honey soothes and promotes healing.

Eating a little cold-pressed-below-96° Fahrenheit fermented coconut oil or stone-pressed olive oil daily, 3 days weekly, helps remove and prevent scars. Eating live red or orange foods helps the body eliminate stored residues and resins from cooked red or orange foods through the bowels (and less through the skin).

Drug residues, like those from cocaine, Novocain and Lydocain, require 200-4000 white and/or fat cells to arrest and eliminate one molecule of toxin. When that large mass is eliminated through a pore, the skin is torn, lesions occur and inflammation results. Consuming 1-2 tablespoons pre-prepared mixed clay in 2 ounces of water or juice, or eating cheese with butter, helps the body absorb those toxins into the bowels and discard them from the rectum rather than through the skin. See Clay, page 181.

My mother, a Registered Nurse, told me that she eliminated her teenage acne by washing her face with her urine (an Ayurvedic medical method that works). The concentration of nutrients and ammonia in the urine aids the cleansing and healing of the skin.

Certain toxins must be removed through the skin instead of through the bowels. Therefore, a few pimples may be unavoidable until those toxins are completely cleansed from the system. Removing them could take many years. *See* Dermatitis, page 254.

ADRENAL EXHAUSTION is characterized by weight loss, fears beyond what is "rational", ridges in the nails in a length-wise direction, apathy toward most forms of effort, unusual loss of hair; and by feeling unable to keep the back straight, feeling that your legs could easily collapse from under you, and feeling chemically unbalanced no matter what you eat. People who have adrenal exhaustion often have an energy drop within 15 minutes of the same time every day.

Eating the Nut Formula (page 194), or, less preferably, a cooked starch, like French, sourdough, and Italian breads with raw fat, 15 minutes before the energy drop is due each day, usually allows for normal energy levels. Eating a raw diet with plenty of fat, fish, vegetable juices and alkalizing foods gradually heals this condition in most cases. *See* Alkalizing Food, page 178.

Also *see* Chronic Fatigue Syndrome, page 247.

See Eating Schedules in my book The Recipe For Living Without Disease, pages 40-42.

AGING in our "advanced" society is basically a process of body-deterioration leading toward disease and death. That deterioration is caused by accumulated toxicity, limited cellular reproduction, cellular mutations, and cellular exhaustion. Aging and deterioration do not have to be synonymous.

Symptoms: loss of hair moisture, dexterity, skin tone, muscle tone, flesh tone, and strength.

Consuming a raw diet in which 40% of calories are raw fat prevents the "normal" process of body deterioration. The body gradually or quickly deteriorates without fat. At least 3% and up to 30% of that raw fat should be from raw milk, that is unsalted raw butter, raw cream, no-salt-added raw cheese, full-fat raw milk and raw plain kefir. Raw full-fat milk soothes tissues best.

About 50% of the human race needs starches to prevent aging. Those people need starches to bind with toxins (including excess hormones) that stress the body. We may obtain that starch by eating a Nut Formula (page 194) once or twice each week. Some people may need to eat a little cooked starch if they cannot digest the Nut Formula. That may be determined by eating the Nut Formula when you are extra-stressed. If you become more self-controlled within 12 hours after eating the Nut Formula, you do not need to eat any cooked starch.

Aging men and women could create and maintain youth by eating meat twice daily, about 1 pound daily. Men do better when they drink 1 cup raw plain kefir, if available, as often as possible with meat.

AGORAPHOBIA is a pronounced fear of leaving a safe familiar home to go anywhere. More often, this is from a severe chemical imbalance due to allergies to pesticides, preservatives, medications and other chemical toxins.

Eating (separately or together) mushrooms, naturally sparkling mineral water, raw baby spinach, fresh raw fruit and 5 raw eggs each day calms this condition. *See* Eating Schedules, in my recipe book The Recipe For Living Without Disease, Chapter 12. In most cases, avoiding chemicals (including household chemicals) and any gases they produce, relieves agoraphobia. Avoid all cleaning compounds and fluids, hairspray, insecticides and aerosol sprays.

AIDS: Owanza, a colleague, has observed that advanced symptoms of AIDS is partially related to the destruction of melanin. Melanin stagnates when the lymph is in poor condition due to chemical inundation and clogging. Melanin also stagnates from lack of enzyme-mutations, lack of lysine in unaltered states, poor retention of phosphorus due to liver damage, and ingestion of swollen, ruptured and corrupted molecules (nutrients) from heat processing. The loss of the melanin creates impairment of oxygen absorption and prevents photosynthesis of light from the sun. Advanced AIDS seems to be a disease of isolation, the person being unable to interact internally and externally, bio-chemically and ecologically. The result is death through cellular suffocation. AIDS is not contagious. For the direct man-made scientific cause of AIDS, *see* the book BIO-ATTACK ALERT, Theodore A. Strecker, LL.D.

I have not had enough nutritional experience with AIDS to be comfortable with my knowledge of it. My observation has been that most of those with HIV positive who developed AIDS-like symptoms developed them only after medical treatment for AIDS. There is overwhelming evidence that the theory that HIV is a precursor to AIDS is flimsy. Individuals who have AIDS lack enzyme-mutations to practically all cooked foods, and extreme allergies to pollution. People with those conditions would improve if they would eat a raw balanced diet daily, including the Nut Formula once or twice weekly. *See* Nut Formula, page 194. If the Nut Formula is not effective, an AIDS sufferer may help her/himself by eating a little cooked white gluten starch (that is, no baked yams, purple potatoes, yellow corn, including yellow popcorn, and other colored starches) with plenty of raw fat. That may stabilize the condition and very gradually reverse it. *See* If I Lack Enzyme-Mutations, What Foods Should I Avoid?, page 174; and HIV, page 272. Lysine in an unaltered state can be found only in unprocessed raw foods, not in supplements.

ALCOHOLISM is a disease that involves compulsively craving and drinking alcoholic beverages. Most alcoholics do not breakdown cooked fat properly, so they crave alcohol to help breakdown cooked fat. However, the side effects are most often traumatic.

When an alcoholic stops drinking, he or she should consider that the liver goes through a drastic temperature drop (liquors artificially heat the liver). The temperature drop causes the liver to go into shock (d.t.'s). Eating at least ¼ pound (4 ounces) of raw fish twice daily for three days helps the liver and most often prevents the d.t.'s. Continuing to eat raw fish for another week helps the transition from alcohol. Processed alcohol destroys liver, pancreas and brain cells by the millions and robs tissues and cells of fluids. Eating raw meats and unheated honey replaces the enzymes and sugars absent in the radical alcohol (distilled or pasteurized liquors) that destroy the membranes around cells. Raw meats and unheated honey also promote the chemical breakdown of radical alcohol. A diet that is 45% raw fat would be the most healing for an alcoholic. Eating ½ cup nonsteamed dates with a raw fat in the mornings restores the thyroid and balances the sugar level. Then eating small amounts of raw meats with raw fat, alternating with very small amounts of whatever fresh fruits (preferably unripe) that are appealing with raw fat throughout the day keeps the blood sugar level balanced. If a craving for alcohol hits, blend a raw drink consisting of the juice of 5 limes, an avocado, 4 kiwis and 4 tablespoons of unheated honey to satisfy the craving. When fresh kiwis are not available, sun-dried non-sulfured kiwis are okay, or substitute 1 cup of live pineapple in place of the kiwis.

Some people crave alcohol because they lack certain enzymes that digest fat - the alcohol helps break down fat. This particular type of individual is prone to hepatitis. For this type, eating a little unripe pineapple with raw fat usually supplies enzymes for fat digestion and stops the craving for alcohol. For those few who cannot produce their own body alcohol, drinking 2 ounces of organic raw wine once or twice weekly supplies the alcohol that is needed. Eating raw cheese or raw fat immediately before drinking alcohol prevents a lot of damage.

ALD is an accelerated deterioration of myelin (the covering over nerve networks) causing loss of concentration, uncommon dazes, convulsions, unmotivated fits, loss of motor control and coma. This is usually diagnosed in an advanced stage in children when the symptoms are very pronounced (as are most diseases). It has been lethal in children because without myelin the nerves have no protection or buffer.

Eating stone-pressed olive oil, fresh raw fish and red meat or poultry at the same meal daily provides the body with the nutrients it needs to regenerate the myelin. The key to these nutrients being properly utilized is drinking 1 drop of homeopathic quinine up to 5 times daily and eating up to 4 ounces of unheated honey daily.

ALLERGIES are disagreeable sensitivities to particular foods, light rays or pollutants (including vapors from magazine and newspaper print, perfumes and colognes). Some allergies are the result of airborne pollutants that the body cannot neutralize or detoxify and eliminate, including fibers from synthetic clothing (plastic). Other allergies result from substances in foods, natural or man-made, that the body cannot digest, assimilate, or utilize. These substances become radical toxins that severely damage tissues with which they come in contact. The same goes for allergies to cosmetics and soaps - if you can't eat it, don't put it on your skin.

<u>Symptoms from airborne allergies</u>: rash, sinus congestion, sneezing, coughing, headache, hay fever, asthma, high blood pressure, abnormal fatigue, dizziness and mental depression, and bleeds from mucus membranes, like nose bleeds and considerable blood in the feces.

Symptoms from food allergies: all of the above plus loss of appetite, nausea, vomiting, stomach and intestinal ulcers.

Eating plenty of raw fat with a Nut Formula, or a cooked starch, unheated honey and fruit (frequently live pineapple) most often corrects allergies. Another reason for allergies is that a body may lack the enzyme-mutations to digest and utilize cooked minerals. People who lack mineral enzyme-mutations often have premature graying. Drinking naturally carbonated mineral waters is helpful. Some people who lack enzyme-mutations for cooked minerals have severe reactions to cooked fish. Eating raw fish with unheated honey heals this allergy. Eating no-salt-added raw cheese with raw fish and honey usually speeds healing. (That does not mean that a person develops a mutation to digest and utilize cooked minerals. It means the toxic minerals that are stored in the body are gradually removed. Then symptoms of allergy subside.)

Another reason for allergies is that some people allow the body to get too cold, causing the body to burn all its blood fat. That leaves radical minerals and toxins free to damage and constrict cells to the extent that they cannot absorb nutrients. Taking care to keep the body warm with clothing or heat, and to feed the body raw fat alleviates this allergy-to-cold-weather condition.

Pollen-related allergies can most often be alleviated by eating up to ½ cup of fresh local pollen daily until symptoms subside. Mix pollen in anything that's appealing, e.g. sprinkle it on a raw salad, or blend it with raw milk or raw juice. *See* Hay Fever, page 268.

ALZHEIMER'S disease is presenile dementia usually occurring in middle age and associated with sclerosis and nerve deterioration. The hardening is in the nerves of the brain that delineate motor impulses, preventing proper association with motor commands. In advanced cases, hardening has extended to ganglia, disrupting sensory as well as motor response patterns. Alzheimer's is mainly the result of low blood protein levels over long periods, such as in vegetarianism or fruitarianism, or in someone who lacks enzyme-mutations for digesting and assimilating cooked or processed protein, or lacks enzyme-mutations for digesting and assimilating cooked or processed sugar, forming calcification along nerves, which erodes nerve tissue. Another factor that causes Alzheimer's is accumulated aluminum from vaccines, canned food and beverages, aluminum cook-wear and chemtrails. Aluminum destroys Zeta Potential causing high sediment in blood and neuro-serums and excessive clotting. That often causes hardening and scarring in the brain.

Avoiding cooked and processed protein, including all meat, eggs, roasted nuts and nut butters, and avoiding cooked and processed sugar, including drinks, jams or jellies, steamed and/or sulfured fruits, any canned food, and deodorants that contain aluminum stops progression of this malady. Usually, by the time Alzheimer's symptoms manifest, hardening and deterioration of nerve tissue is too advanced to reverse. However, recent indications lead me to believe that frequently eating fresh raw coconut cream with cucumber dissolves the hardening of nerves that causes Alzheimer's, effecting reversal in its early stages. Eating fresh raw coconut cream with banana, or eating 1 tablespoon daily of cold-pressed-below-96° Fahrenheit peanut oil with 5 drops of quinine water, gradually dissolves hardening of the arteries that feed the brain. Also, drinking moldy water from rinsing moldy raw grains every 3 weeks for the rest of one's life, and eating moldy grains once every 6 months for the rest of one's life removes some hardening. Eating a raw-food diet with plenty of raw meats, especially fish, fresh raw fruit and Nut Formula strengthens mental functions.

Moldy grains are made by soaking 1/3 cup of one or more kinds of grain in a glass or ceramic vessel containing 6 ounces mineral water for three days, then pouring off the fermented water and drinking it immediately. Then let the fermented grains stand for 6-8 days in a place with little natural light with a cloth covering the vessel. After 6-8 days, pour ½ cup distilled water over the moldy grains and stir until the mold is mixed into the water, pour off and drink. Once every six months, moldy grains may be eaten after blending only 3 ounces of moldy grains with ½ cup distilled water.

ANEMIA is a low red blood cell level or weak red blood cells that cause oxygen deficiencies. That results in carbon dioxide accumulations in cells, decreased blood and general body efficiency, general weakness, paleness, brittle nails, loss of appetite, fatigue, abdominal pain, and lower rates of bodily processes. If affecting the brain, anemia causes dizziness. If a person is exhausted all of the time, usually she or he is anemic.

Choosing whichever meat is appropriate for a person's type and eating it raw daily, or at least three times weekly, usually corrects anemia. (*See* Appendix P, page 150, for your type.)

ANGER is emotional feedback that something in a person's life needs to change. Realize what is making you angry and resolve it rationally. Leaving a situation that is inappropriate for you, or is irresolvable, may be the best choice. Letting go of concepts, desires, things and people that are not good for you and that you can't change with love and compassion, opens doors for better opportunities. An overly acidic system causes irritability that can evolve into anger and violence. Cooking meat forms heterocyclic amines and lipid peroxides that irritate nerves in many people. I suggest that you eat raw white meats. Anger expressed as violence usually perpetuates violence and fear. Therefore, be certain that violent words or actions are constructive and the only option.

Nutritionally, eating a Nut Formula, or cooked starch with raw fat and raw fresh fruit helps eliminate excess adrenaline, calming anger in about 20-40 minutes. Exercise is extremely helpful, especially one you enjoy. *See* Appendix G, page 138.

ANGINA PECTORIS is the cramping of muscles in or around the heart. Most always, the cramps are a natural process by which the body tries to increase circulation and remove toxins and hardened fat from muscles and arteries. A lack of enzyme-mutations for digesting, assimilating and utilizing cooked green foods and mostly vegetable oils are responsible for most hardening of the arteries that causes heart muscle spasms. Avoiding cooked green foods and vegetable oils stops the accumulations. *See* If I Lack Enzyme-Mutations, What Foods Should I Avoid?, page 174`

Eating raw green foods (salads) with a fat-free dressing as the last meal of the day helps remove the resins and residues that cause this type of hardening of the arteries. A preferred dressing would be raw unpasteurized apple cider vinegar, or a mixture of fresh lemon juice and raw unpasteurized apple cider vinegar. Some people would benefit from using a raw wine/vinegar dressing, that is, an organic raw wine (pesticide-free, chemical fertilizer-free and preservative-free) and an organic raw unpasteurized apple cider vinegar. Eating raw fat with other foods, especially with a little lemon juice, helps lubricate the hardened arteries. *See* Drink for Moisturizing and Lubrication, page 210. Eating raw coconut cream with cucumbers helps remove hardened resins. Eating bananas, nonsteamed dates, tomatoes, melons or unripe pineapple with plenty of raw fat, especially raw coconut cream helps to relieve the lactic acid build-up and the resulting soreness from muscle spasms.

ANXIOUSNESS expressed as unsettled desire or fear is often caused by excess adrenaline or other hormones or toxins.

Eating no-salt-added raw cheese and/or the Nut Formula, or small amounts of cooked starch with plenty of raw fat usually calms this condition. Drinking naturally sparkling mineral waters helps to calm the adrenals. Eating salt is especially toxic here and should be avoided. Eating raw meats, especially white with red and plenty of raw fat helps mitigate and soothe this condition. Eating unheated honey or a few nonsteamed dates with raw fat help maintain enzymes and blood-sugar level during anxious times when tremendous amounts of blood sugars and enzymes are utilized. *See* Anger, page 224, and Appendix G, page 138.

If accompanied with the shakes, anxiety is often caused by a low protein level. Eating raw meats, especially white meats, no-salt-added raw cheeses or cooked starch with raw fat calm this condition.

APPENDICITIS is an inflammation in the appendix.

Symptoms: pain in the lower abdominal area that graduates to severe is most common; also nausea, sometimes high fevers with sweating, and feelings of failure accompanied with feelings of low self-esteem.

Drinking a large glass of raw fresh tomatoes (for some people the Roman variety is more effective) blended with at least 5 tablespoons of unheated honey and 5 teaspoons of the fresh juice of lemons neutralizes this volatile toxic condition and calms the infection without antibiotics. Drinking this concoction every four hours until symptoms are gone usually relieves pain and heals this condition quickly. Also, eating 1 tablespoon raw unsalted butter with 1 tablespoon of no-salt-added raw cheese every hour helps absorb toxins discharged from the appendix. If nervousness is experienced, eating some French bread with avocado (or other raw fat if avocado is not available) usually settles the body's systems. Drinking 2 ounces of fresh raw lime or beet juices every 4 hours and/or eating fresh raw corn, on or off the cob, helps to regulate infection and control toxins.

See the Shakes, page 310.

ARTERIOSCLEROSIS is a condition of mineral build-up in the arteries.

Symptoms: frequent nausea, sharp pains without apparent cause, feelings of deep fear and despair, pronounced indignation on all subjects, quivering hands and feet and life is viewed as stressful.

Eating ½-1 cup unripe pineapple with ¼ cup coconut cream daily for up to 7 days in a row helps digestion, assimilation, and utilization. However, pineapple often causes over-emotionality. Therefore, be aware of your moods and eat pineapple cautiously. Raw fats are soluble, easily soothing and lubricating to the entire body. Eating plenty of raw fat ensures that mineral toxicity is very gradually removed from the body, not reabsorbed. Eating fresh raw coconut cream with banana gradually dissolves hardened mineral build-up. This can also be achieved, more slowly, by eating raw citrus and raw fat together, such as live pineapple with avocado, or live pineapple with raw cream, or raw eggs with raw orange juice, or raw orange and avocado, or raw orange and raw cream.

ARTHRITIS is inflammation in the joints or the connective tissue that is accompanied by soreness or pain. Arthritis is usually caused by volatile toxins that cause decay in the joints. Often, bacteria results that try to help the body remove joint toxicity by eating decayed cells.

Drinking a blend of 2 raw tomatoes with 4 tablespoons fresh raw lemon juice most often relieves pain within several hours. All foods which help alkalize the blood are helpful in this condition, especially raw unpasteurized apple cider vinegar. *See* Alkalizing Food, page 17840.

If you have a taste for cherries, eating raw cherries helps to prevent uric acid deposits in joints. Or eating raw celery or drinking raw celery juice does the same.

Drinking 6-8 ounces of raw milk blended with 1 tablespoon of cold-pressed-below-96° Fahrenheit flax seed oil, peanut oil, or unheated-above-96° Fahrenheit fermented coconut oil helps lubricate and strengthen joints. The best recipe for lubricating and strengthening joints is the Drink for Moisturizing and Lubrication, page 210.

Applying a poultice made of 1 raw celery stalk blended with 2 tablespoons grated raw horseradish root to a painful joint most often reduces pain within 20 minutes.

ASPHYXIATION occurs when high levels of pollutants are breathed causing exhaustion, shortness of breath, claustrophobia, headache, dizziness, fainting, choking, nausea, and vomit. Even a so-called minor asphyxiation - breathing air in a theater or office building that uses gaseous formaldehyde in the ventilation system to retard molds - produces nausea, claustrophobia and headache in some people.

Eating whatever raw fats that are appealing to you, with raw meat or a little unripe fresh raw fruit clears toxins from the blood. Avocado and no-salt-added raw cheeses are two raw fats that are especially helpful. A raw diet in which at least 40% of calories are from raw fat (including no-salt-added raw cheese) eaten for at least 10 days has produced the best results. Drinking 2 cups of naturally sparkling water daily helps restore the electrolyte balance and oxygen level of the blood.

ASTHMA is a chronic respiratory condition that is both allergy and emotionally related. It often occurs in individuals who are, or feel that they are repressed. Finding a way to express yourself creatively and to communicate helps to heal asthma.

Symptoms: chest tightness, frequent coughing, wheezing or whistling sounds that, all together, make a sufferer feel as if he or she is suffocating.

Avoid processed cheeses and caffeine in any form, such as coffee, chocolate, medications, soft drinks and teas, all of which are especially poisonous to an asthmatic condition. Avoid store-bought mayonnaise and mustard - they prevent proper digestion and the metabolism of certain minerals.

Eating plenty of raw fish, plenty of raw eggs, and plenty of tomatoes helps heal asthma. Raw tomatoes may be juiced or made into a raw sauce. When available, drinking raw milk with eating raw fish, or drinking raw milk with raw eggs speeds the healing process. Getting plenty of sunshine, fresh air and enjoying open places also helps.

These foods help relieve asthmatic symptoms: eggs, unripe raw apricots, fresh raw garlic, fresh raw horseradish, raw Jerusalem artichokes, and sunflower seeds used as the nut in the Nut Formula, or a little raw potato juice. Eating 1-2 eggs every hour relieves asthmatic fits.

ATHEROSCLEROSIS is hardened fat build-up in the arteries.

Symptoms: high blood pressure, pink or flushed complexion, deep grooves across the nails, difficulty urinating; feeling very bloated, making faces at sour foods, viewing life as overwhelming, making or seeming to make little headway although working hard, and fussing over nothing.

The Drink for Moisturizing and Lubrication, page 210, should be consumed daily.Drinking 2-4 cups of good mineral water and eating plenty of raw fat with most foods gradually correct this problem. Frequently eating fresh raw coconut cream with unripe banana gradually dissolves hardened fats. Sometimes the body manifests muscle spasms to help increase circulation, and the dissolution and removal of hardened fat accumulations, for example, the muscle spasms experienced with angina pectoris. If spasms occur, it is best to sit, eat some unheated honey and relax. Eating plenty of raw fat, especially coconut cream, with any of the following: unripe bananas, nonsteamed dates, unripe melons or unripe pineapple, helps to relieve the lactic acid build-up that causes muscle soreness.

ATHLETE'S FOOT is a fungus under and in the skin characterized by itchy, peeling skin that has a sour odor. I have found two basic causes for it: high adrenaline level, or accumulated volatile toxins (including vaccines and antibiotics).

Coffee, chocolate, cooked soups, cooked teas, and cooked meat create volatile toxic conditions in most people, as well as overstimulate adrenals, causing decay to cells. The fungus tries to help by eating decaying cells or the decaying parts of cells. Avoiding those foods and all medications usually stops a tendency to produce foot fungi.

However, as long as toxins remain in the area causing the decay, the fungus will continue to do its job unless it is poisoned by medication.

Eating foods that alkalize minimizes discomfort. *See* Alkalizing Food, page 178. Letting fungus run its course increases health, but if that is not possible, coating the feet with unheated honey and covering them with clean white cotton socks for four consecutive nights smother and stop fungus for awhile. *See* Fungus, page 265. Also, applying the Primal Facial Body Care Cream (recipe from the book The Recipe For Living Without Disease) soothes itching and usually allows fungus to work without excessive discomfort.

BACKACHE: There are many causes for this, from spinal detoxification and tension, to accidents. Often, backaches happen in conjunction with emotional exhaustion.

Drinking plenty of raw milk, a little good mineral water (*see* Appendix M, page 143, about water) and, when available, plenty of raw cream help relax the spine. During a backache, eating several smoothies daily made with 2-3 raw eggs, ¼ cup unheated honey, either 2 tablespoons unsalted raw butter or 5 tablespoons raw cream or coconut cream, and either ½-1 cup unripe papaya or unripe banana helps remove toxicity and soreness. Eating nonsteamed dates or pineapple helps remove soreness. Eating no-salt-added raw cheeses with equal amounts of fat, especially raw butter, helps strengthen the back. (Note: Eating too many papayas can cause intense back detoxification and therefore too much pain.)

Hot baths and very gentle back massages are helpful. Lying on one side and applying a hot water bottle propped between your spine and a pillow speeds circulation and nutrients to the effected area, relaxing muscles, and taking pressure off nerves, especially while sleeping.

Also, enjoying one's self speeds healing.

BACTERIAL FOOD-POISONING that causes disease is caused by cooked or processed food. The belief that raw food causes bacterial food-poisoning is nonscientific myth and hysteria. All epidemic food-poisoning that has occurred was caused by bacteria feeding on cooked food. The bacteria feeding on cooked and/or chemically treated food develops disease and mutates. The mutant/diseased bacteria excrete volatile toxins that cause poisoning that result in vomit and/or diarrhea and intestinal damage, including decay. The Jack-in-the-Box epidemic was caused by cooked meat, not raw meat. No one ate any of those burgers raw. For bacterial food-poisoning data regarding pasteurized milk products, *see* Chapter 31, Infant Safety, Health Benefits, Propagandized False Risks From Feeding Raw Milk, And The Harm Of Feeding Infants Pasteurized And Processed Milk, in my book The Recipe For Living Without Disease.

Symptoms: nausea, vomiting, diarrhea, headache, high blood pressure, abnormal fatigue, dizziness, mental depression, and loss of appetite.

The myth that raw foods cause bacterial disease was ingrained into society when two giant food manufacturers paid fortunes in research from 1928-1938 to prove that bacteria in food causes disease. They wanted to prove that their cooked and processed foods were cleaner, healthier and safer than raw foods. Animals were separated into two groups. Several groups were fed raw food and others were fed cooked, processed food. The companies' officers released to the press, the conclusion based on mere speculation and belief that the theory that bacteria in raw food caused disease. When the long-term results of that research proved that the raw-food-fed groups did not develop any disease, and that the cooked/processed-fed groups developed most of the diseases that humans suffer, the two companies burned all of the research and hid the results from the public in 1940.[38]

Only bacteria feeding on cooked, non-organic foods are likely to turn pathogenic. E. coli feeds rapidly on frozen meat but is not dangerous if eaten raw. The worst that could happen from eating raw meat with a high bacteria count is vomit or diarrhea, yet that response is very rare, and not from poisoning. Instead, it is a radical detoxification of the liver, pancreas or intestines. The toxins are potentially damaging and so the body must flush them quickly.

Eating raw food, including raw meats, with or without high bacterial counts has proved to promote good health and not cause disease in humans. (Ripley's Believe It Or Not, July 17, 2002, featuring Aajonus

---

[38] That information was reported to me in 1975 in Louisiana at the home of one of the retired scientists who worked on the project at one of the companies. He stated that he felt great remorse for not coming forward to contest the propaganda. He did not because he feared for the life of his family.

and 3 patients.) *See* the book The Recipe For Living Without Disease, Chapters 25-31.

BAD BREATH: *See* Halitosis, page 267.

BALDING is the rapid or gradual loss of hair growth, usually occurring from metal-poisoning from canned foods, aluminum cooking utensils, deodorants, shampoos, soaps, and medication. Poor oxygen utilization is sometimes causative. It is also believed that poor thyroid function is causative, but my experiments disproved that theory.

Eating raw berries with raw coconut cream, a little unsalted raw butter and a little raw cream helps bind with the metals so that they do not cause as much damage to follicles. Topically, rubbing into the scalp a blended mixture of 1 ounce fresh raw aloe vera gel (directly from the inside of the leaf) and 2 ounces never-been-heated-above-96° Fahrenheit fermented coconut oil helps protect the scalp and follicles. That usually stops hair loss and sometimes promotes hair growth within several weeks, unless you have an allergy to shampoo. Drinking naturally carbonated waters helps oxygen absorption. Drinking some parsley juice with celery juice helps oxygen absorption. Eating non-steamed dates helps thyroid functions. Eating 2 ounces of stone-pressed olive oil with meat 3 times each week helps remove dead cells in and around follicles. A good shampoo is whipped raw egg. Wet hair, apply and rub whipped raw egg to hair and scalp, let stand for 1-5 minutes and rinse.

BEDWETTING is the inability to control the bladder during sleep because of nutrient losses during stressful waking hours, usually when toxic blood conditions exist. Blood sugar problems are commonly causative, such as in childhood diabetes.

Drinking the combination of 3 ounces fresh raw cabbage juice, 2 ounces fresh raw cucumber juice, 2 ounces fresh raw carrot juice, 2 ounces fresh raw parsley juice and 3 tablespoons unheated honey supplies nutrients for nerves and bladder control. Drinking that juice combination once early in the day every 3rd day, and eating unsalted raw cheeses, raw eggs blended with unripe banana (or other appealing unripe fruit), raw fish and celery daily usually correct this condition within several weeks.

BELL'S PALSY is paralysis of some facial muscles, resulting from facial nerve damage.

This is most often due to excess adrenaline produced from toxic diets and/or environmental pollution. When adrenaline utilizes all of the blood fat, it seeks other fats. For example, adrenaline may eat at the nerve coatings (myelin), and leach fat from the myelin. The result is neural lesions and scarring.

Eating the Nut Formula (*see* page 194) every other day, or very small amounts of cooked starch with plenty of raw fats, especially avocado, unsalted raw butter, or raw cream, helps neutralize excess adrenaline and prevents nerve damage. Eating raw fish with raw red meat or with raw poultry helps heal and restore nerves and replenish myelin.

BERIBERI is a form of severe malnutrition. Correcting beriberi requires adherence to a well-balanced dietary regime for a long time. *See* Eating Schedules, pages 40-42 in the book The Recipe For Living Without Disease.

Symptoms:

<u>In adults</u>: appetite and weight loss, diarrhea, edema, fatigue, heart failure, nerve dysfunction causing paralysis and wasting of limbs.

<u>In children</u>: abdominal discomfort, constipation or diarrhea, nausea, respiratory difficulties and vomiting.

Eating plenty of tomatoes with raw mushrooms, some fresh whole raw parsley in the late afternoon with a little French bread with plenty of avocado, 3 ounces unheated honey each day, and raw milk, when available, helps detoxify the digestive system in preparation for handling a balanced diet.

BITOT'S SPOTS are white, foamy elevations on the whites of the eyes.

Drinking raw fresh parsley juice helps to prevent and correct this condition. Parsley juice should be consumed with celery and can be combined with a mixture of other juices to make it more palatable. A drop of filtered fresh parsley juice dropped in the eyes is helpful to reverse this condition. A balanced healthy diet, such as this Primal Diet helps remove toxins and rebuild the eyes.

BLADDER INFECTION is a detoxification of the urinary bladder characterized by pain in the lower abdomen and back, sometimes fever, and an urgent, most often painful, frequent need to urinate.

Drinking raw fresh grapefruit juice throughout the day, and eating the butter/honey mixture every ½ hour for as long as it takes to calm the bladder, relieve bladder infections. For people prone to bladder infections, drinking 4 ounces of raw fresh beet juice twice weekly, or 4 ounces fresh raw lime juice blended with 2 tablespoons unheated honey added to 4 ounces of good mineral water keeps bacteria levels low and helps detoxify the bladder a little every day so that discomforting, exorbitant infection is rarely, if ever, necessary. *See* Kidney Infection page 282, Kidney Stones page 282, Urethra Infection page 319.

BLOOD PRESSURE:

High blood pressure: Fresh raw grapefruit or fresh raw grapefruit juice lowers blood pressure. One half of a grapefruit may be adequate, but some people may need more. Eating raw cucumbers or fresh raw cucumber juice helps soothe stretched arteries, veins, capillaries and nerves. Eating fresh raw garlic helps stabilize high or low blood pressure. High blood pressure is the body's method of stretching, cleaning and healing congested arteries and veins. Unlike what is said in the media and portrayed on television, many heart attacks occur during times of low blood pressure and low cholesterol levels. High blood pressure is necessary to vital arterial health when blood passages are congested from overweight or hardened arteries and veins. I suggest that high blood pressure should not be suppressed with drugs.

Low blood pressure: Fresh raw garlic, or fresh raw onions, or fresh raw hot peppers raises blood pressure. A small amount of any of those is usually adequate, although some people will need to eat substantial amounts.

BLOOD SUGAR:

High: *See* Diabetes, page 258.

Low: *See* Hypoglycemia, page 274.

BODY ODOR indicates that putrid gases have formed inside the body by toxic chemical changes, or by eating foods with strong odors, for instance, garlic or broccoli. Avoiding foods that easily putrefy in your body (cooked and/or processed foods) eliminates body odor. Putrid gases produced by the body when dissolving and eliminating old toxic storages can be eliminated, or at least mitigated, by eating fresh raw parsley, or ginger, or peppermint, or spearmint, or fresh raw juice from any of them. Celery juice and unripe pineapple relieve foul body odor.

BRITTLE BONES is a condition of the bones where there is little or no flexibility. It is caused by a lack of utilizable fat (and other nutrients as a result of a fat deficiency).

Symptoms: fear of jumping short heights, and easily breaking bones.

Drinking fresh full-fat raw milk gradually corrects this problem. If raw milk isn't available, eating 4 ounces fresh raw organic carrot juice with avocado, or with unsalted raw butter, or with another raw fat daily will be effective but may take a little longer. Eating fresh and unfrozen organic bone marrow with raw beef speeds healing. The texture and taste of beef bone marrow is similar to butter. It is best eaten with a raw meat meal. It may be made as part of a meat sauce. *See* the book The Recipe For Living Without Disease for raw meat sauces.

BROKEN BONE: Make sure bone is properly set for healing.

Unripe pineapple has enzymes that help heal bone. Eating ½ unripe pineapple each day for 1 week, and then every third day for 5 more weeks works the best, especially in conjunction with a balanced raw diet and the foods recommended for Brittle Bones.

BRONCHITIS is an inflammation (cleanse) of the air passages to the lungs because of toxin-damaged bronchial cells. It is exacerbated by suppression of what needs to be said, that is, suppressed emotions turned against one's self. The resultant tension in the chest is often secondarily causative because it spends fat in the bronchi, drying them. It is then difficult to produce protective mucus and the bronchi become susceptible to irritation from airborne substances.

Symptoms: back and muscle pain, sore throat, dry coughs that are followed by coughing up mucus.

Finding a form of artistic expression that suits a person's nature begins a more expansive approach to life and health.

Eating raw fats, especially unsalted raw butter, raw cream and raw eggs, soothes this condition. Drinking fresh raw carrot juice mixed with raw cream or raw eggs soothes and nourishes the bronchi very quickly. Smoking and other airborne pollution worsen this condition.

See Anger, page 224; and the Dink for Moisturizing, page 210.

BRUISE is ruptured veins and cells causing internal bleeding in small or large damaged areas of the body that turn black/blue. As the blood in the tissues is dissolved, absorbed or excreted, the bruised area turns yellow and finally clears to normal. Applying a thin slice of raw beef to a bruise for at least 5 hours and up to 24 hours helps soothe, reduce swelling and speed healing. If a large area is bruised, like a foot, you may apply ground beef. Thinly pack the area with sliced or ground red meat and cover with a sock or bandage.

Eating raw eggs blended with unripe banana or unripe pineapple helps clear damaged cells and toxicity from injury. Eating raw meat helps heal and replace damaged cells. *See* Appendix P, page 150.

BURNS: Eating avocados and fresh raw aloe vera gel directly from the leaf for several days helps soothe burned cells and eliminate scars.

For SUNBURN, topically apply the Primal Facial Body Care Cream from the book The Recipe For Living Without Disease, or make a mixture by stirring 2 tablespoons fresh raw aloe gel (best taken directly from leaf), 1/6 teaspoon fresh royal jelly, ¼ teaspoon sun-dried powdered clay and 1 teaspoon stone-pressed olive oil. Or simply apply raw egg white to sunburn. Any of those will often make sunburn disappear magically. They quickly soothe and heal other first degree burns. They increase relief and healing to second-degree burns. Another remedy for sunburn is to bathe as soon as possible in a bath with at least 1 cup of raw unpasteurized apple cider vinegar and, if available, 2 cups raw milk stirred into the bath water. Then, very gently rub plain raw kefir, raw milk, or egg white into sunburn every 2-6 hours and let it stay on the skin. That soothes the skin and relieves pain.

SECOND AND THIRD DEGREE, OR DEEPER BURN OR ABRASION may be quickly healed WITHOUT skin-grafts. First, remove as much burned tissue or dirt-filled abrasion as possible and apply a thin layer of unheated honey over burn or abrasion. That may cause 2-5 minutes of intense stinging. Over the layer of unheated honey, apply a thin slice of raw beef and cover with a damp cotton cloth to prevent the meat from drying quickly. Then wrap a bandage to hold the meat and damp cloth in place. Remove the dressing and reapply the same way every 24 hours for 2 days. On the 3rd day, eliminate the honey layer and continue to apply raw beef, damp cloth and bandage every 24 hours for at least 14 days. If pus appears in areas, clean those areas before reapplying the layers. Do not let the wound dry between applications. Usually, if a person has been following the Primal Diet for 2 or more years, a third-degree or deeper burn or abrasion will heal in approximately 3-4 weeks. If a person has recently begun eating the diet, it may take as long as 4-6 weeks to completely heal a serious third degree burn or abrasion.

James had been on the diet approximately 6 years when he was in a truck accident. His skin was scraped from his right wrist to nearly his shoulder. The abrasion was deep enough to expose his muscles, and in some areas his tendons. He instinctively designed and utilized the procedures in the above paragraph for 14 days. In 14 days, his body completely refilled the abrasion with healthy live cells without skin-grafts. After three weeks, I witnessed that the abrasion looked as if it had never occurred. The skin looked slightly pinkish at the spot that had been scraped deepest. There was no scar whatsoever. That proved to me that medical treatment for burns and abrasions was harmful, disfiguring, physically and psychologically crippling, expensive, and in many serious cases caused long-term pain from skin-grafts and scars.

BURSITIS is an inflammation of the sacks (bursas) that lubricate joints, muscles, tendons, and bronchi.

Symptoms: swelling and tenderness of the hip, shoulder, elbows or feet. Symptoms during infection: extreme tenderness and sharp severe localized pain.

During inflammation, eating beef with avocado at least twice daily soothes the condition. Eating small amounts of food more often is better unless you have a healthy appetite. Consuming the Drink for Moisturizing/Lubrication after meat meals speeds healing of bursitis (see page 210). Adding 1 tablespoon of bee pollen to that drink, and eating 1-2 tablespoons of no-salt-added raw cheese with the drink helps relieve pain quicker and for longer periods.

Drinking live orange, lemon or lime juices no sooner than two hours after having meat and avocado mitigates detoxification and alkalizes blood and lymph. Waiting at least one hour after drinking citrus juice before eating beef is better for digestion.

CANCER is basically the body's inability to discard dead cells. The body gathers those cells in a particular area, called a tumor, until it can later dissolve those cells.

Whether before or after a tumor forms, dead and degeneratively toxic cells must be dissolved and neutralized. Then the waste must be excreted and secreted. The body has two basic methods for dissolving those cells. The body's natural and first choice is the action of bacteria, parasites and/or fungi. Its second choice seems to be through the action of viruses. Bacteria, parasites and fungi can consume degenerated or dead cells quickly, and the volume of the waste products produced by their cleansing action constitutes a mere fraction of the volume of the original toxic cells. It is then relatively easy for our bodies to eliminate that waste. The opposite is true with the action of viruses because viruses are crystalline solvents manufactured within poisonous toxic cells. The waste from viruses is magnified and grossly distributed throughout the body.

Here, I will explain why the body develops and employs viruses. Poisonously degenerative cells often kill bacteria, parasites and fungi. When that occurs, our bodies no longer have the preferred assistance of those helpful agents in dissolving toxically sick or dead cells for elimination. Resultantly, our bodies resort to manufacturing viruses to do that job. Unlike the reduction of waste produced by bacteria, parasites and fungi, the waste produced by viruses increases because viruses utilize volumes of H_2O to dissolve and dilute dead and degenerative cells. That grossly toxic wastewater contaminates the various circulatory systems (blood, nervous and lymphatic), spreading the toxicity throughout the body. The actions of bacteria, parasites and fungi are always the most natural and preferred methods used by the body to detoxify dead and degenerative cells.

When our bodies are overly contaminated with pollution and too deficient in vital nutrients, bacteria, parasites, fungi, nor viruses can dissolve all the dead and degenerated cells. So our bodies must embalm those cells and contain them. First, the embalmed cells are dispersed throughout our bodies, intermixed with live cells, sometimes creating thick fibroids. When our bodies reach the limit of their ability to tolerate so much dispersed dead cell structure, our bodies must construct tumors to contain the embalmed (dead) cells. Building tumors is a means of isolating dead cells into a localized area so that the dead cells will have less impact on the functions of living tissue and bodily functions.

Tumors are built as benign or malignant. In the case of malignant tumors, our bodies sparsely intermix live young mutated cells with many times more of the embalmed cells. The young mutated cells are phenomenally designed to produce and contain potent solvents within themselves. Those young mutated cells have been termed by medicine as *cancer* cells. In the case of benign tumors, our bodies do not incorporate those young mutated cells that produce and contain solvents.

The difference between benign and malignant tumors is dramatic. Our bodies, with the help of those young mutated (cancer) cells, can dissolve tumors rapidly, in 2 days to 5 years, depending on the size and number of tumors. Without the help of cancer cells in benign tumors, most often our bodies must manufacture extra-cellular solvents to dissolve those benign tumors, from the outer edges inward, slowly. Often, that can take from 5-40 years or never, if our bodies do not receive proper nutrients. Therefore, idealistically, malignant tumors are preferable to benign tumors, as long as our bodies receive enough nutrients to neutralize and eliminate the tremendous amount of acrid waste that results from the quick dissolution of malignant tumors. If our bodies cannot neutralize that acrid waste, the waste will injure, damage and dissolve adjacent living cells, such as in the case of an open cancerous lesion that grows and stinks. *Read* Appendix O *now*, pages 145-150, and return here.

According to the conclusions of Dr. Harbin B. Jones, emeritus professor from University of California, Berkeley, cancer is like the flu: Let it run its course, and 76% of the time it will reverse itself, even if you do not improve your diet or lifestyle. He made that statement in

1972, when we were less inundated with carcinogens. Nowadays, we may have to change our diets and lifestyles to reverse cancers. Dr. Jones said that although you may temporarily stop cancer, we cannot heal the body with medical treatments for cancer. He testified before the congress that medical treatments were dangerous and always harmful long-term.

There are three factors to address when eliminating and healing cancers. The first is to stop eating cooked, processed and contaminated food that weakens or kills cells with toxicity and debris. Avoiding fried foods is imperative because so many active and volatile toxins are by-products of frying. (For identified toxins, see the book, The Recipe For Living Without Disease, Chapters 17 and 18.) The second is to fill the blood and body with raw fats that will dissolve and bind with dead cells and carry them from the body, or at least will neutralize toxicity, so that tumors will cease to grow. A very high blood-cholesterol level (between 250-400) made of raw fats, is almost always necessary. The third is to dissolve tumorous tissue as safely as possible by eating fresh raw citrus or other fruit that is appealing. However, if the tumor has broken the skin and is festering, it is already in the process of dissolving too rapidly. In such a situation, restricting fruit and consuming large quantities of honey would be best to reduce acidity.

Following a balanced raw diet as suggested in the book, The Recipe For Living Without Disease, Chapters 8-12, has helped hundreds of people develop a high rate of cancer reversal if the cancer has not broken the skin. The lowest reversal rate for cancer on the Primal Diet for people who did not receive any medical treatments has been approximately 90% for all cancers except lung and esophageal. The reversal rate for lung and esophageal cancers has been approximately 60% without any medical treatments. With medical treatments, sadly, reversal rates decrease astoundingly.

To reverse cancer, the best results have been obtained by keeping the diet simple, even though, at times, it is monotonous. (The exceptions were in cases that involved cirrhosis of tissues. Then the diet had to be more complex.) Usually, indications of reversal were achieved within three months of beginning the diet. Some cases took as long as thirty months; they were 4 cases of breast cancer. Only 1 of 239 cases did not achieve indications of reversal. Of those 239 cases, 223 have survived.

Fourteen of those who died were malnourished and very thin. They either refused to eat because of nausea or were unable to eat enough because of pain medication that destroyed their appetites and/or made them nauseous. Vomit is a very healthy aspect of cancer reversal in many instances. Vomit indicates that toxins dump into the stomach and our bodies want to expel them immediately. As I mentioned, Owanza intermittently vomited up to 11 times daily for up to a 5-weeks cycle. She recovered from 63 tumors. It took her 11 years. She is living and happy to this day, 24 years later.

Raw fats, including some oils, are tantamount for eliminating cancers and should be 30-45% of caloric intake. Raw dairy products are very soothing to cancerous conditions, especially raw cream and unsalted raw butter. Although fats are 80% responsible for eliminating the accumulated dead cells that cause cancer, fats do not work alone. Protein, unripe fruit and green vegetable juices are essential catalysts. Eating fatty raw ground beef, and raw unripe oranges or fresh raw unripe orange juice (but not meat and oranges at the same meal) have brought about excellent results toward healing, as well as detoxifying cancers that have not broken the skin. Unripe pineapple, or any unripe fruit that is appealing, can often be substituted for orange. For some people, drinking fresh raw vegetable juices may be more healing than oranges. If experiencing anxiety, eating raw fish with whipped raw cream acts as a calmative. Also, consuming the Nut Formula twice weekly helps to calm anxiety. If those are not immediately available, eating raw fish with a little cooked starch and raw butter or with avocado or with another raw fat or raw oil works as a calmative.

In one case, breast cancer continued to advance to the point it broke the skin, becoming overly acidic. I suggested an alkaline raw milk diet for 3 days with extra raw cream and unheated honey. Also, I suggested fresh raw green vegetable juices. The patient became severely painful, unable to move. Her voice quivered from intensity of pain. Prior to that dietary experiment, her pain had been isolated mainly to the chest and arm. Afterward, the pain moved to her back and then all over her body. I suggested that she immediately resume eating the normal Primal Diet suggestions for cancer and her pain mitigated within hours.

Through circulation, the body gets its nutrients. Swimming or gentle movement on a regular or daily basis increases circulation to cancer-congested areas of the body. Applying heat to tumorous areas with a hot water bottle helps blood and lymph circulate to those areas, and once there, to cleanse and heal. (Electrical heating pads emit electromagnetic fields that can interfere with neural functions and healing.)

For health's sake, have some fun on a regular basis, even if you have to work at it at first. Focusing on the positive, even if it's fantasy, promotes creativity, satisfaction and well-being. Sex is good fun and is good exercise as long as it is not accompanied with anxiety.

Tomatoes contain lycopene that shrinks tumors, including prostate cancer, in cases when cancers have not broken skin. Owanza discovered that eating 1 tablespoon of cold-pressed-below-96° Fahrenheit flax seed oil each day helps prevent tumor development. I noticed that she drank 2 ounces of fresh raw lemon juice blended with 2 ounces of unheated honey and mixed with 4 ounces of naturally sparkling water 3-4 days weekly. None of her cancers broke the skin. Remember, cancers that break skin are already too intensely dissolving tumors, so the object with those cancers is to slow the dissolution process by alkalizing the body with non-acidic and non-detoxifying foods. That eliminates oils and reduces fruit consumption.

Along with what is suggested above, full-fat raw milk is very helpful for people who have cancer in and around the spine. I suggest adding 3-4 tablespoons raw cream and 2 tablespoons unheated honey to each quart of milk for spinal problems, including cancer.

For cancers in the groin area, such as prostate and lymph, eating raw fish with a Nut Formula, or a little cooked potato, as well as all that is suggested above, can be more effective.

It has been Owanza's experience that breast cancer in people who have consumed aspirin, other medications, and food additives and preservatives, or have been exposed to toxic chemicals for many years, requires surgical removal. I have not yet come to that conclusion, even though I know that in many people, certain chemicals, like the compounds in aspirin, turn some cells into cement. It is sometimes impossible to dissolve those cells to removable substances. Unlike most tumorous tissue, cement-like cells cannot be dissolved and eliminated by the body.

I have lost only two clients to breast cancer who refused surgery. One was in her sixties and was 135 pounds overweight. For a period of 43 years, she had consumed several bottles of aspirin each week for headaches. As soon as she began the Primal Diet, her headaches stopped and never returned, and her weight normalized within 4½ years. But her breast cancer could not be stopped because of 43 years of accumulated cemented cells. When she died, her chest was overgrown with tumorous sores. The other client was in her forties and in advanced stages by the time she came to me. She was consuming appetite-suppressing dosages of morphine for pain. After four months of eating as much as she could of what I suggested, her tumors began to dissolve (by more than 35%). But she could not eat enough to get strong enough. The one client who Owanza lost to breast cancer was in her late thirties when she died. She was raised and played next to a farm where the crops were dusted with pesticides. A biopsy done and specifically analyzed for toxic substances that occur in many pesticides showed a very dense ratio of those compounds. It had been about eighteen years since she had lived on that farm.

Another client I lost to cancer (not breast) was in her seventies and would not stop taking chemotherapy. She went into a coma on the colonic table (I cautioned her about chemotherapy and colonics). She was the first and last cancer-sufferer I accepted as a client who took chemotherapy and radiation during the experimental period where over 3,000 people tired the effectiveness of my Primal Diet (1984-2005). Chemo- and radiation therapies are toxic and cause cellular genocide, amassing dead cells that are likely to be built into tumors throughout the body (metastasis), usually within 7 years of treatment. *See* pages 22-25.

When cancer occurs in an individual who has progressed cirrhosis of tissues throughout his or her body (or in one or more areas), it indicates that tissues are unnaturally polluted with compounds that cannot be easily eliminated. If the body were to dissolve those tissues (cells), the by-products could be so poisonous that the body's systems could be severely damaged or the person could suffer anaphylaxis. Under such conditions, cancer remission has been questionable, and reversal (cure) has remained doubtful. That is often the case in cancers that have broken the skin. However, two such cases surprised me after six years, by at least beginning to dissolve hardened tissues and creating soft new tissue.

Bone deterioration that is sometimes found in conjunction with some cancers is not directly part of the cancerous process (the process of containing - tumor - and then dissolving dead cells). Bone deterioration results from a severe fat and mineral deficiency that is exacerbated in cancerous cases. In those cases, the body leaches minerals and fat from bones to facilitate the isolation and neutralization of the waste from dissolved cells. Eating unsalted raw cheese with unsalted raw butter (or other raw fat) and raw ocean fish, especially raw scallops, oysters, clams and urchin, supplies fats and concentrated minerals so that the body does not have to leach them from bone. Also, *see* Clay, page 181.

CANDIDA is a yeast-like condition (detoxification) that eats little stagnant pools of blood that result from internal lesions caused by dryness and cracking of the tissues within the body. Candida fungus cleans the system by eating degenerated tissue damaged by accumulated cooked carbohydrate-based, adrenaline- or insulin-related chemicals. Candida is helpful and should have its cycle. The worst thing anyone can do if he or she wants to improve his or her health is to destroy Candida. Smoking puts a person at higher risk of developing Candida. If a person has a high adrenaline level and drinks alcohol, he or she is putting herself at great risk of developing Candida.

Symptoms: a somewhat pallid complexion, sensitive and swollen extremities, dry skin, extreme lethargy, critical attitude, a general dislike for people, and a tendency toward isolation.

Soft drinks with caffeine, salt, alcohol, smoke, coffee, teas, and aspirin are all poisonous because they overstimulate the adrenals and pancreas, causing excess adrenaline and insulin that spends fat, creating the dryness that causes lesions, the storage of volatile toxins in tissues, and disturbing blood sugar levels.

When experiencing extreme symptoms, eating half of a Nut Formula once daily in the afternoon for 3 days helps remove toxic adrenalin and insulin.

Eating a raw diet with cooked starch in combination with plenty of raw fat eliminates high adrenaline and insulin levels. Eating raw tomatoes, fresh or nonsteamed unsulfured sun-dried figs, fresh raw green vegetable juices, raw unpasteurized apple cider vinegar and fresh unripe pineapple neutralizes and soothes the condition over a period of years. Eating raw fish or organic raw chicken or turkey helps heal and restore damaged and dead nerve tissue and skin. Raw beef and other red meat may be eaten when the condition is neutralized enough. A sign that a person is too toxic to eat beef is severe itching and irritability, accompanied with nausea after eating beef.

Drinking the freshest raw juice of 1 yam once every 4 days helps produce hormones that reduce the swelling and soreness in the joints as a result of Candida. Yam juice should be consumed within 10 minutes after juicing. To re-lubricate the joints and body, I suggest daily consuming the Drink for Moisturizing and Lubrication, page 210, but made with only 1-3 teaspoons of fresh raw lemon juice.

To temporarily reduce rampant Candida, I suggest that you blend 4 tablespoons fresh lime juice, 1-2 tablespoons unheated honey and 1-2 tablespoons raw unpasteurized apple cider vinegar together, add that to 4 ounces of naturally sparkling water, and drink 2 ounces every 4 hours for no more than 3 consecutive days. In some individuals, that may cause increased symptoms for the several days but ultimately it reduces Candida proliferation.

CANKER SORE is an open sore on the mouth that usually burns and tingles.

Topically, it is best not to apply anything. Cankers heal best when left to air. Sometimes though, the burning and sensitivity can be too much. Applying a thin layer of unheated honey soothes this condition.

CARBUNCLES are deep pus-filled infections under the skin.

Topically, make a poultice with 1 tablespoon powdered mustard seeds, ¼ teaspoon powdered sun-dried clay, 2 drops of royal jelly (optional), and 1 ounce of good mineral water. Applying it to the carbuncle and surrounding area and letting the poultice remain on for 80-90 minutes once or twice daily until it subsides, attracts and absorbs toxins and soothes the tissues.

CATARACTS are the collection of organic waste clouding the cornea and/or crystalline lens of the eye. Most blindness is a result of cataracts. Cataracts are usually found in hyperactive individuals with high adrenaline levels who constantly exhaust blood and body fat levels, or in diabetics as a result of improperly assimilated sugars and medicinal insulin. Their eyes are completely deprived of certain utilizable fats. The body can't clean debris from the eyes properly and cataracts form.

Consuming 1-3 tablespoons of stone-pressed olive oil every day for the rest of a person's life stops further development of cataracts, and sometimes reverses cataracts. Eating plenty of raw fat and the foods suggested in Alkalizing Food, page 178, soothes the overall toxic condition of the body due to excess adrenaline. Eating raw salmon several times weekly, and drinking a combination of 2 ounces carrot and 2 ounces beet juices 3-4 days weekly speed healing.

CELIAC DISEASE is said to be the inability to digest gluten. That is part fallacy. Most often, Celiac is caused by the chemicals created from combining certain foods with foods containing gluten.

Symptoms: diarrhea, flatulence, abdominal pain, anemia and weight loss.

If a person with celiac <u>avoids</u> eating the following foods cooked or raw in combination with wheat or corn, celiac will usually be eliminated: tomatoes (including catsup), strawberries (including jellies and jams), apples (including sauces and pies), pineapple, citrus and apple cider vinegar. Starches are usually necessary for people with celiac disease. Therefore, eating a Nut Formula (page 194) at least twice weekly usually prevents extreme anxiety. However, if the Nut Formula does not satisfy starch cravings or settle extreme anxiety, try eating bread or pasta made with refined unbleached nonfortified wheat. People with celiac may become extremely anxious without the Nut Formula or cooked gluten. When starch cravings strike and the Nut Formula fails, eating small amounts of breads with plenty of raw fat and avoiding the foods listed above in combination with breads usually resolve the problem.

CHICKEN POX is a viral detoxification in the lymph and skin, particularly detoxifying the nerve endings characterized by rashes, and is sometimes accompanied with headache and slight fever. The skin eruptions eventually break and fluid leaks, turning crusty. Usually, the nerve damage results from metal toxicity.

Raw hormone- and antibiotic-free chicken eaten with avocado soothes, heals and regenerates the tissues. Getting a lot of sleep is best.

Eating the foods suggested for Fever eases discomfort (*see* page 262). Eating fresh raw unripe pineapple or unripe banana with unheated honey relieves soreness. Eating raw eggs before sleep helps cleanse toxins from tissues.

CHOLESTEROL LEVEL, HIGH AND LOW: Cholesterol are necessary fatty-based substances that help fuel (for example, cholesterol needed for the body to develop sex and adrenal hormones) clean, lubricate, and protect the entire body. Cholesterol that the liver forms from raw fat, or cholesterol that we consume in raw foods like meat, dairy and coconut are all beneficial. It is necessary and desirable for our bodies to produce and consume cholesterol in large quantities. It is the cholesterol that the liver makes from cooked fat and cooked cholesterol we consume that is the problem. On a raw diet with plenty of raw fat, a high cholesterol level is wonderful and desirable, indicating that we are digesting, cleansing, lubricating, fueling and protecting the body. *See* Appendix O, pages 145-150, and Appendix W, page 162, to understand why most people have problems with cooked cholesterol.

In all cholesterol problems, whether high or low, there is a deficiency in utilizable blood fat, lacteal fat and lymphatic fat. Usually, those conditions are due to eating cooked oils, especially safflower, margarine, vegetable oils, and any hydrogenated oil. Those oils readily harden and crystallize, turning into rock-like substances, such as amber stone that was once tree oil.

Eating plenty of raw fats, like unsalted raw butter, raw eggs, raw cream, no-salt-added raw cheeses, fresh raw coconut, avocados, stone-pressed or small amounts of below-96°-pressed oils provide health-giving raw fats, making a high cholesterol level beneficial. Many years of eating those fats, raw meats and fresh unripe pineapple gradually remove stored cooked cholesterol (toxins) from body tissues. Note that while a person detoxifies the stored toxic cholesterol, the blood cholesterol level soars because some toxic cholesterol enters the blood to be carried to the bowels and dumped there, or through the skin.

There is no cause for alarm; it is cause for celebration. That process rids the body of cellulite and other toxic fatty storages.

CROHN'S DISEASE is an inability to digest many cooked foods and the inability of the body to prevent undigested food from entering the blood, lymphatic and nervous systems. When undigested food particles enter those systems, they cause extreme reactions, such as painfully swollen and enlarged joints, fibromyalgia and chronic fatigue. Most cooked grains and potatoes are poisonous in cases of Crohn's. Crohn's disease is usually caused by medicinal antibiotics, especially in infancy and childhood, and vaccines. When antibiotic and vaccine toxins enter the intestines, they destroy the healthy bacterial environment of the intestines. That chemical damage to intestines may reach as deeply as intestinal DNA, preventing the natural bacterial environment of the intestines from perpetuating digestive bacteria. In such a case, unless a raw food diet is continuously consumed, symptoms of Crohn's will persist throughout life.

Eating an all raw food diet is vital to reversal and recovery. Raw animal products, with their natural beneficial bacteria and enzymes have helped restore digestion in all cases, but did not completely reverse Crohn's in a few cases where chemicals had caused genetic damage to the intestines.

Eating 1-2 cage-free raw eggs every 1-2 hours followed by ¼ teaspoon unheated honey for 3-5 days usually restores some digestion. Then, daily, adding early morning and evening raw meat meals, an afternoon raw custard (*see* custard recipe page 56, footnote), and 1-2 cups fresh raw celery juice, 4 ounces at a time helps restore strength and bring life to normalcy.

CHRONIC FATIGUE SYNDROME is an almost constant feeling of physical, emotional and mental weariness. Often chronic fatigue syndrome is from not having the enzyme-mutation to digest cooked green foods. Avoid cooked green foods. *See* If I Lack Enzyme-Mutations, What Foods Should I Avoid?, page 174.

Eating raw meat 2-4 times daily on a balanced raw diet corrects this condition, sometimes quickly but most often gradually. *See* the book The Recipe For Living Without Disease, Chapter 12.

CIRRHOSIS OF THE LIVER is a condition of degeneration and hardening of the liver. Although it may not have been caused by the usual volatile toxic condition of excess hormone-related toxins, it is a volatile toxic condition, usually accompanied by frequent nausea.

Early symptoms: indigestion, diarrhea or constipation, fever, yellowish complexion, liver pain and spasms.

Progressed symptoms: anemia, edema, spider-shaped bruises (i.e., internal bleeding) and heaviness throughout the liver area.

For those who experience extreme nausea, eating plenty of raw tomatoes or fresh raw tomato puree throughout each day for as many days as it takes to quiet nausea works best. After that, and for those who have lighter nausea, drinking the fresh juice from about 6 lemons, and at other times of the day, eating plenty of raw fat (especially raw eggs) with small amounts of cooked starches every day helps clean and tone the liver. Eating fresh raw coconut cream with cucumbers dissolves hardening the quickest. Healing the liver is a very long process because, similar to the heart, it is almost constantly working. Eating raw meat twice daily with raw fat also helps restore the liver and liver functions.

Usually, eating unheated honey with every food that is consumed provides the liver with a supply of enzymes to make its work easier. Most often, it is vital that raw fruit, or raw vegetable juice or unheated honey is eaten with raw fat. That is because the liver's most complex task is preparing fat that will lubricate, clean, protect and fuel the body. Raw fruit, especially unripe fruit, raw vegetable juices and unheated honey supply enzymes to make those processes as easy as possible.

When lacking an appetite for any food, eating the butter/honey mixture satisfies the liver's frequent need for fresh nutrients. Eating a little live parsley helps cleanse the blood and liver, and increases appetite. Eating a little live ginger helps liver functions, and increases digestion and appetite.

Nausea may occur frequently, accompanied by mild or extreme depression. Eating small amounts of no-salt-added raw cheese with equal amounts of raw fat, raw fruit and unheated honey throughout each day, and, alternately, eating raw tomatoes or raw lemon juice reduce nausea and depression. If the raw cheese with raw fat does not reduce nausea, try a little cooked starch with plenty of raw fat.

Also, developing and enjoying a creative distraction is helpful.

COLITIS: This inflamed intestinal condition is medically diagnosed far too often among people with intestinal problems. Most often, I have found that people who are diagnosed with colitis have a poor intestinal environment and ineffective intestinal fluids. Colitis is caused by cooked food byproducts and chemicals, including household cleansers that contacted food, absorbed through skin or inhaled.

Early symptoms: abdominal cramps or pain, and frequent diarrhea.

Progressed symptom: rectal bleeding.

Eating raw fresh grapefruit juice, raw tomatoes or raw fresh tomato puree, and small amounts of no-salt-added raw cheese or cooked pasta with a raw fresh tomato sauce made with raw tomatoes and unsalted raw butter and/or stone-pressed olive oil neutralizes volatile substances in intestinal walls and improves intestinal environment. As intestinal discomfort subsides, larger meals may be eaten. Pasteurized milk and its products of any kind can cause mild to severe intestinal discomfort.

Drinking raw plain kefir, when available, or soured raw milk helps restore intestinal flora. (Drinking raw milk that is not soured or predigested by kefir bacillus sometimes causes a problem with colitis.) *See* the book The Recipe For Living Without Disease for the recipe for making natural raw kefir from raw milk. Eating the fresh raw gel from aloe vera plants is very soothing to intestines.

When volatile and ineffective fluid conditions have been corrected, colitis subsides. Then eating a smoothie made with eggs and unripe pineapple once daily helps to cleanse other toxins from intestines. If the combination of pineapple and eggs continually causes flatulence, eating them separately usually resolves the problem.

COLD, COMMON, is mainly a bacterial detoxification (yellow to clear mucus) that is sometimes accompanied by fungi (green to clear mucus) and very little or no virus. Cold detoxification cleanses the respiratory system, connected lymphatic glands and nodes, and brain.

Bacteria and fungi stir from hibernation to consume damaged, decaying and dead cells. That is the natural function of bacteria and fungi in the human body. After they complete their natural function of consuming degenerated organic matter, our bodies enter an intense healing cycle, usually indicated by fever. When that is complete, our bodies have finished a cycle of improvements. Let colds run their course by supplying nutrients that best facilitates cleansing and healing.

Symptoms: chills, cough, fever, headache, muscle soreness, nose and throat draining, sore throat, temporary loss of smell and taste, and watery eyes.

Drinking a blend of 4 tablespoons raw unpasteurized apple cider vinegar, juice of ½ lemon and 4 tablespoons of unheated honey the first thing in the morning helps neutralize toxins. Eating smoothies that are made by blending 2-3 raw eggs and ½-1 fresh raw unripe banana or ½ cup raw fresh orange juice helps the body make this detoxification through the mucous membranes easier. Unheated honey may be added if desired. Getting plenty of sleep allows the respiratory system to rest and clean and if that means taking a day or three off work, all the better for excellent health. Eating the butter/honey mixture soothes membranes. Mixing and drinking 1 tablespoon grated raw horseradish root and 2 tablespoons fresh raw lemon juice helps thin mucus that is too thick to cough up. *See* the book The Recipe For Living Without Disease, Chapter 15, Diet During Symptoms Of Cold, Flu Or Severe Pain.

As soon as fever begins, taking warm baths relaxes us and stimulates perspiration and circulation to cleanse and nourish us.

CONGESTIVE HEART FAILURE is a condition where the heart is unable to pump blood through the body properly. Seek medical help to stay alive. Eating a strict raw diet that includes a little cooked starch eaten with plenty of raw fat gradually cleanses and heals the heart. Eating two Nut Formulas weekly helps restore heart nerves.

Eating two smoothies daily (one made with unripe pineapple) helps cleanse and tone the heart. Eating the honey/butter mixture helps soothe it. Eating unheated honey with meat strengthens and gradually restores the heart.

CONJUNCTIVITIS, also called "pink eye', is an inflammation of the whites of the eyes and eyelids.

Sipping 2-3 smoothies (each made with 4 raw eggs blended with 3/4 cup of fresh unripe pineapple and 8 tablespoons of unheated honey) throughout the day for several days helps the eyes cleanse during this radical detoxification. Getting rest, relaxing the eyes and avoiding sunshine make this process tolerable. Then for ten days more, eating a balanced raw diet and drinking one pineapple smoothie once daily ensure healing.

Topically, applying a poultice made by blending 1 raw apple and ½ teaspoon unheated honey, or a poultice made of 1 red potato or yam by itself on your closed eyes and letting it stay there for at least 20 minutes soothes and relaxes the condition while the diet heals the eyes.

CONSTIPATION is a condition where fecal matter collects, dries out and is difficult to expel.

For temporary relief: Blending a green apple with 5-8 tablespoons of cold-pressed-below-96° Fahrenheit oil, the juice of ½ lemon or lime and 1-2 tablespoons unheated honey usually gets fecal matter moving quickly. Owanza's remedy is to drink raw fresh grapefruit juice. Another is to drink the mixture of 6 ounces hot water (no hotter than a finger can stand when immersed for 3 seconds), 4 tablespoons unheated honey, 3 tablespoons raw unpasteurized apple cider vinegar and the juice of ½ lemon or lime. A less comfortable remedy would be to eat unripe pineapple while drinking 5-8 tablespoons stone-pressed raw olive oil, or 4 tablespoons cold-pressed-below-96° Fahrenheit raw flax seed oil.

Constipation indicates that a person is not eating enough fat, or that he or she is eating too many cooked foods that are drying and hardening because they are indigestible, inassimilable and unutilizable. Eating plenty of fresh raw foods, including plenty of raw fat, usually eliminates constipation.

Chronic constipation results from too little E.coli bacteria in the digestive tract, usually caused by antibiotics, vaccines, food additives and preservatives. *See* the book The Recipe For Living Without Disease, Chapter 15.

COUGHS are the body's way of loosening and eliminating toxic mucus, or increasing circulation to the torso, including respiratory and cardiac systems, intestines and gonads. However, if the mucous membranes cannot produce enough mucus to bind with the toxins, they become dry, and convulsive coughs may result.

Drinking smoothies made of 2-3 raw eggs, ½ cup fresh raw fruit and 2-4 tablespoons unheated honey supplies the nutrients to form healthy mucus and lubricate mucous membranes. Eating equal portions of grated raw horseradish root or ginger root and fresh raw lemon juice helps thin toxic mucus so coughs don't have to be as violent.

CROUP is a high-pitched cough that is accompanied by difficult breathing. A sore throat usually precedes the cough. This type of cough generally affects children under age five. The cough is necessary to bring circulation to toxin-blocked tissue of the lungs, heart and throat.

Eating honey/butter mix soothes the tissue and eases difficult breathing. Drinking smoothies and eating citrus fruits help cleanse the mucous membranes. Eating antibiotic-free and hormone-free raw chicken or turkey helps to strengthen and rebuild the affected tissue.

CYSTIC FIBROSIS is a hardening and thickening of glands, such as gallbladder, lungs, pancreas, and sweat glands, similar to keloidal tissue. It is thought to be an hereditary inability to digest foods, causing failure of normal growth and development. (It is only hereditary in that the genes have lost access to the plan for synthesizing many enzymes.) The enzyme-mutations for digesting, assimilating and utilizing cooked green and red fruits and vegetables are not produced, causing dryness, lesions and scarring, eventually producing thick mucus in an attempt to harness and eliminate the resultant toxicity.

Symptoms: poor circulation, respiratory difficulties (especially in the later part of the day), sour palate, mustard taste in the mouth, eyes that have difficulty focusing in bright light, difficulty in communicating, and a feeling of isolation.

Avoiding cooked green foods, and cooked red and orange fruits and vegetables, stops the general hardening of glands. *See* If I Lack Enzyme-mutations, What Foods Should I Avoid?, page 174.

Eating raw green salads with a raw unpasteurized vinegar dressing helps cleanse the residues and resins that have scarred the glands. Eating all foods raw, except some cooked starches if necessary, supplies the body with plenty of enzymes for digestion. Eating plenty of raw fat and unheated honey with everything, especially with cooked starch if necessary, supplies the body with the nutrients to lubricate the body and make and replace most enzymes that may be missing in glands and throughout the body.

CYSTITIS: *See* Bladder infection, page 232.

DANDRUFF is one layer or more of dry dead skin on the scalp that cracks and flakes. Hardened fat or unutilizable fluid fat are the cause. The bacteria that usually accompanies this condition are a result of the body trying to detoxify the fat. Some people use antibacterial shampoos. These shampoos poison the scalp. The poisons are often absorbed into the body/brain, causing impatience, discontent and irritability.

Eating plenty of raw fat and alkalizing foods usually ends dandruff within 1-2 months. Occasionally it may return for a week or two as the body discards old stored unutilizable fat and other toxins through the scalp. Those toxins cause the scalp to dry and the upper layer to flake. During these times, a topical remedy can be applied. Once every second or third day, massage 1½ tablespoons of cold-pressed-below-96° fermented coconut oil or stone-pressed olive oil blended with 1 teaspoon fresh cucumber into the scalp and let stand over night. Then wet hair, wash hair and scalp with a whipped raw whole egg, let egg remain for 3-5 minutes, and rinse hair and scalp thoroughly.

DEHYDRATION is a deficiency of H_2O in cells. Drinking water does not supply cells with absorbable H_2O. Drinking water causes cellular drying and bloating in the body's fluid systems. For H_2O to be properly absorbed, H_2O must be bound to nutrients other than minerals in water. The only way to properly hydrate the body, is to eat and drink raw foods. Eating tomatoes hydrates cells best. Or blending 3 cups tomatoes, 1-2 teaspoons raw unpasteurized apple cider vinegar, 2-4 tablespoons unheated honey and either 4 tablespoons unsalted raw butter, or 6 tablespoons raw cream, or 4 tablespoons raw coconut cream, or 8 tablespoons avocado, and drinking it throughout the day hydrates cells wonderfully. A less desirable alternative would be to drink the mixture of at least 2 tablespoons of unheated honey, 2 tablespoons fresh raw lemon or lime juice and 1 cup naturally sparkling water. *See* Water page 202.

DEPRESSION: **Transient depression** is most often caused by low blood sugar. Drinking a blenderized mixture of ½ cup of raw fresh fruit (such as orange, or pineapple, or whatever fruit appeals to you) and ½ cup unheated honey usually brings immediate relief. Drinking a little and then sipping the rest over a 1-to-2-hour period often creates better results. If hypoglycemia or diabetes is involved, 1-3 ounces raw cream or ½-1 avocado or other raw fat (e.g., raw coconut cream, unsalted raw cheese) should be blended in or eaten with the fruit and honey mixture. To handle repeated and extended spells of depression, *see* Appendix H, page 138, and Appendix L, page 141.

Chronic depression is most often caused by low bacterial levels in the digestive tract and/or protein deficiencies. Eating at least 1 pound of raw meat and ½ cup raw cream daily helps ease chronic depression. To completely resolve it, I suggest eating "high" meat. (*See* the book The Recipe For Living Without Disease, High Meat, Chapter 15.

Doing something creative inspires creative thinking for problem solving instead of worrying. Concentrating on creating positive things and experiences helps create a better future. Then making choices based on yourself experiencing a more suitable future makes your future a better reality. Believing in sayings like "too good to be true" closes the door to wonderful experience. Inventions are rarely made by proving something can't be done. Inventions are made by focusing on the possibilities that something can be done. If I had believed what the doctors said about my probabilities, I would be dead. If I had listened to what most of my teachers and counselors told me my aptitudes were, I would not have been able to read a book, much less write this one. What will you invent or create of your future? For suggestions on creating happiness, *see* Awareness, page 325, and Mental illness, page 290.

DERMATITIS applies to various inflammations in the skin. These inflammations are detoxification of the lymph and the skin.

Eating 2-4 smoothies daily blended with red or yellow fresh raw unripe fruit (like tomato, or papaya, or pineapple) and getting plenty of sunshine assist this detoxification. If the taste of tomatoes blended with eggs is repulsive, the smoothie can be made with another fruit. Then, in between smoothies, eating plenty of raw tomatoes or a raw tomato drink (2-5 tomatoes blended with 1-4 tablespoons unheated honey and 1-2 tablespoons of raw unpasteurized apple cider vinegar) neutralizes toxins that cause this condition.

Topically, rinsing the skin with a mixture of 2 ounces water and 1 tablespoon raw unpasteurized apple cider vinegar provides the skin with nutrients to detoxify more easily so that large skin eruptions are not as necessary, if at all. *See* Acne, page 216, and Fever blister, page 263.

DETOXIFICATION is the metabolic process by which toxins are changed into less toxic or more excrescent substances. Bacteria, parasites, fungi and virus perform many types of detoxification. Stopping detoxifications will cause toxic build-ups that become disease. It is much healthier in most circumstances to let detoxification run its course while we nurture our bodies with the best raw diet.

I don't suggest that anybody force any type of detoxification, including by fast or colonic (*see* Colonic, page 330, and Fasts, page 334 and page 70). Everybody will have enough colds, flu, occasional vomit and/or diarrhea, skin eruptions and sores, and short-term aches and pains (which are all detoxification) throughout his or her lifetime without forcing any more. However, if someone is feeling extra strong, has 30 days when he or she can afford to be lethargic, and wants to rid himself or herself of some of the mutant antibodies caused by vaccines, eating moldy raspberry juice as mentioned in Appendix D, pages 132-137, frees many blood proteins to speed his or her journey to optimal health instead of being utilized by needless mutant antibodies. An orange, or lemon, or lime, or strawberries may be molded and the juice drunk instead of raspberries - whichever is more appealing to you will be the one that is right for you. Note that if lethargy strikes, usually it strikes 3-4 weeks after drinking the moldy juice, and lethargy can last for at least 30 days and, in rare cases, up to 1 year. Sometimes lethargy is accompanied by mild to severe depression. If anyone is going to drink moldy juice he or she should be prepared.

DETOXIFICATION, STOPPING IT. A person who needs temporary relief from a continually heavy painful detoxification may discourage that detoxification by taking 102°-107° Fahrenheit, 1-1½-hours baths 3 days apart. Immediately before each bath, the bather should drink a blended mixture of ¼-1 cup unripe lime juice, 3-7 tablespoons coconut cream, 1-6 teaspoons raw dairy cream or 2-6 tablespoons avocado. Measured ingredients should be equal for suggested amounts, that is, for a person who is 4'-4'6" the smallest amounts of each ingredient to be blended is 1/3 cup lime juice, 3 tablespoons coconut cream, 1 teaspoon dairy cream or 2 tablespoons avocado. A person who is 4'6"-5'2" should blend ½ cup lime juice, 4 tablespoons coconut cream, 2 teaspoons dairy cream or 3 tablespoons avocado. A person who is 5'3"-5'9" should blend 2/3 cup lime juice, 5 tablespoons coconut cream, 3 teaspoons dairy cream or 4 tablespoons avocado. A person who is 5'10"-6'2" should blend about ¾ cup lime juice, 6 tablespoons coconut cream, 5 teaspoons dairy cream or 6 tablespoons avocado. A person who is 6'3"-6'10" should blend about 1 cup lime juice, 7 tablespoons coconut cream, 2 tablespoons dairy cream or 7 tablespoons avocado. After the bath, the bather will be weak. The bather should move slowly from the bath, and sit to dry. Bundle in very warm natural clothing and take a 30-45-minute easy walk.

The hot-bath routine above works by instigating the healing cycle that relaxes bacteria, putting them in hibernation, and discouraging cells from producing virus. Those are the same effects produced by fever. Fever is an important and beneficial feat of the body. Fever ends microbe and viral proliferation and initiates intense healing (cellular division/reproduction). Usually, fever is accompanied by necessary lethargy that transforms into tiredness. Rest, relaxation and sleep are important because most healing occurs during those states.

Or a less beneficial alternative for stopping painful persistent detoxification for the elderly, is to eat a cooked meal once weekly. A cooked meal discourages continual detoxification of old stored toxins. One cooked meal of baked chicken once weekly usually stops and prevents extreme detoxification of old toxins stored in the body.

DETOXIFICATION OF DRUGS is characterized by coating on the tongue, sour taste in the mouth, chemical-smelling urine, skin eruptions, nausea and/or headache, and often by the returning of symptoms that had occurred at the time a drug had been taken. *See* Detoxification, page 255.

Drinking a mixture of 2 tablespoons of unheated honey per 1 cup of raw fresh orange juice helps the body neutralize drugs. Here are the foods that have helped to bind with the following toxic substances and remove them from your body:

Amphetamines, caffeine - carob powder, raw kefir, unheated honey.

Antibiotics - fresh parsley.

Antihistamines - sun-dried powdered clay (twice daily, drinking 2 ounces of good mineral water with ¼ teaspoon clay mixed in, works best). *See* Clay, page 181.

Aspirin, cocaine (including Novocain) - avocados.

Cough medications, sedatives - yellow banana pepper (yellow chili) eaten with ½ avocado and some raw meat.

Drugs in general - smoothies made with raspberries. *See* Smoothies, page 200.

Nail polish on nails - (very toxic!) 25% more fat, fresh parsley (15 sprigs daily), and put coconut or olive oil on nails instead of nail polish.

Salt - naturally sparkling mineral water, ripe tomatoes.

Vitamin C supplements - oranges.

DETOXIFICATION OF RADIATION is characterized by nausea, nervousness, and a feeling of extreme sensitivity in the body. Radiation-poisoning can come from medication, medical testing, X-rays, fluorescent lighting, television, computer monitors, laser printers, cellular phones, Bluetooth tech, irradiated food, microwaves, scanners, industrial pollution, jewelry, building material, and EMF's from improperly grounded electrical connections and operating machinery.

Eating avocado with orange, or with melons facilitates the body's ability to discard stored radiation. If a person received barium or iodine as an x-ray contrast, eating a combination of raw meat with plenty of beef fat, and in the afternoon, eating 3 ounces coconut cream blended with either ¾-1 cup dark berries (such as blue, black and boysenberries) or 1/3 cup raspberries and 1/3 cup dark berries helps detoxify it. For individuals who have taken radioactive medication, drinking raw milk with unheated honey helps detoxify it. *See* Radiation Burn, page 306.

DIABETES is an impaired ability to utilize carbohydrate blood-sugar or protein blood-sugar (pyruvate) because of insufficient production of insulin or faulty insulin manufactured by the pancreas.

Symptoms: frequent hunger and urination, impaired vision, muscle cramps shortly after eating sweets, and wounds that heal slowly and poorly.

Medicinal insulin causes poor sugar assimilation and metabolism, and causes the pancreas to further deteriorate. The poorly assimilated and metabolized sugars most often store in the extremities, causing deterioration of tissue and eventual gangrene and amputation.

Eating tremendous amounts of unheated honey (about 3/4 cup throughout each day) replaces the functions of insulin missing in the blood while it heals the pancreas and encourages pancreatic functions. The best honey for this is a partially crystallized completely unheated honey. Unheated honeys naturally crystallize within a year, unless exposed to hot weather conditions. Refrigerating honey speeds crystallization but remove from refrigeration when crystallization begins.

Eating plenty of raw fat strengthens glandular cells. Eating plenty of the particular meats that are right for you rebuilds the pancreas over a period of 2-5 years. If diabetes is accompanied with other ailments, rebuilding the pancreas may take many more years. If a person is suited for eating red meat, eating raw red fish (like tuna or salmon) with raw beef at least once weekly helps rebuild the nerves in the pancreas. (*See* Appendix P, page 150.)

When a pronounced decrease in energy occurs, eating avocado (or other raw fat) with raw fresh unripe fruit and unheated honey raises the energy level.

When clients had been taking insulin for at least two years, he or she did best by weaning himself gradually off insulin over a long period - up to two years; it usually took that long before the pancreas worked well enough. When an insulin-taker started experiencing itching of the skin, it was an indication to decrease his or her insulin intake.

DIARRHEA is the frequent elimination of watery fecal matter. Diarrhea should be welcomed (*see* Detoxification).

Eating plenty of raw fats, especially no-salt-added raw cheeses or raw eggs with raw unripe banana and unheated honey absorbs radical toxins causing diarrhea, soothes membranes and replenishes lost nutrients. One to three tablespoons of raw carob powder may be added to that combination if it is a smoothie. Avoid apples; they have a tendency to overstimulate the adrenals which often causes more diarrhea. Drinking soured milk such as raw plain kefir helps restore intestinal flora lost in diarrhea.

DIVERTICULITIS is inflammation in one or more of the sacs of the intestines. It can result from food that has collected and adhered to the sac, or toxins within the intestinal walls in a given area. It most often results from a fat-deficiency, usually accompanied by protein deficiency. Often that results in the body's inability to produce proper or enough mucus to protect intestinal walls. There may be several reasons for fat deficiencies; *see* Appendix O, pages 145-150.

Symptoms: abdominal cramps or pain, irregular bowel movements, gas, lethargy and continued abdominal bloating.

Eating 1-2 eggs every 1-2 hours following that with ½ tablespoon of butter/honey mixture for 3-7 days calms this condition. Afterward, eating more raw fat with everything that is eaten, and eating raw meat corrects diverticulitis. Eating vegetable salads often slows digestion and irritates the intestines; it is healthiest not to eat salads except as the very last food of the day. Drinking raw fresh vegetable juices soothes intestines. If experiencing intestinal cramps, eating ½ raw papaya with ½ avocado, or other raw fat (except cheeses) usually relieves cramps. Eating whichever raw meats that are appropriate for you will strengthen and tone your intestines.

DIZZINESS is most often from low blood sugar; *see* Hypoglycemia, page 274. Dizziness may be caused by swelling in one ear and not the other ear; *see* Ear Infections, page 260.

DRY SKIN & GENERAL DRYNESS: *See* Fat deficiency, page 262, and Aging, page 218.

DYSPEPSIA: *See* Indigestion, page 275.

EARACHE: *See* Ear infection, below.

EAR INFECTION: Resting a hot-water bottle next to the entire side of the head increases circulation, speeds nutrients to the area and soothes pained tissue during this detoxification. Eating tomatoes reduces fever and minimizes swelling. Eating citrus (as well as tomatoes) helps neutralize toxins in the effected area so that healing progresses more quickly.

If experiencing severe pain, eating a golf ball-sized amount of ground meat with ½ tablespoon unsalted raw butter and ½ teaspoon unheated honey every 4-6 hours helps relieve pain and speed healing. Drinking a mixture of raw milk and bee pollen, or raw carrot juice and bee pollen (*see* Pain, page 297), also relieves pain. More immediate relief may be obtained by pressing the juice from fresh garlic or onion, mixing 4 drops into 1 teaspoon of room temperature unheated-above-96° Fahrenheit fermented coconut oil, or cold-pressed peanut oil or stone-pressed olive oil, slowly putting drops into the ear and gently plugging the ear with a puff of cotton. Then apply heat with a hot water bottle (not an electric heating pad). Electric pads generate electromagnetic fields that may interfere with neural function and healing.

ECZEMA is an inflammation of the skin accompanied by itching and scales. *See* Dermatitis, page 254.

EDEMA is the retention of fluids in the body. It is sometimes a mineral deficiency or mineral imbalance where cells are unable to utilize water.

Avoid salt! *See* Appendix M, page 143. Drinking honey mixed with fresh raw vegetable juices or fresh raw tomato puree, and eating no-salt-added raw cheese at the same time correct many mineral imbalances. Eating raw fish and getting fresh air and sunshine are helpful.

Nowadays, a major contributing cause of edema is volatile compounds and fluids collecting in the body. They must be diluted or they will irritate, burn and kill cells. *See* Overweight, page 296, on how to neutralize volatile substances. Read all of: Specifics About Particular Foods, pages 178-207, to know what foods to avoid that create volatile toxins, for instance, coffee, canned food, pesticides and household chemicals.

EMPHYSEMA is swelling and destruction of the sacs in the lungs, usually brought on by airborne pollution (for instance, tobacco smoke, including secondary smoke, smog, and prolonged inhalation of dusts – such as lint from synthetic fibers from bedding, clothing, carpets and rugs, and coal dust). The lungs have become loaded with garbage that they cannot easily detoxify and discharge. If a person stops smoking, stays away from airborne toxins, including synthetic fibers, and eats a raw diet with plenty of raw fat and raw meat, he or she may have a good chance of living with emphysema. *See* the book The Recipe For Living Without Disease, Chapter 12.

EPILEPSY is characterized by sensory seizures (change in sensation or loss of consciousness) or convulsive seizures (involuntary muscle movement). This is an ailment that mainly results from a lack of enzyme-mutations, to digest, assimilate, and utilize both cooked fat and proteins. It is dangerous for people with epilepsy to eat cooked meat and cooked fat. In infants and children, I have observed that antibiotics caused frequent or constant grand mal and petite mal seizures.

Eating plenty of raw fat and raw meat has corrected this problem within 9 months to 2 years (that is, unless a person continued to eat cooked fat and meat and take medication). When a person had taken medication for a longtime, it worked best to wean herself or himself over a comfortable period of time by reducing the dosage every three to four months. In infants, I suggest that medication be immediately discontinued and 1 teaspoon of the mixture of 2 parts unsalted raw butter to 1 part completely unheated honey be given every 20-40 minutes until seizures subside. It was best for infants to receive meals of only raw milk blended with unsalted raw butter and completely unheated honey (2 tablespoons butter and ¼ teaspoon honey to 7 ounces milk). In one case, an infant experienced seizures only when she nursed from her mother; her mother took medication.

EYE INFLAMMATION AND IRRITATION: The same remedy suggestions for Conjunctivitis has soothed and healed those conditions. *See* Conjunctivitis, page 250.

EYESTRAIN: Getting sleep, plenty of sunshine, and eating red and orange live foods, such as raw fresh tuna, salmon, tomatoes, raw carrot juice, oranges, watermelon, and cantaloupe soothe and heal eyestrain. Eating unsalted raw butter is also helpful. Blurred vision accompanying eyestrain is often a red-meat deficiency. Eating red meat with unheated honey corrects blurred vision.

FAT DEFICIENCY results from either not eating enough fat or lacking the enzyme-mutations for digesting, assimilating and utilizing cooked fat.

Eating plenty of raw fat with unheated honey eventually and properly lubricates and strengthens cells. For a quick body-lubricating drink *see* the Drink for Moisturizing and Lubrication, page 210.

FATIGUE is the "normal" feeling of physical, emotional and mental weariness at the end of a day. However, if fatigue happens during the day, it frequently results from self-criticism. Focusing on one's talents and accomplishments develops and continues them. (If you don't know you have a talent, you could develop one to which you are attracted.) Also, *see* Depression, page 254, and Mental illness, page 290, about creative suggestions.

Drinking a mixture of ½ cup raw fresh juice mixed with ½ cup unheated honey usually brings immediate relief. Sleep is both healing and energizing. *See* Stress, page 313, and Chronic fatigue syndrome, page 247.

FEVER is a body temperature above the body's normal temperature. Fever ends proliferation of bacteria and other detoxification microbes, stops cells from producing virus and initiates intense healing (cellular division/reproduction). Usually, fever is accompanied by necessary lethargy that transforms into tiredness. Rest, relaxation and sleep are important because most healing occurs during those states.

Getting plenty of sleep, fresh air, and eating red and orange live foods, such as raw fresh tuna, salmon, tomatoes, carrot juice, oranges, unripe watermelon and cantaloupe soothe tissues and prevent cellular destruction. If blood-sugar problems exist, add 4-6 tablespoons raw fat to any high-carbohydrate fruit. Eating fresh raw aloe vera gel also soothes tissues, especially mucous membranes, and prevents cellular destruction. Consuming raw cream or unsalted raw butter also helps. If there is not an appetite, drink the freshest raw juices mixed with unheated honey. Raw cream mixed in equal proportions with the freshest raw carrot juice, or cream mixed with orange or watermelon juice is often the most soothing. If a fever rises above 105° Fahrenheit, drink chilled fresh blended raw tomatoes, or fresh raw fruit purees of red and orange raw foods. Don't panic; when eating a predominantly raw diet convulsion and irreversible brain damage has not happened from fever.

Night fevers - night sweats - are usually a combination of friction from mass cellular division (cellular reproduction) and cessation of intense detoxification. That is cause for joy. It is a time of intense rejuvenation when an individual becomes more alive with new cells. Sleeping more, getting fresh air and sunshine, and eating plenty of raw meat during and after these cycles bring youth and strength. Eating 1/8 teaspoon of royal jelly with raw meat and with raw fat daily during those cycles increases the body's ability to reproduce and strengthen cells.

FEVER BLISTER is a sore in or around the mouth characterized by inflammation, swelling and sensitivity. Fever blisters are the result of too many free volatile toxins in the serums in the mouth (including blood). This results from a deficiency of nutrients that neutralize and bind with toxins. A person not getting enough sleep can cause fever blisters and acne because the body spends all available nutrients on physical activity, resulting in excessive accumulated toxins throughout the body.

Drinking the following mixtures usually has healed fever blisters within 36 hours but in a few instances has taken up to 5 days. First food in the morning: heat good mineral water until it is no hotter than an immersed finger can tolerate for 3 seconds. Stir in 2-5 tablespoons unheated honey. Then stir in 1-2 tablespoons raw unpasteurized apple cider vinegar, 4-6 tablespoons fresh raw lemon or lime juice, and 2 tablespoons raw cream (if available). Last food before sleep: blend 1 tomato, 1-2 tablespoons raw unpasteurized apple cider vinegar, 2-4 tablespoons unheated honey and 4-6 tablespoons fresh raw lemon or lime juice, and 2 tablespoons raw cream (if available). *See* Acne, 216, Dermatitis, page 254, Preservatives and pesticides, page 196.

FLU: *See* Influenza, page 278.

FOOD ADDICTION is the frequent craving for a particular food or foods. Most people can't digest, assimilate, and utilize what their bodies need from cooked foods, so they overeat.

It is almost impossible for a person to overeat when on a raw diet that includes meat. The body loses its appetite when its needs are satisfied. If someone deprives her or his body of what it needs, she will experience emotional deprivation (depression), or anxiety (anxiousness and irritability) and malnutrition. Eating the foods a person craves fresh and raw brings on a degree of physical and emotional satisfaction that would not have ill repercussions. For people who crave chocolate, I have included a recipe for a substitute (*see* Chocolate Substitutes, page 181).

Everyone should trust his or her cravings. Cravings are the body telling a person that it needs the nutrients in the food(s) craved. If a person craves ice cream and raw cream is not available, she or he could eat other raw fat with unheated honey, such as avocados and unheated honey, or fresh raw coconut cream with unheated honey.

Owanza, a nutritional colleague, has found a relationship between emotional needs and physical needs. She has found that people who are overaggressive - trying to sink their teeth into things - have a protein deficiency and need to eat more raw meat, especially white meat. People who crave sweets have a need for a sweet life. Finding and interacting with sweet people will be as emotionally nourishing as raw fresh fruits and unheated honey will be physically nourishing.

FOOT PROBLEMS:

Aching or burning feet: Drinking a combination of raw tomato, raw cucumber and raw carrot juices helps soothe the feet. Applying cold slices of fresh raw tomato, or cucumber or potato to the soles of your feet soothe and relax the feet. Or soaking your feet alternately for two minutes in cold and then in warm water as many times as you like stimulates circulation and relaxes the feet.

Athlete's foot: *See* Athlete's foot, page 228.

Cold feet: Drinking a combination of raw tomato, raw spinach, raw carrot juices with the juice of ½-1 hot fresh raw pepper (chile, jalapeño, etc.) and 2 tablespoons unheated honey increases body temperature. Alternately standing on your toes for 1-2 minutes and then on your heels for 30 seconds increases circulation to the feet, warming them.

Corns: Alternately rubbing stone-pressed olive oil twice daily for 1 day and then rubbing cold-pressed-below-96° Fahrenheit peanut oil twice daily for 3 days gradually causes the corn to let go. Peel off the corn and you will find smooth skin. Or, bandage a piece of fresh raw lemon peel or pineapple peel on the corn (inside of peel against the corn) overnight for several nights until the corn comes off leaving smooth skin.

FRACTURE: *See* Brittle bones, page 234, and Broken bone, page 234.

FROSTBITE: The remedy suggestions for burns are effective for frost-bite. *See* Burns, page 235.

FUNGUS is characterized by itching and peeling of the skin. All fungi naturally appearing in the body are beneficial. They consume intercellular toxicity, including toxicity caused by antibiotics. Consequently, fungi detoxify antibiotics.

Eating foods that alkalize facilitates the cleansing and healing processes (*see* Alkalizing food, page 178), reducing the need for fungi. Cooked acidic foods, like coffee, chocolate, teas (including herbal), soups and meat should not be eaten. It is best to let a fungus run its course, usually in 5-6 weeks. If that is impossible, coating the area with unheated honey and covering it with a clean cotton cloth will smother the fungus and stop it for a period of time.

GALLSTONES are deposits of crystallized resins and minerals, the same as kidney stones but combined with bile in the gall bladder.

Along with the suggestions for Kidney Stones, *see* page 282, eating foods containing a lot of minerals, that is, fresh raw vegetable juices, raw eggs, raw milk (preferably full-fat), raw plain kefir, tomatoes, melons, no-salt-added raw cheeses and fresh raw fish, especially raw oysters and clams with raw fat soothes the condition. Drinking 2 ounces of fresh raw beet juice mixed in other vegetable juices and eaten with no-salt-added raw cheese once daily speeds the process. A raw milk eggnog made by blending 2 raw eggs, ½ cup raw milk and ¼ banana (nutmeg isn't necessary) works just a little bit slower but sometimes is more soothing.

GASTRITIS is inflamed stomach walls. If a person is paunchy, he or she lacks the enzyme-mutations to digest, assimilate, and utilize cooked green foods. Avoid eating cooked green foods. *See* If I Lack Enzyme-mutations, What Foods Should I Avoid?, page 174.

Another cause is drinking alcohol, *see* Alcohol, page 178. Other causes are eating processed sugars, and taking antibiotics.

Eating plenty of unheated honey and raw fat has corrected this condition, that is, as long as cooked green foods and alcohol were not ingested.

GINGIVITIS is an inflammation of the gums. *See* Pyorrhea, page 305.

GLAUCOMA is edema in the eyeball and hardening of the conjunct-tiva. Eating raw red meat daily helps reverse glaucoma.

Avoid all cheese for 6 months. Eating ¼ cup stone-pressed olive oil daily, several fresh raw tomatoes blended into puree with plenty of unheated honey and a little fresh live hot pepper once or twice daily, and fresh raw fish at least once daily usually heals this condition in several months. If you are diabetic, glaucoma is probably due to poorly assimilated or metabolized sugars (*see* Diabetes, page 258).

GOITER is the enlargement of the thyroid. Eating raw fish everyday for five weeks has corrected this mineral-imbalanced condition and helped fortify the thyroid gland. *See* Thyroid problem, page 315.

GONORRHEA is an inflammation of the urethra and or vagina accompanied with pus. It is a necessary detoxification of the tissues that is usually caused by the inability to utilize caffeine and cooked green foods. Avoiding caffeine and cooked green foods stops the accumulation of these toxins. *See* If I Lack Enzyme-mutations, What Foods Should I Avoid?, page 174.

It is best to be celibate for 10 days. Getting a lot of sunshine and drinking 2 quarts of raw fresh orange juice throughout the first part of the day and then a balanced raw diet for the remainder of the day has brought this detoxification to a quicker end.

GOUT is a condition in which volatile substances (e.g., uric acid) collects in the blood and around the joints, causing swelling, especially in the fingers and toes. Gout occurs in people who can handle very little, if any, uric acid. Cooked and processed meats produce tremendous amounts of volatile toxins; avoid cooked and processed meats.

Eating plenty of raw meat with raw fat, however, helps remove the saturation of volatile toxins and strengthens the body. Eating raw fresh tomatoes, pineapple and melons, and drinking raw fresh carrot juice mixed with other raw fresh vegetable juices alkalize, cleanse and soothe this condition. *See* Alkalizing food, page 178.

GUMS, SORE: *See* Pain, page 297, and Pyorrhea, page 305.

HAIR PROBLEMS: *See* Balding, page 231.

HALITOSIS is a foul odor emanating from the mouth. In hygienic people, only 1% of "bad breath" comes from decaying teeth. The other 99% of "bad breath" comes from a toxic intestine where foods have putrefied. Some putrid gases in the intestines pass into the blood and expel from the lungs.

Eating unheated honey often (and, when available, plain raw kefir) supplies enzymes necessary for better digestion. Eating fresh raw parsley, or other fresh raw aromatic herbs, or fresh raw vegetable juices or fresh raw pineapple or papaya aids digestion and sweetens breath. Very seldom does anyone on a raw diet have bad breath, and only during detoxification.

Some people are ill-effected by the putrid gases of bad breath that are emitted by other people. Those people get a headache when they are within two feet from someone who has bad breath. Many people who drink alcohol have a destructive chemical reaction that causes their breath to smell like airplane glue. Many people who do not drink alcohol have breath that smells like airplane glue. Some people get nauseous, claustrophobic and headachy when enclosed in an unventilated room with someone whom has breath that smells like airplane glue. Following the same suggestions above alleviates the gaseous ill effects suffered from someone else's bad breath.

HAY FEVER is an extreme sensitivity to airborne substances that irritate the mucous membranes of the air passages and eyes.

Immediate relief can be obtained by eating a little honeycomb. Eating plenty of raw fat daily, especially eggs, with red and orange fresh raw foods eventually resolves this problem. For example, a fresh raw orange, carrot or tomato smoothie (*see* Smoothies, page 200) soothes and sets a condition for healing the sinuses. Fresh raw meat, like tuna and swordfish, help heal and strengthen sinuses.

Also, eating fresh local bee pollen can help reverse this condition. If a person starts by eating ¼-½ teaspoon unheated bee pollen at a time, six times daily, there will be only a remote chance of the rare incidence of anaphylactic shock. If hay fever is severe, working up to ½ cup of unheated bee pollen daily with at least 1/3 teaspoon royal jelly and 1 tablespoon unheated honey mixed with 12 ounces of fresh raw vegetable juice (including carrot) and sipping it throughout the day may be a more palatable form to consume the pollen. Drinking 1/6 of this mixture 6 times daily has stopped sneezing and headache. Avoid cheeses during hay fever season; they can cause dryness of the sinuses.

HEADACHES: The common headache is from either high blood pressure (most often caused by eating salt), or low blood circulation, or toxic blood stream.

<u>High blood pressure headache</u>: Mix 2 ounces of naturally sparkling water with 2 tablespoons of unheated honey and the juice of 1 lemon. Add 6 ounces more of naturally sparkling water and drink. Usually, that relieves this headache in 20-40 minutes.

<u>Low blood circulation headache</u> is accompanied by sluggishness: Mix

2 ounces of naturally sparkling water with 2 tablespoons of unheated honey. Add 6 ounces more of naturally sparkling water and drink. Usually, that relieves this headache in 20-40 minutes.

Toxic blood stream headache is accompanied by nausea: Drinking 1 cup fresh raw orange juice mixed with 3 tablespoons unheated honey usually relieves this headache in 20-40 minutes. Or drinking 6 ounces good mineral water mixed with 2 tablespoons of raw unpasteurized apple cider vinegar, fresh raw juice of ½ lemon and 3 tablespoons unheated honey usually relieves this headache in 20 minutes.

Cluster headaches (also called "suicide headaches") are successively occurring headaches that grow in intensity, usually immobilizing the sufferer. Cluster headaches occur in a body laced with volatile toxins, usually from excessive adrenaline, accompanied by low blood fat and low body fat levels. Cluster headaches are somewhat allergy related. Avoiding the following foods and substances usually solves the problem: caffeine (including aspirin, coffee, chocolate, and sodas), alcohol, processed sugars, cheddar and jack cheeses (even if cheeses are raw), salt and anything made with baking soda. For cluster sufferers over age 25, following these suggestions for at least 3 days weekly for several months before the cluster season begins usually prevents reoccurrence: abstain from the foods listed above and eat cooked starches with plenty of raw fat and tomatoes, and eat fresh raw fish (salmon is more often the most effective).

Migraines are sudden headaches that fluctuate in intensity, usually occurring on one side of the head. Sleeping is the best relief. When awake, eating a little spoonful of unheated honey every five minutes and avoiding all other food, especially avoiding meat and dairy, eventually relieves migraines. If thirsty, sipping some good mineral water, or some fresh raw orange juice with an equal amount of unheated honey is helpful.

HEART ATTACK: Get medical help to stay alive. Then, eating a healthy raw diet gradually restores the heart. *See* Heart disease, below; Angina pectoris, page 224, Arteriosclerosis, page 226, and Atherosclerosis, page 228.

HEART DISEASE: Eating plenty of raw meat, raw eggs, raw dairy, stone-pressed olive oil, raw pineapple, raw fresh onions and unheated honey very gradually restores the heart. *See* Angina pectoris, page 224, Arteriosclerosis, page 226, Atherosclerosis, page 228.

HEMOPHILIA is an inability to properly coagulate blood, characterized by bleeding easily and difficulty in stopping a bleed. Heredity or taking medications causes this condition.

Eating a high raw meat diet, preferably a combination of fish with another raw meat of choice, restores health to platelets, and strengthens tissues. Hemophiliacs do not digest, assimilate, or utilize cooked fat properly. The thyroid is sometimes at fault. *See* Thyroid problem, page 246. Eating plenty of unheated honey and pineapple with raw fat and with raw meat helps digestion, assimilation, and utilization.

During a bleed, drinking 1 cup of raw white cabbage juice mixed with 7 tablespoons of honey helps coagulation. The juice mixtures suggested in Hemorrhage sometimes work better. *See* Hemorrhage, below.

Aspirin and aspirin-based medications prevent blood clotting, damage platelets and cause skin to easily tear. Avoid those poisons.

HEMORRHAGE is profuse bleeding from a ruptured blood vessel, wound or discharge. To promote and speed clotting: drink 1 cup of raw white cabbage juice blended with 7 tablespoons unheated honey. Consuming white cabbage will stop hemorrhage even without unheated honey, however, unheated honey speeds general healing. (If you are alone and unable to juice the cabbage, eat the whole cabbage. Eat the honey before, while or after you eat the cabbage.) Mixing 3 ounces of fresh raw carrot juice and 5 teaspoons lime juice to the cabbage juice and honey mixture improves taste for some people as well as speeds healing. Lime juice is the key to preventing excessive infection. Drinking over a period of 16 hours, a blend of 18 raw eggs, 2 small tomatoes and 2-4 tablespoons of unheated honey usually prevents re-hemorrhage.

HEMORRHOID is a distended or ruptured vein in or around the anus. This is a condition caused by the accumulation of volatile toxins.

Eating alkalizing foods soothes and gradually heals the condition. *See*

Alkalizing food, page 178. Avoid black pepper, marshmallows, and store-bought mustard, because they often cause chronic hemorrhoids.

The most effective remedy for speeding detoxification and healing the rectum has been to insert a small-finger-sized slice of raw beef into the rectum, leaving only $^1/_8$ inch protruding from the anus day and night until hemorrhoids disappear. A fresh slice of meat should be inserted every 24 hours.

HEPATITIS is an infection in the liver. This severe liver detoxification occurs in people who lack a particular fat processing enzyme, and is usually brought on by drinking alcohol, or taking legal or recreational drugs (including vaccines, eating cooked marijuana or smoking marijuana).

The missing enzyme can be replaced by eating raw fresh unripe pineapple often. Getting plenty of rest and sunshine, and eating no more than two foods in combination (like a smoothie made with 2-3 raw eggs and 3/4 cup pineapple), and no more than one cup of food at a time, make the liver strong again. Eating pineapple twice daily as often as possible supplies the liver with enzymes that make its work easier while it cleanses and rebuilds itself. Eating fresh raw fish at least three times weekly for the first three weeks, then at least twice weekly for another 6 weeks, helps regenerate nerves in the liver.

HERPES is an inflammation of the skin or mucous membrane, characterized by clusters of blisters that seem to spread. This is sometimes a condition that results from taking medication during chicken pox. Sometimes it is a condition resulting from taking the small pox vaccine. Another cause is very high adrenaline saturation (volatile toxic condition) in the nerve endings.

For six weeks, drinking 1 level teaspoon of powdered sun-dried clay mixed in 2-6 ounces of good mineral water or raw fresh juice helps attract and absorb toxins that cause herpes. Eating raw fresh fish and raw chicken several times weekly with no-salt-added raw cheese and an equal portion of unsalted raw butter for eight weeks helps soothe and heal the nerves. Eating fresh raw unripe pineapple with unheated honey relieves soreness. For many years thereafter, and in general, following a balanced Primal Diet, mainly utilizing alkalizing foods, helps heal the liver and other affected areas. *See* Alkalizing Food, page 178.

HICCOUGHS are spasms of the diaphragm muscles causing abrupt short inhalations with a slight gasping sound.

Sipping 1 cup of very warm good mineral water mixed with 3 tablespoons unheated honey relaxes the diaphragm muscles within a few minutes.

Applying warmth with a hot-water bottle and gently massaging the diaphragm and the upper spine just below the neck helps relax the affected muscles.

HIV is toxic and exhausted condition affecting lymphatic, nervous and blood systems that are failing, caused by caffeine, medical and recreational drugs, alcohol, smoke tars and other chemicals (including from cooked food). HIV is not AIDS which involves a different virus. The one client who I followed the longest did very well living with HIV positive for almost ten years. He followed my raw food suggestions only sporadically but they were always helpful. Then he panicked during a three-month bout with tiredness and exhaustion. He underwent chemotherapy that thinned him of his healthy constitution. Consequently, he died from medical-poisoning within a year. Owanza has found that eating 3-6 tablespoons of cold-pressed-below-96° Fahrenheit flax seed oil a day several days weekly helps strengthen all systems. Adhering to a balanced raw diet makes living with HIV easy and asymptomatic.

HIVES: *see* Itchy skin, page 281.

HYPERACTIVE individuals are unusually active and are unable to relax, often feeling anxious.

I hope by now people realize that children are not hyperactive because they are deficient in sedatives, drugs, or abuse. Children who are hyperactive lack the enzyme-mutation for digesting, assimilating and utilizing cooked proteins, especially in cooked and processed meat and eggs. Also, hyperactive children lack the utilizable proteins necessary to deal with irritants like mustard, alcohol, caffeine, preservatives, additives and pesticides. Many tests from Canada and the USA show that preservatives and malnutrition cause hyperactivity in children that leads to violence in adulthood. Avoiding cooked and processed meat and eggs, mustard, alcoholic and caffeine beverages (including sodas), preservatives, food coloring and other additives help settle this condition.

Eating raw fresh meat with raw eggs, or raw meat with lots of raw fats alone, usually makes hyperactivity disappear. Also, getting lots of sunshine and fresh air helps the body utilize proteins.

If people are hyperactive because they have high adrenaline levels rather than because of the cooked-protein allergy mentioned above (children of this type are usually thin until at least teenage), eating a Nut Formula at least twice weekly subdues the excess adrenaline. If the Nut Formula fails to subdue hyperactivity, try eating some cooked starch with plenty of raw fat. Eating 3-4 ounces of the Nut Formula or cooked starch with raw fat thirty minutes before homework time, or a test, allows the mind to work without being distracted by excess adrenaline. A hobby, creative pursuit or sport is also helpful for high adrenaline types.

All hyperactive children have potential genius, but unless they can utilize proteins or harness adrenaline, their genius may turn into antisocial behavior. If the excess adrenaline is not spent in physical activity, the body will spend it in anxiety, irritability, bullying or arrogant bravado.

HYPERTENSION is either from high blood pressure or the same causes as hyperactivity. High blood pressure is mainly caused by the lack of enzyme-mutations to digest, assimilate, and utilize cooked fats. Eating plenty of raw fats with raw fresh tomatoes, eating other raw foods, especially unheated honey, and following the suggestions for high blood pressure, alleviate hypertension. *See* Blood pressure, High, page 233. *See* Hyperactivity page 272.

HYPERTHYROID: Hyperthyroid is a condition where the thyroid overproduces hormones.

The same causes and suggestions as hyperactivity usually works. *See* Hyperactive, page 272.

HYPOGLYCEMIA (low blood sugar): This is very often a condition where the pancreas over-secretes insulin. The excess insulin binds with sugars and turns them into glycogen (a storable sugar), causing low blood sugar, and is often the precursor to diabetes because the pancreas becomes exhausted from overproducing insulin. This in turn overworks the liver. Along with the suggestions in Appendices H and L, eating 3-4 ounces of unheated honey daily supplies enzymes to regulate and heal the pancreas and liver. Also, eating small amounts of food frequently, instead of normal meals, makes the entire body work more easily and efficiently. Eating raw meat, including raw fish, gradually rebuilds the pancreas. *See* Appendix H, page 138, and Appendix L, page 141.

IMPETIGO is an inflammation in the skin characterized by itchy sores that tend to spread and ooze yellow pus that turns crusty. Impetigo usually results from a loss of melanin, resulting from metal and chemical toxicity, especially from injections such as dental and vaccines. Following the suggestions in Diabetes (for different reasons) heals this severe skin infection (*see* Diabetes, page 258).

IMPOTENCY: Owanza says, "Relax."

Most often this is not just a physiological problem. If a person finds himself or herself in a relationship where sex is no longer exciting, letting the imagination run wild with fantasy before and during sex usually gets the juices going again. In some relationships it may be best not to tell your mate your imagined fantasies because your mate may become insecure or offended. For some people, telling a fantasy ruins its potency. For others, sharing your fantasies is exciting and causes sexual arousal.

Physiological impotency occurs from deterioration in the nervous system, medication that lowers blood pressure, psychotherapeutic drugs, genital-related problems, including prostatitis and vaginitis, childbirth, and surgeries or injuries that have damaged nerves. Spermicides, lubricants, birth control pills and chemical douches absorbed into vaginal and uterine walls cause poor mucus formation and/or production, and nerve damage. A pure unheated-above-96° Fahrenheit fermented coconut oil is the best lubricant that will not cause side effects.

Eating plenty of raw fat with raw fresh unripe fruit (non-steamed dates may be included) and having at least ¼ cup of unheated honey daily stop nerve deterioration. Eating, or blending and drinking, 4-8 tablespoons raw coconut cream with ½-1 cup peeled cucumber helps dissolve hardened nerves. Regularly, eating raw fresh fish heals and rebuilds deteriorated nerve tissue over time.

Another reason for physiological impotency is an intolerance for milk heated above 100° Fahrenheit (pasteurization is about 160° Fahrenheit). If a person suspects that he or she may have a milk intolerance, abstaining from drinking and eating milk products for 2-3 months usually restores potency. Then, for most of those people, drinking and eating only room-temperature or warmer raw milk products will not affect potency as long as unheated honey is eaten with them (for example, up to 2 tablespoons of honey per 1 cup of raw milk or raw plain kefir).

See also pages 123-124. In cases of low sexual hormone production, eating plenty of raw shell fish, like oysters, clams, scallops, and urchin with other raw fats often increases hormone production and sexual appetite. Another aphrodisiac is 2 ounces of cold-pressed-below-96° Fahrenheit peanut oil, 1 raw fertile egg, 1 tablespoon raw carob powder and 1/8- ¼ teaspoon vanilla extract. Eating enough raw meat and 1 cup unheated honey daily usually sustains erection for an hour or more. Drinking 2 cups of hard peeled cucumbers blended with 2-3 ounces fresh raw coconut cream and 3 ounces of unheated honey usually helps to develop and sustain erections. Adding 1 teaspoon bee pollen to the cucumber/coconut cream mixture strengthens erections for many men but not for others. Experiment and discover for yourself. For some men, raw garlic or red onion is also effective in maintaining erection; for others, garlic has the opposite effect.

INDIGESTION is poor digestion accompanied by a feeling of fullness, discomfort, and any or all of the following symptoms: pain, cramps, heartburn, nausea, belching, flatulence.

Eating a diet of unheated honey with warm or room temperature raw milk for 2-6 weeks quickly aids digestion. If raw milk is problematic, eat a diet of 1 raw egg every 1-1½ hours followed with 1 teaspoon raw cream and 1/8 teaspoon unheated honey for 2-6 weeks, until symptoms subside. If more fluid is needed, see Dehydration page 253. Someone who does not synthesize enzymes well would be much healthier if she or he would eat a balanced raw-food diet only.

INFANT PROBLEMS: There is a terror among doctors about babies under 1 year old eating honey. One-point-one percent of all babies have been known to react badly to honey, causing a few deaths. However, I was unable to find one scientifically proved infant death that was attributed to honey. Those that claimed honey responsible were mere conclusions from surveys that noted the infant had been fed honey. The cause of death was probably medicinal but the doctors were not going to accept responsibility. I wish doctors would react that way with all of their medications and vaccines because the risks of side effects from pharmaceuticals are astronomical. *See* Vaccine Induce Diseases, page 319.

Since unheated honey is such an energizing and healing food in our fast polluted environments, we would be negligent to deprive our infants of completely unheated honey. If there were any ill reaction to honey in infants, it was probably from heated honeys. A rare infant may have a slight allergy to unheated honey but I have never seen any conclusive evidence of an ill reaction from unheated honey in over 120 infants. To test this without risk, I have put 1 drop of honey in 3 ounces of raw milk or good mineral water. In only one instance, a baby cried continuously for 15 minutes. I tried the 1-drop-of-honey test in a week and there was no ill reaction.

Colic: When an infant enters this world he or she does so as a raw-food eater. The mother's blood has not been cooked or sterilized even though the mother may have been eating cooked foods. However, babies always developed better when drinking raw cow or raw goat milk because those animals ate only raw food. When a baby had colic and continuous diarrhea for 36 hours with raw cow or goat milk, blending 2 tablespoons unsalted raw butter and ½-1 teaspoon unheated honey into every cup of warm raw milk usually corrected colic. Sometimes, blending ¼ teaspoon of raw ginger root juice (pressed with a garlic press) with every cup of raw milk helped. If colic persisted even after unsalted raw butter, or unheated honey or raw ginger juice was added, feeding the baby 1 raw fertile egg blended with 2 ounces of good mineral water nourished the baby. However, the immature protein from eggs does not supply much body-building material. Therefore, after a week of raw eggs and water, raw cow or raw goat milk was tried again.

Diaper Rash: Applying a little of the mixture of ½ cup good mineral water and 1 tablespoon unheated honey has usually promoted healing. When rashes had persisted, applying salves for rash usually relieved discomfort immediately (see Rash, page 306). Getting a little direct sunshine discourages the yeast involved in diaper rash. Letting baby's skin breathe without a diaper as often as possible also discourages yeast.

Diarrhea: Feeding 2-3 tablespoons unripe banana blended with 2-3 ounces raw plain kefir or raw milk stops diarrhea and replaces nutrients lost as a result of diarrhea. If raw plain kefir or raw milk is not available, replace the kefir with good mineral water. Do not feed apples in any form to a baby suffering diarrhea because apples overstimulate adrenaline production, which often causes diarrhea in infants.

Fever: It has been my experience that fevers below 104.5° Fahrenheit are important to healing and do not result in brain damage when babies are eating a raw-food diet; that is, mother's or raw cow or raw goat milk. Feeding a blend of 2 ounces fresh raw celery juice, 1 ounce fresh raw carrot juice, 1 ounce fresh raw tomato puree and 1 raw egg keeps fever at a comfortable temperature without danger. Feeding that drink slightly chilled or applying moist cool compresses (not cold) to the forehead reduces fever in the head if fever reaches 104-105° Fahrenheit.

Hiccups: *See* Hiccups, page 272.

Teething: Feeding ½ teaspoon of the butter/honey mixture every 20-30 minutes during obvious gum pain eliminates or reduces pain to bearable. Drinking a blended mixture of 1 cup raw milk and ½ teaspoon bee pollen, or ½ cup raw milk, ½ cup raw carrot juice and ½ teaspoon bee pollen has relieved teething pain. Gently rubbing unheated-above-96° Fahrenheit fermented coconut oil or peanut oil on the gums soothes them. *See* Pain page 297

INFERTILITY is the inability to produce offspring. If a woman's reproductive organs are properly formed, infertility generally results from poor mucus production in the ovaries and uterus. The mucus or its fiber is too sparse, or too thin, or too short, or weak. Fertility clinics are usually unnecessary. Spermicides, lubricants, birth control pills and chemical douches absorbed into the uterine walls cause poor mucus formation and/or production, and damage ovaries and ovum quality and production. An unheated-above-96° Fahrenheit fermented coconut oil is the best lubricant that will not cause side effects.

Drinking 2 smoothies daily, 5 days weekly for 6 months, or 1 smoothie daily, 5 days weekly for up to 2 years, along with a healthy raw diet that includes raw meat, corrects the mucus formation and ovum problems. Foods and substances to avoid that interfere with mucus and ovum productions and quality are: coffee (including decaffeinated), caffeine, aspirin, sodas, teas, horseradish and mustard. Caffeine also disturbs the spermatozoa's swim. *See* Eggs, page 184.

Occasionally, simply douching with a raw fertile egg at fertility time will suffice. If the mucus quality remains insufficient during pregnancy, miscarriage may result.

I have had clients who had not been able to get pregnant for up to 16 years. They became impregnated after two years or less on a healthy raw diet that included raw meat.

INFLUENZA (FLU): This is mainly a viral detoxification of the respiratory, intestinal and/or lymphatic systems, like cleaning the carbon from a car's engine. Influenza flushes the body of many accessible stored toxins and allows for a fresher, cleaner-running body. Rejoice and see them through. Increased vitality follows if flu are not stopped with drugs and a healthful diet is eaten that helps the flu process.

Viruses are not living organisms. They are solvents manufactured within cells. They do not self-replicate as believed. Viruses are body soaps. They cleanse contaminated cells, or parts of cells, from the body. When damaged, decaying or dead cells are so polluted that microbes, such as bacteria, parasites and fungi, cannot eat and eliminate the contaminated damaged, decaying or dead tissue, cells manufacture viruses (solvents) to dissolve and dilute the chemically contaminated waste for elimination through mucous membranes, skin, tear ducts, ear wax, gums and tongue.

I reiterate, when damaged, decaying and dead cells are too toxic from chemical pollution (from shampoos, cosmetics, medication, preservatives and pesticides in food, processed foods, and pollution of water, air and land), bacteria and fungi cannot survive to eat and discard those contaminated damaged, decaying and dead cells. The body almost exclusively uses viruses (solvents) to dissolve, and hopefully neutralize and eliminate those contaminated damaged, decaying and dead cells. Science knows that viruses are NOT living organisms. They cannot reproduce so, the belief that they self-replicate is preposterous. Cells manufacture viruses. Viruses are solvents. Saying that viruses self-replicate is the same as saying soap self-replicates.

Eating plenty of smoothies all day long for as long as flu endures facilitates that detoxification process. *See* Smoothies, page 200.

Stomach flu: Drinking plenty of naturally carbonated water with plenty of unheated honey for a day or so allows the stomach and intestines to cleanse. Then drinking plenty of smoothies, such as eggs blended with unripe banana, facilitates the detoxification and elimination processes.

INSECT BITES: Applying raw fresh raw lime juice helps dissolve and neutralize insect's saliva. Applying a mixture of ½ teaspoon powdered sun-dried clay, 1½ tablespoons of water and 1 drop of stone-pressed olive oil, attracts and absorbs poisons and soothes the area. Or, if fresh raw corn on the cob is available, simply chew some and apply it to the bitten area. If the bitten area continues to swell, make a poultice with 1 tablespoon corn starch, 2 teaspoons good mineral water, 1 pinch of powdered mustard, 2 drops stone-pressed olive oil and ½ pinch of fresh self-grated nutmeg.

If it is a poisonous bite, apply a poultice made of 1 teaspoon fresh shredded and minced beet, 1½ teaspoon fresh raw lime juice and ½ teaspoon powdered sun-dried clay.

Another poisonous bite poultice is: 1 teaspoon normally cooked moist coffee grounds, 1 teaspoon fresh raw lime juice and ¼ teaspoon powdered sun-dried clay. (I never suggest that anyone drink coffee of any sort, but topically it works for poisonous bites in an emergency.)

INSOMNIA is the inability to sleep soundly characterized by frequent waking and restlessness.

For those who had raw milk available, slowly drinking a blended mixture of 1 cup warm raw milk and 1-3 tablespoons unheated honey immediately before bedtime relaxed them for the night. For those who did not have fresh raw dairy, a smoothie made with 2-3 raw eggs, ½ to 1 whole unripe raw unripe banana and as much unheated honey as desired usually took them through the night. If bananas were not appealing, another fresh unripe raw fruit mixed with 3-4 tablespoons unheated honey worked. (Do not make a smoothie with berries or apple. Berries mixed with raw egg often causes drugs and toxic minerals to detoxify from glands, and apple excites adrenals. Either combination may interfere with sleep.)

For people who felt wired, eating raw fish a few hours before bedtime, and then drinking one of the suggestions in the paragraph above near bedtime got them through the night.

Another choice was a piece of toast with plenty of raw jam made of equal parts fresh raw berries and unheated honey. (Berries, especially raspberries, eaten with the Nut Formula made without egg, or eaten with unheated honey and toast supplies minerals that relax the body, and do not cause detoxification as berries do when eaten with egg or coconut cream.)

INTESTINAL CRAMPS: Eating ½ an avocado with ½ a papaya usually stopped cramping within 20 minutes. Eating honey/butter mixture (1 part honey to 4 parts butter) often throughout the day soothes the intestines. Eating raw custard once daily improves digestion and intestinal ease. *See* custard recipe page 56, footnote. *See* Colitis, page 249.

INTESTINAL INFECTION (a detoxification) is characterized by abdominal swelling and discomfort, poor digestion, flatulence, cramps, diarrhea and sometimes headache.

Eating 1-2 smoothies made with ½ raw unripe banana and 1-3 raw eggs, 1 tablespoon unheated honey and, when available, 2-4 tablespoons raw cream daily, and 2 raw custards daily soothes and heals the intestines during infection. Avoid any whole vegetables, lettuce, spinach, carrots, parsley, etc., until several days after the intestinal discomfort has subsided. However, drinking the raw juice of predominantly low-carbohydrate vegetables such as celery and parsley promotes a healthier intestinal environment, but not in children under 15 years of age. *See* also Peritonitis for the tomato drink, page 36-43.

ITCHY SKIN: This is a condition usually caused by high adrenaline, drugs (medical or recreational), pesticides, preservatives and condiment salt including sea salt (Celtic or other). The excess adrenaline, salt and chemicals utilize all available fats, or fats are not available because they are not eaten, or fats are not digested, assimilated or utilized properly and leave the skin dry. As toxins leave through the skin, they cause excessive dryness that results in itchy skin and sometimes hives.

Eating plenty of raw fat gradually lubricates the skin. Topically, blend ¼ cup of good mineral water, 1 small tomato, or ¼ cup of melon with 1 tablespoon unsalted raw butter, unheated-above-96° Fahrenheit fermented coconut oil or 1 tablespoon stone-pressed olive oil. So that the oils are properly homogenized, blend until ingredients are warm to the touch. Pouring this mixture into a hot bath - no hotter than the body is comfortable in - and soaking for 15-30 minutes usually bring immediate relief.

If suffering with hives, pour into a not-too-hot bath the mixture of tomato or melon blended with butter, coconut or olive oil (recipe given above), then add ½ cup sun-dried clay or corn starch, and soak in the bath for 20 minutes. That will draw the toxicity from the skin as well as soothe it. The warmth of the bath increases circulation and hydrates the skin which is usually dehydrated from excess adrenaline or drugs, pesticides and preservatives. *See* Baths/Sauna/Steam, page 326.

Some people would be relieved of itchy skin simply by pouring 1/3 cup raw unpasteurized apple cider vinegar into a hot bath and soaking for 15-30 minutes. To lubricate the skin, add 3-4 tablespoons of raw coconut cream to the bath water.

For people with overactive adrenals (hyperactivity), eating a Nut Formula (page 194) usually resolves itchy skin caused by excess adrenaline. Or a less healthy alternative that works is eating a combination 1-2 pieces of toast, a jam (made by blending 4 ounces raw fresh fruit with 2 tablespoons unheated honey and 2-4 nonsteamed dates) and a fat (½-1 avocado, or 4-8 tablespoons unsalted raw butter, or 4-6 tablespoons coconut cream).

JAUNDICE usually results from liver contamination, exhaustion and malfunction from pasteurized dairy, most medication and chemicals. Sometimes kidney dysfunction causes jaundice, and sometimes the inability to digest cooked lactate (the milk sugar in pasteurized milk) is responsible. Undigested lactate strains the liver. The same applies to carbohydrates in grains, such as rice, that cannot be completely digested or assimilated, and collect in the liver and kidneys.

Avoid medication, chemicals, including foods grown with pesticides and herbicides, food treated with additives and preservatives, and avoid drinking any milk that has been heated above 100° Fahrenheit for the rest of your life. Avoid drinking raw milk for 3-7 days while the liver gets cleansed and alkalized. Drinking ½ cup of raw fresh carrot juice, preferably with 2 tablespoons raw coconut cream or raw dairy cream the first thing every morning for 3 weeks supplies the liver and blood with missing nutrients during this disorder. *See* the foods suggested in Alkalizing food, page 178.

KIDNEY INFECTION (a detoxification) is characterized by pain originating in the middle back that reaches around to the lower abdominal area, frequent urination, sometimes blood or pus in the urine, nausea, and vomit.

Throughout each day of infection, drinking a large glass of good mineral water with 3 tablespoons fresh raw lime juice and beet or ½ cup raw fresh vegetable juices (that includes 1 ounce beet juice) with 3 ounces of good mineral water ½ hour before eating has nurtured and soothed the kidneys. (The juice and water were mixed or drunk separately.) Raw lime and beet juices and fresh raw corn on the cob regulate bacteria levels so that infection does not become excessive. If there is blood in the urine, it is best to stay off the feet and remain sedentary.

KIDNEY STONES are crystallized cooked vegetable-fat resins and crystallized hydrogenated fats and oils, and mineral salts that collect and form into clusters and clumps in the kidneys. I have had many kidney stones analyzed. Most were composed of food additives such as flavor and fragrance oils. Many were composed of crystallized oils from syrups and candies.

Most stones are formed during sleep. Kidney stones cause pain originating in the middle back that reaches around to the lower abdominal area, increased urination that sometimes contains blood or pus, sometimes sharp pains in the kidneys, and nausea and vomiting.

Two to three hours before sleep, abstaining from solid food and drinking a mixture of 1 cup warm raw milk with 4 tablespoons raw cream and 2 tablespoons unheated honey relaxes kidneys during sleep. Drinking a blended mixture of ½ cup raw unripe pineapple, 1 tablespoon raw unpasteurized apple cider vinegar, 3 tablespoons fresh raw lemon juice and 4-6 tablespoons raw coconut cream helps gradually dissolves kidney stones. Or 6-8 tablespoons of fresh raw lemon or lime juice mixed with 6 tablespoons fresh raw beet juice, 2 ounces fresh raw carrot juice and 4-6 tablespoons raw coconut cream 2-3 hours before sleep gradually dissolves kidney stones. Eating at least ½ cup of raw fat (for instance, avocado or unsalted raw butter) daily usually prevents large kidney stones.

When stones are being dissolved, there may be some discomfort. Drinking plenty of raw milk to which you have added 4-6 tablespoons raw cream and 2 tablespoons unheated honey per 28 ounces of raw milk, and staying in bed for 1-2 days allows the body to use all of its accessible nutrients and energies for dissolving stones, making the process easier.

KWASHIORKOR is another severe form of malnutrition. It occurs in people who live primarily on starches and sugars, especially cooked.

Symptoms: diarrhea, edema, loss of appetite, nervous irritability, poor skin and hair conditions; and in children, the symptoms are retarded mental and physical growth.

Eating a balanced raw diet with plenty of raw fish and/or raw fowl for 3-6 months settles that condition. *See* the book The Recipe For Living Without Disease, Chapter 12. If after 6 months (when the protein levels are built-up or restored) lethargy continues, eating red meat, like beef, corrects the problem (anemia).

LICE: There are several ways of dealing with these little creatures. It is difficult to ascertain which will work for whom. Use your instincts and intuition.

Vigorously oiling the body, especially the hairy areas, with a mixture of 1 tablespoon raw apple cider vinegar with 4 tablespoons unheated-above-below-96° Fahrenheit fermented coconut oil or stone-pressed olive oil or cold-pressed-below-96° Fahrenheit flax oil, and leaving it on thickly for several hours and then wiping excess (without washing) and leaving it on for twenty-four hours smothers lice and retards the eggs from hatching. (Clothes and bed sheets might get stained.) After twenty-four hours, slicing the oily part of the rind of a lime, eliminating the white pulp, and juicing or blending the rind with the meat of the lime, and then rubbing the oily lime juice over the entire body, vigorously over hairy areas, removes lice and eggs.

In case the oil and lime don't work, simply applying urine three times daily without washing at all for twenty-four hours gets rid of lice and eggs easily. (The odor can be endured.)

The standard chemical attack of poisoning the skin along with the lice may be easier for some people but I certainly do not recommend it. If you use a chemical to rid lice, after use, rinse with a mixture of ½ cup raw unpasteurized apple cider vinegar and 4 cups water to remove the loose chemical. Then whip 2-3 raw eggs and vigorously rub the eggs into the skin and let them remain on the skin for 20-40 minutes; the eggs will absorb some of the chemical poison that has penetrated the skin. Rinse again with the mixture of apple cider vinegar and water. Then apply unheated-above-96° Fahrenheit fermented coconut oil or stone-pressed olive oil to help soothe chemically poisoned and burned skin.

LYME DISEASE seems to be another smokescreen to blame nature for disease that is actually created by accumulated toxicity from medical and industrial chemicals, and poor diets. There are only conflicting reports and far-fetched stretches of scientific fantasy that support claims that Lyme Disease exists and comes from ticks. The debilitating symptoms that are attributed to Lyme Disease are common symptoms of severe toxicity. Since the medical community is unwilling to acknowledge that medicine and industry cause most diseases, they search for any relationship between us and other creatures. If they find anything similar, they vigorously attempt to blame that for a disease that they have no success identifying, labeling and treating.

Many desperate people believe the medical community's weak explanations of the varied tests for and symptoms of Lyme Disease and accept poisonous medication. I have observed approximately 14 people who were medically diagnosed with Lyme Disease and adhered to the Primal Diet. All of them reversed their symptoms within 2½ years. Most felt much better within 3 months on the balanced Primal Diet. *See* the book The Recipe For Living Without Disease, Chapter 12 for balanced diet.

If you truly have an allergy to the saliva of a tick, following the recommendations for bites would help. Also, blend a mixture of 10 ounces of lime juice, 10 ounces unheated honey and 3½ ounces of raw cream or never-heated-above-96° Fahrenheit fermented coconut oil or stone-pressed olive oil. Drinking 4 ounces at a time every 3-4 hours daily for 10 days usually resolves any allergy to insect fluids.

LIVER PROBLEMS: Alcohol, caffeine, chocolate, sodas, coffees and teas complicate liver problems and should not be consumed.

Eating ½ pound nonsteamed dates with 12 tablespoons unsalted raw butter or with 1 cup raw cream or with 9 tablespoons never-heated-above-96° Fahrenheit fermented coconut oil or stone-pressed olive oil each day until problems cease, helps the liver work easier. (Dates and oil can be eaten together or at separate times.) Then eating plenty of unheated honey with everything, and in between, supplies the liver with plenty of enzymes for its work. Eating 10-15 raw tomatoes for 1-2 days weekly alkalizes the liver. Normally, eating a balanced raw diet with plenty of raw meat over many years rebuilds the liver.

When feeling nauseous, it is helpful to eat 1-2 teaspoons of no-salt-added raw unheated cheese with an equal quantity of fat, especially unsalted raw butter every 2-3 hours.

See suggestions for Cirrhosis of the Liver, page 248, and Hepatitis, page 271.

LOW BLOOD SUGAR: *See* Hypoglycemia, page 274.

LYMPHATIC CONGESTION is caused by toxicity accumulated in the lymphatic system, especially glands and nodes. The lymph system feeds every cell in the body except red and white blood cells. Additionally, the lymphatic system is responsible for neutralizing toxins, reducing toxins to smaller substances and eliminating them through tear ducts, ears (wax), mucous membranes, bowels, vagina, urinary tract and especially skin. Reversing lymphatic congestion takes time.

Symptoms: muscle and/or bone soreness, skin problems including psoriasis and eczema, chronic fatigue and chemical sensitivity.

From laboratory analysis, I observed that much lymphatic congestion results from chemicals such as medications, preservatives, pesticides and herbicides, in combination with hydrogenated oils such as margarine, soy, flavoring additives, safflower oils, and peanut butter. Those oils and combinations harden over time (5-20 years) and are not fluid at body temperature. Eating a balanced Primal Diet is important for slowly reversing lymphatic congestion (*see* the book The Recipe For Living Without Disease, Chapter 12).

To help our bodies melt and dissolve hardened lymphatic congestion, I suggest taking 1-1½ hours hot baths every 3-4 days. Drinking the following blended mixture immediately upon entering a hot [102° F (39° C) to 105° F (41° C] bath helps prevent the melted lymphatic congestion from hardening as much when the body temperature later normalizes: ¼-1 cup of unripe pineapple, 3-6 tablespoons coconut cream, 1-3 tablespoons unsalted raw butter, and 1-2 tablespoons raw dairy cream. Measured ingredients should be equal for suggested amounts, that is, for a person who is 4'-4'6" tall, the smallest amounts of each ingredient to be blended are ¼ cup pineapple, 3 tablespoons coconut cream, 1 tablespoon butter, and 1 tablespoon cream. A person who is 4'6"-5'2" tall should blend ½ cup pineapple, 3 tablespoons coconut cream, 1 tablespoon butter, and 1 tablespoon cream. A person who is 5'3"-5'9" tall should blend 2/3 cup pineapple, 4 tablespoons coconut cream, 1½ tablespoons butter, and 1½ tablespoons cream. A person who is 5'10"-6'2" tall should blend about ¾ cup pineapple, 6 tablespoons coconut cream, 2 tablespoons butter, and 2 tablespoons cream. A person who is 6'3"-6'10" tall should blend 1 cup pineapple, 6 tablespoons coconut cream, 3 tablespoons butter, and 2 tablespoons cream. After the bath, the bather will be weak. The bather should leave the bath slowly, and sit to dry. Then bundle in very warm natural clothing and take a 30-45-minute easy walk.

Standard lymphatic massages that are offered by alternative practitioners are brutal, causing internal lacerations, and dried and hardened lymphatic networks to break and leak into connective tissue. The best lymphatic massage is to touch the skin so lightly that it almost tickles, causing great neuro-stimulation between the brain and whole body that stimulates and relaxes all circulatory systems.

MALNUTRITION: Practically everyone is suffering to some extent from eating cooked and processed foods and pollution. Eating a raw diet of fresh fruit with plenty of raw fat, raw vegetable juices, and raw meat strengthens the body. *See* the book The Recipe For Living Without Disease, Chapter 12.

MEASLES are viral infections that detoxify the lymph system and strengthen the whole body. Measles should be allowed to run their course.

Common measles: Early symptoms are fever, cough and eye inflammation. Within 48 hours, red spots appear on the cheeks. Within 5 days from the early symptoms, a rash forms that usually starts on the neck and spreads to the rest of the body. Fever declines as the rash spreads.

To prevent any damage to organs and cells during measles, it is important to drink good mineral waters with fresh raw lemon juice. Drinking smoothies made of raw eggs blended with fresh raw fruit and unheated honey and, if available, raw milk helps to speed this detoxification. After measles have run their course, eating plenty of fresh raw tomatoes soothes and relaxes membranes. Eating a balanced raw diet with plenty of raw fat and raw meat feeds, rebuilds and strengthens the lymph.

German measles (this is the milder of the measles detoxifications): Symptoms may include fever, headache, stiff joints, and a rash that lasts about three days appearing on arms, chest and forehead. German measles is a thyroid detoxification that causes localized lymph glands to detoxify simultaneously.

Making a poultice of 3 tablespoons powdered sun-dried clay mixed with 2 ounces good mineral water and applying it to the entire neck, especially the thyroid area, for 35 minutes supplies minerals to facilitate detoxification. It is best to rap a damp cloth around the neck to keep the clay pack moist. *See* Clay, page 181.

Drinking raw milk helps this condition best. However, if raw milk is not available, drinking smoothies made of raw eggs blended with raw unripe banana and unheated honey speeds this detoxification. After this detoxification has run its course, eating plenty of fresh raw tomatoes soothes and relaxes membranes. Eating a balanced raw diet with plenty of raw fat and raw meat feeds, rebuilds and strengthens the lymph.

MEMORY LOSS AND OTHER SIMPLE MENTAL MALFUNCTIONS: Drinking fresh raw carrot juice or other fresh raw vegetable juices with raw milk, if available, daily, restores mental functions. Drinking fresh raw ginger root blended in raw juices or grated and eaten with other foods helps to stimulate mental functions. Drinking fresh raw asparagus juice with other vegetable juices helps mental functions. A lot of memory problems result from concentrations of accumulated toxins, especially aluminum from vaccines, cooking utensils, canned food and drinks, and packaging, including aluminum foil. Eating ½-1 cup organic raspberries blended with 4-6 tablespoons raw coconut cream, 1 tablespoon unsalted raw butter, 1½ tablespoons raw dairy cream and 1 tablespoon unheated honey helps remove aluminum from the body. Adding ½ teaspoon clay to that drink increases its effectiveness. If you do not like the taste with clay added to it, you could put the clay in your mouth and wash it down with the raspberry drink. *See* Clay page 181.

See Hypoglycemia, page 274.

MENIÈRE'S SYNDROME is a disease of the labyrinth of the ear characterized by recurrent deafness, ringing in the ear, dizziness, nausea and vomiting. It is chiefly caused by lack of enzyme-mutations for assimilating and utilizing minerals in cooked and processed foods.

Eating plenty of full-fat raw milk, no-salt-added raw cheeses and raw meat heal this mineral imbalance in time. *See* Mineral Deficiency, page 291.

MENINGITIS is a detoxification of the two inner coatings of the brain (cerebral), or spinal cord (spinal), more commonly occurring in children. Meningitis detoxifications are either bacterial or viral, and are mainly caused by metal toxicity that settled in the brain or spinal cord. Often, they are caused by the mercury, aluminum and formaldehyde in vaccines. The reason so many children develop meningitis is because they receive vaccines that damage nerve and brain cells.

Symptoms: fluctuating high fever, chills, headache, stiff neck, nausea, vomiting, drowsiness, sometimes pneumonia-like symptoms and temporary excruciatingly crippling pain in back and/or legs, and rarely coma.

Eating ½ cup unheated honey in good mineral water every hour for 8 hours has eased congestion. Then eating 4-6 tablespoons of Pain formula every 2-3 hours remarkably eases pain. Eating a little alkalizing food and raw meat, especially fish, every 2-3 hours (between Pain Formulas) has healed the membranes. *See* Alkalizing Food, page 178. *See* Pain, page 297 for recipe, and Pain Formula in the book The Recipe For Living Without Disease, Chapter 15.

MENOPAUSE is the cessation of the menstrual cycle. There is so much psychological baggage with this change (for instance, women fear loss of hormones, youth and sexual appeal), but the only natural loss in this life cycle is the ability to have children.

As long as a woman can digest properly, if she eats a predominantly raw diet with full-fat raw milk (when available), 2-4 raw eggs, raw meat twice daily, and no-salt-added raw cheese, her body will continue to produce hormones and keep her glands and organs from drying. Eating fresh raw peppermint leaves or fresh raw cucumber (or the fresh raw juice of both) soothes, relaxes, helps digestion, and rids her of the bloated feeling. Eating raw melons, including unripe banana, eases the ill side effects of hormonal changes. If available, drinking 1-2 cups of raw yam juice with 3 tablespoons raw coconut cream with each cup of yam juice once every 3-8 days ensures hormonal production that balances mineral levels after menopause. Yam juice should be consumed within 1 hour after juicing.

For some women, having sex is beneficial because it flushes hormones and expedites the hormonal changes of menopause (not hormonal cessation). If lacking a sex partner during this cycle, self-sex is helpful for some people. Although a woman may have completed menopause, she may occasionally experience menstruation. That is a healthy function where the body cleanses those tissues.

MENSTRUAL CRAMPS are abdominal muscle contractions that sometimes accompany menstruation, and are usually painful. These cramps are directly related to a lack of utilizable proteins in the blood. Either a sufferer is not eating enough meat or she doesn't digest, assimilate, or utilize cooked meat.

Eating at least 5 raw mushrooms daily for 5 days before menstrual onset with a raw green salad, and eating raw red meat, like tuna, beef, or lamb, usually prevents these cramps. (Raw mushrooms contain enzymes that facilitate protein utilization.) *See* Premenstrual Syndrome, page 304. Drinking the blended mixture of raw milk and bee pollen, or raw carrot juice and bee pollen relieves pain. *See* Pain, page 297. For another Pain Formula, *see* the book The Recipe For Living Without Disease, Chapter 15.

MENSTRUATION, LATE: Drinking 1 cup of fresh raw beet juice with 2 tablespoons unheated honey helps bring on and regulate menstruation unless you are pregnant; or eating grated fresh raw ginger root or fresh raw horseradish root with other foods usually brings on and regulates menstruation.

MENTAL ILLNESS is a condition in which a person has tremendous difficulty dealing "rationally" with problems and stress. Although the problems may be normal, the emotionally challenged individual is overwhelmed by them. Some people react antisocially. That usually occurs in very sensitive, overly criticized individuals who are in constant fear of making disastrous decisions. I have found that the resultant stress overtaxes the nervous and glandular systems. Neural and glandular irritation and exhaustion result in actual physiological imbalances, such as: hypoglycemia, diabetes, thinning of neural membranes, and thyroid malfunction. Unless physical health is restored, psychotherapy of any kind is not likely to be complete or long-lasting.

Eating a raw diet that includes some cooked starch with plenty of raw fat and some raw unripe fruit 1-2 times daily helps balance hormonal levels. Eating plenty of raw fat, including no-salt-added raw cheese and raw cream (when available), and meat, especially fish, gradually restores health to glands and nerves.

A fun deficiency is also the cause. If you are not having enough fun you are probably criticizing yourself and others. Be a cheerleader for yourself. Trust and encourage yourself and others in whatever is right for each of you as individuals. Although education and science try to formulate everything and everybody, no two people will ever think or act alike, or have the same tastes. Just as two flowers on the same stem are different, both are beautiful and right. Only machines that have no choice follow formulas. If you try to validate yourself by comparing yourself to other people's thinking and talents, you will always be confused and insecure. When you have a taste (a need) for strawberries and someone else has a taste (a need) for oranges, each of you is right for yourself.

Listening to one's self, discovering one's likes and dislikes, and trusting one's choices based on those likes and dislikes are important to liking yourself. Finding an appealing creative outlet, not comparing one's creativity to anyone else's, and pursuing that creative outlet help build self-esteem. *See* Depression, page 254, and Awareness, page 325. *See* the book The Recipe For Living Without Disease, Chapters 12 and 15.

MIGRAINES: *See* Headaches, Migraines, page 268.

MINERAL DEFICIENCY is the lack of minerals needed to provide for proper body development and/or functions.

Symptoms: very warped and grooved nails, chapped lips, reserved attitude toward people, and lots of fecal matter produced because food doesn't digest well.

For several days weekly, drinking ¼ teaspoon clay with a little mineral water, usually corrects mineral deficiencies. Most people have benefited best by drinking this in the mornings. Although fresh raw juices, especially vegetable, are high in minerals, the body uses most of those vitamin-coupled minerals in solution to transport glucose to the brain and bind with toxins. Therefore, drinking clay in water, rather than in juices, works best.

Some people need to eat several fertile raw eggs with good mineral water to correct this deficiency. Drinking two eggs and chasing them with mineral water may be an easier way of taking this combination. Another way would be to blend and drink a combination of 2-3 fertile raw eggs with ½ cup good mineral water, juice of ½ fresh raw lemon, 1-2 tablespoons unheated honey and 1 teaspoon clay. *See* Clay, page 181.

Some people need to eat fresh raw celery too, to correct this imbalance. Whole celery, not just the juice, should be eaten. Eating no-salt-added raw cheeses also supplies needed concentrations of minerals.

MISCARRIAGE: To stop bleeds or hemorrhage, *see* Hemorrhage, page 270.

Eating eggs, even when raw, more than 5 days in succession sometimes causes uterine mucus to thin, becoming watery, and increases the possibility of miscarriage. However, eating raw eggs (as in milk shakes and smoothies) for 5 days, then not eating eggs for 2 days, and repeating this cycle helps build and sustain the strong stable mucus needed to maintain pregnancy. Eating a balanced raw diet helps support stable pregnancy. *See* the book The Recipe For Living Without Disease, Chapter 12.

Too much horseradish may cause mucus to thin and should not be eaten too frequently by women prone to miscarriage, unless they crave it.

Sexual intercourse with orgasm during the eighth month often makes the blood too rich in hormones for the fetus to properly establish brain functions. Sometimes this results in miscarriage. Kissing and petting without orgasm are good. (It might be a sensitive gesture for the man to refrain from having orgasm also.)

Moldy foods and moldy environments can cause miscarriage.

Women who are prone to miscarriage can maintain pregnancy better by remaining flat on their backs as much as possible. Doing Hatha yoga stretch exercises (except for the Sun-salutation) stimulates circulation and tone while being sedentary.

MONONUCLEOSIS often coincides with depressed states of being. Finding a creative outlet, or doing something that is enjoyable everyday, enriches life. Food-poisoning is often misdiagnosed as mononucleosis because the maladies sometimes produce similar virus.

Eating plenty of raw meat helps correct this mineral-imbalance-related virus, that is, detoxification. Drinking raw milk, when available, at the same meal with raw meat helps mineral absorption.

Avoid smoking for the rest of life and try to avoid smoky places. Smoking is especially harmful for people who have had this detoxification. The best healing results are achieved by not exercising for a 5-weeks period during mononucleosis, and afterward exercise plenty.

MOTION SICKNESS is intense nausea caused by involuntary constant fluctuations of the fluids in the inner ear, as experienced in the motion of an airplane, boat or car.

Drinking a blend of 6 ounces warm good mineral water, the fresh juice of a whole lemon and 2 tablespoons unheated honey every 1-2 hours helps relax this condition. Deep slow breathing also helps. Applying gentle pressure to the insides of the wrists gives immediate relief. You may have to continue the pressure for awhile.

MULTIPLE SCLEROSIS is a disease that deteriorates the protective coating of the nerves in the brain and spinal cord, causing scars or lesions and hardening of the affected nerves. This is similar to ALD which occurs in children, but multiple sclerosis usually develops more gradually in adults between the ages of 25 and 40. It is chiefly caused by metal- and chemical-toxicity, and by lack of enzyme-mutations for digesting, assimilating and utilizing cooked and processed green and red foods.

Symptoms include bowel and bladder problems, dizziness, loss of balance and coordination, emotional, visual and speech disturbances, and paralysis.

Avoiding cooked and processed green and red foods, and eating plenty of raw fats, like raw cream, full-fat raw milk, no-salt-added raw cheeses, 4 tablespoons of stone-pressed olive oil with each of 4 meat meals weekly, and at least ½ avocado daily, eventually stops the progression of multiple sclerosis. Eating fresh raw fish, antibiotic-free and hormone-free raw poultry, raw red meat, and raw eggs provides the body with the nutrients it needs to regenerate nerves and myelin tissue. Physical activity is important to dissolve scar-blocked circulation to nerves. Eating ½-1 cup cucumber with 4-6 tablespoons raw coconut cream and 1 tablespoon unheated honey helps dissolve hardened nerve cells.

Drinking 2 cups of naturally sparkling mineral water daily for 5-10 days restores the electrolyte balance and oxygen level, and reduces adrenaline production that often deteriorates myelin.

MUSCLE CRAMP ("Charley Horse") is a muscle contraction, or spasm, that is most often painful. Arch your foot or hand backward while gently rubbing your leg or arm. There are a variety of deficiencies that cause cramps, but usually cramps occur when there are high concentrations of uric acid in the muscle accompanied with low blood fat or sugar or mineral levels. Eating concentrated carbohydrate foods without fat can cause cramps in hand, legs and feet.

Eating a combination of fresh raw unripe fruit (especially banana or pineapple or melon or tomato), raw fat, unheated honey and no-salt-added raw cheese quickly alleviates cramps. Or drinking 6-8 ounces of raw milk blended with 2 ounces bee pollen, or fresh raw juice blended with 2 ounces bee pollen or good mineral water blended with 3 tablespoons grated fresh raw ginger root quickly alleviates cramps. *See* Clay, page 181. Simply drinking ½-1 cup raw cream eases a cramp.

MUSCULAR DYSTROPHY is a condition chiefly caused by the lack of enzyme-mutations for eating cooked meat and cooked proteins, resulting in atrophy. Antibiotics and vaccines often cause loss of enzyme-mutations or the inability to produce enzyme-mutations.

Physical therapy in conjunction with hot baths and a diet consisting of plenty of raw eggs, raw meat (including raw fish), raw milk before sleep, and at least ½ cup unheated honey daily has stopped and often reversed degeneration. Drinking raw milk, when available, along with eating raw meat (including raw fish) has helped mineral absorption in this disease. Eating ½ unripe banana with 4-6 tablespoons raw coconut cream and 1½ tablespoons unheated honey helps dissolve hardened muscle cells. Getting as much sunlight as possible without sunblocks (lotions) and without sun glasses speeds the healing processes. *See* Fresh Air and Sunshine, page 334.

MUSCLE SORENESS usually results from uric acid concentrations in muscles from lack of enough utilizable blood and lymph nutrients, especially enzymes, fat, minerals and fruit sugar.

Taking long hot baths, and eating plenty of raw fish with raw avocado, and eating raw unripe bananas and melons relieve muscle soreness.

NAIL BITING is caused by mineral deficiencies or severe mineral imbalance. A person eats finger and/or toenails, instinctively, to recycle minerals in the nails. Eating any or all of the following usually corrects this mineral deficiency within 3 months: no-salt-added raw cheeses with an equal quantity of fat, especially unsalted raw butter, fresh raw ocean fish (including scallops, oysters or clams), whole raw milk, and, occasionally, ¼ teaspoon of clay. *See* Clay, page 181.

NAIL PROBLEMS: Avoiding salt most often settles this condition. Salt dries cells and interferes with mineral and fat utilization and the process of building nails. Ridges in the nails mainly result from mineral deficiencies. *See* Mineral Deficiency, page 291.

Drinking fresh raw milk within 2 hours after eating raw meat helps mineral assimilation and utilization, and consequently this condition.

Topically, making a balm of 5 parts unheated-above-96° Fahrenheit fermented coconut oil or stone-pressed olive oil and 1 part unsalted raw butter, when available, and rubbing it into the nails 2-3 times daily is helpful.

NAUSEA is the result of toxins dumping into the stomach to be neutralized or vomited. Drinking ½ cup unheated honey mixed with ¼ cup naturally sparkling mineral water helps ease nausea. The next best remedy is drinking the fresh juice of 1 lemon mixed with 4 tablespoons unheated honey and ¼ cup good mineral water. When experiencing frequent nausea, eating a little no-salt-added raw cheese with an equal quantity of raw fat, especially unsalted raw butter, and a little unheated honey will absorb toxins that dumped into the stomach.

NEURAL PROBLEMS: *See* Pain, page 297.

NIGHT BLINDNESS is distorted vision, including depth perception, in dark or dim light.

Drinking a blended combination of fresh raw lemon juice, 2-3 raw eggs and 1-3 tablespoons unheated honey alkalizes fluids in the eyeballs. Generally, though, this condition mainly results from low protein levels in the blood. Eating raw red meat gradually improves vision, including depth perception. Drinking raw carrot juice improves the general health of the eyes. Adding a little raw watercress juice to raw carrot juice increases healing of this condition. For better eye health, add 4 tablespoons raw cream or 2 tablespoons unsalted raw butter to 1 cup carrot juice.

OBESITY: *See* Overweight, below.

OVEREATING: *See* Food Addiction, page 264.

OVERWEIGHT: Being fat is not a "bad" condition. Fat storages are protective to all body systems and provide stamina. But if stored fat cannot be utilized, it can be burdensome, as it overtaxes the entire body, causes general exhaustion and may harden, causing build-ups, dryness and blockages.

Low thyroxin production often results from overweight. Overweight often results from the inability to utilize fat, resulting in dry skin and listless hair. *See* the suggestions for Thyroid Problem, page 315.

Overweight often results from the lack of the enzyme-mutations for eating cooked green foods. People who have that enzyme-mutation deficiency often have little white spots on the finger nails or toe nails. *See* If I Lack Enzyme-Mutations, What Foods Should I Avoid?, page 174.

Some people who have excessive insulin production have very watery fat (if slapped, it jiggles like gelatin). The extra water in their fat dilutes the toxicity produced by excessive hormones. Two foods that are especially helpful in reducing watery fat storages are fresh raw lime juice with good mineral water, or fresh raw lemon juice with good mineral water. Raw lemons and limes alkalize the tissues and neutralize volatile substances, reducing the need for edema.

Eating 40% of the daily calories consumed as raw fat supplies the body with healthy fat that gradually cleanses the system of useless fat or fat that has bound with toxins and stored by the body. *See* Fat For Great Health, page 185, Appendix O, pages 145-150, and Appendix W, page 162.

For people with firm or solid corpulence, eating ½ raw unripe pineapple daily for 2 weeks supplies the liver and pancreas with the enzymes they need to remove hardened fat properly. That regime may cause over-emotionality, so be certain to consume enough raw cheese with unsalted raw butter, raw cream and lots of raw meat. It takes 2 weeks on a raw diet before the liver and pancreas are balanced enough to begin gradually removing hardened-fat storages. Years are required to cleanse those glands of hardened fat. Eating plenty of raw fat ensures that hardened fat will be removed from the body. *See* Edema, page 260.

PAIN: Avoiding salt helps prevent the swelling and pressure on nerves that increase pain. A very effective pain remedy has been a blended mixture of 7-8 ounces full fat raw milk, 2 ounces fresh bee pollen and 1-2 tablespoons unheated honey. Drink 2-4 ounces immediately and refrigerate remainder. Sip 1-2 tablespoons every 20 minutes until pain is gone. Shake each time before drinking. Repeat the entire procedure if pain returns.

General pain will also be alleviated by eating raw butter, or raw eggs, or any other raw fat, especially when combined with unheated honey. Eating eggs is usually necessary during pain for binding with toxins and removing them from the body. Released toxins cause swelling and therefore pain. However, sometimes eating eggs causes more detoxification, which increases or prolongs pain. If pain increases rather than decreases 20 minutes after eating eggs, stop eating eggs until pain has ceased. After pain has stopped, wait 2 days before eating eggs again.

Pain from broken bones: Alex was a seven-year-old boy who completely broke and dislocated both bones in his forearm and experienced a lot of pain. To make his pain tolerable, he ate a golf ball-sized amount of fresh antibiotic-free and hormone-free ground turkey with unheated honey and unsalted raw butter, then waited 2 hours and ate some unripe banana, then waited 2 hours and ate raw turkey, honey and butter again, and 2 hours later he ate banana. He continued eating like that and within 12 hours, his pain was minimal.

Tooth pain: Eating plenty of fish and avoiding citrus and ripe fruit, avoiding exercise and avoiding strenuous activities speed this detoxification and reduce pain.

However, once when I had an excruciatingly painful toothache, to make the pain tolerable, I ate ½ cup of raw ground beef with honey and butter, waited two hours and ate ½ unripe banana. Like Alex did for broken bones, I alternated those foods continuously for eight hours until the pain subsided. If a person is acidic, eating beef can increase pain rather than alleviate it by raising the adrenaline level and blood pressure. If a person is high in adrenaline (an indication that a person is inclined to be acidic), eating beef may increase pain. Therefore, drinking full-fat raw milk blended with fresh bee pollen, and eating raw fish, butter/honey mix, and no-salt-added raw cheese mitigate pain.

Gum sensitivity is most often the result of low blood protein level accompanied by low blood sugar level. Eating plenty of unheated honey and drinking raw milk with raw meat (or within 2 hours after eating raw meat) mitigate gum pain.

Chest pains around the heart: *See* Angina Pectoris, page 224.

Growing pains are mitigated by drinking plenty of full-fat raw milk, and getting fresh air and sunshine.

Muscular pain: Drinking plenty of full-fat raw milk, unripe bananas, fresh raw unripe pineapple, unripe melon, non-steamed dates and figs, and plenty of raw eggs most often mitigates muscular pain.

Pain caused by fissures in the finger tips: Drinking a quart of raw cream daily for 1-2 weeks, when available, then ½ cup daily until the condition stabilizes, relieves fissures and pain. If raw cream is not available, drinking the juice of fresh whole coconut meat (raw coconut cream) mixed with unheated honey gradually relieves the pain and heals the fissures.

Pain behind the knees is often related to anemia. Eating raw meat mitigates that pain.

Pain in the temples is indicative of toxic blood. Drinking the fresh raw juice of lemons between meals mitigates that pain. *See* Headache, page 268.

Pains in hands and feet are very often from low blood mineral absorption. Consuming plenty of unheated honey with food and in between eating foods, most often mitigates hand and foot pain. Eating raw fish and no-salt-added raw cheeses with an equal quantity of unsalted raw butter help correct mineral balances. *See* Clay, page 181.

Pain in the eyes and throat is often from a cooked lactose (pasteurized milk) intolerance. Drinking full-fat raw milk mixed with plenty of unheated honey and avoiding raw eggs until pain is gone mitigate those pains. If raw milk is not available, eating raw meat and drinking the fresh raw coconut cream with unheated honey mitigates pain.

Pain from shingles: *See* Shingles, page 310.

General tightness in the body often occurs from deteriorated nerve coatings (myelin). Eating plenty of raw fat, raw fish and as much unheated honey as possible with all food mitigates this pain and gradually restores the myelin.

For a general pain formula that has worked for almost every type of pain, *See* Pain Formula in the book The Recipe For Living Without Disease, Chapter 15.

PARANOIA is an exaggerated fear that someone, something, or life in general is going to destroy you. The psychological cause is cynicism. The physiological cause is low blood pressure, caused by allergies to pollutants, including medical or recreational drugs and pollution, and/or poor diet.

Eating the Nut Formula (page 194) or fresh raw garlic with a cooked starch and/or raw meat usually raises blood pressure within minutes and dissolves paranoia within 40 minutes. If drugs are continued, garlic has a limited effect on raising blood pressure and removing paranoia.

PARASITES that live in the body are friendly and should be allowed to run their course. They eat weak, damaged and decaying tissue. Parasites usually occur in individuals lacking enzyme-mutations for eating cooked green and red fruits and vegetables. *See* If I Lack Enzyme-Mutations, What Foods Should I Avoid?, page 174. Caffeine causes weakening and decaying of tissue.

If you get too weak during a tape worm detoxification, eating plenty of fresh raw onions with meat usually forces a tapeworm to evacuate with feces. Drinking lime juice usually prevents or minimizes any parasite's ability to reproduce. Avoiding cooked green and cooked red fruits and vegetables (including caffeine) and eating plenty of fresh raw red, orange and green foods, raw vegetable juices, unheated honey and fresh raw lemon juice cleanse the tissues and stop future need for parasites.

PARKINSON'S DISEASE is the slow destruction of an essential type of nerve cell. Overproduction of adrenaline, accompanied by metal toxicity, is often the major cause. Nerve cells spend too much fat trying to protect themselves from the high adrenaline acidity. Consequently, nerve cells are left deficient and vulnerable to toxins. Compoundedly, adrenaline often leaches fat from nerve cells.

Symptoms: rigidity, cramps and involuntary movements.

Eating a Nut Formula (page 194) or small amounts of cooked starches with plenty of raw fat at least three times daily reduces the high adrenaline that leads to nerve damage. Avoid cooked meats (except cooked chicken once weekly if necessary; *see* page 255-256). For Parkinson's, eating cooked meat creates too many volatile toxins, causing irritation to nerves and glands, dryness and overproduction of adrenaline. Eating plenty of raw meat, especially fresh raw fish and/or raw fowl, allows for healing and regeneration of nerve tissue. Processed sugars very often cause adrenaline and insulin overproduction. Therefore, avoiding cooked and processed sugars is essential in correcting Parkinson's disease.

PELLAGRA is severe malnutrition that is most common among people who mainly eat corn. However, low-grade pellagra is common with all people who have not developed enzyme-mutations for eating cooked or processed greens.

Early symptoms: anxiety, depression, loss of appetite and weight, reddened and swollen tongue, and weakness.

Progressed symptoms: skin changes, severe nerve dysfunction, and diarrhea.

Pellagra can most often be alleviated if the sufferer avoids eating or drinking cooked green foods. *See* If I Lack Enzyme-Mutations, What Foods Should I Avoid?, page 174.

Eating fresh raw greens or the juice of raw greens, if desired, helps flush the accumulated resins that are a major factor in this disease.

Eating a raw diet restores health.

PERITONITIS: *See* pages 36-43.

PERNICIOUS ANEMIA is the gradual reduction in the numbers of blood cells because the bone marrow fails to produce mature red blood cells. Pernicious anemia most often develops from low blood sugar, usually because of the inability to digest or utilize cooked and processed sugars.

Symptoms: weakness, gastrointestinal problems, sore tongue, sallow skin, and tingling extremities.

Avoid cooked and processed sugars. Eating raw meats, a little raw unripe fruit, and a minimum of ½ cup unheated honey daily supplies the nutrients necessary to reverse that condition. Since many other malfunctions are the result of pernicious anemia, eating small amounts of raw foods every few hours, instead of large meals, keeps the body freshly supplied with nutrients. Eating raw meat, especially beef, at least once daily with a Nut Formula (*see* page 194) or a little cooked starch with plenty of raw fat inspires healing. When the body begins to have hot flashes, pernicious anemia has begun to reverse. During hot flashes it is beneficial to consume unheated honey in good mineral water, or in raw milk.

PHLEBITIS is inflammation of vein walls, most commonly occurring in the legs. This is a fat and protein deficiency most often resulting from the inability to digest or assimilate or utilize cooked fat and cooked proteins. In many cases oral (birth control pills) and injected contraceptives cause phlebitis. Many cases are results of sulfa drugs or other medications taken to reduce water retention, and aluminum-poisoning (*see* Edema, page 260).

Symptoms: swollen and reddened veins, increased pulse rate, slight fever, and pain.

Consuming plenty of raw meat, including raw fish with raw milk, no-salt-added unheated cheese with an equal quantity of raw fat strengthens the veins. Pain can be minimized by eating the honey/butter mixture or raw milk blended with bee pollen. If feeling nervous, drinking a raw fertile egg by itself is calming.

PNEUMONIA is inflammation of the tiny air sacs in the lungs that fill with fluids and mucus. This usually happens following a severely stressful detoxification or medical procedure that has consumed all available nutrients. Consequently, mucus cannot be properly constructed to protect the lungs. Then, even a particle of dust or lint in the lungs causes fluids to collect, trying to cleanse the lungs. Pneumonia is always associated with internal or airborne toxins that irritate lungs and result in allergy.

Symptoms: fever and chills, more mucus, fatigue, rapid respiration, cough, sharp chest pains and sometimes headache.

Eating a little raw fish every couple of hours and drinking plenty of orange smoothies, that is, 2-4 raw eggs blended with raw fresh orange juice usually has ended this severe detoxification in two days. Continuing to drink the raw orange smoothies daily and eating only 1 cup of raw meat for one week has brought the mucous membranes to a healing state. After that, eating a balanced raw diet that included raw eggs and plenty of raw meat, including raw fish, strengthened and restored the mucous membranes to very good health.

POISON IVY, POISON OAK, and POISON SUMAC are itchy skin rashes that ooze when those plants' oils contact the skin. They do not bother everybody. Those easily vaporized oils land on the skin or enter the respiratory system and burn the skin, causing blisters that ooze, itch and seem to spread. The body absorbs, dilutes and distributes the oils over the largest area necessary to exhaust the volatility of the oils. The way to remove the oils is to absorb and dissolve them.

Firstly, rubbing raw unpasteurized apple cider vinegar into affected and surrounding areas helps neutralize the oils. Secondly, applying clay thickly to affected and surrounding areas, letting it dry and rinsing helps draw the oils from the skin. Thirdly, the Ayurvedic and tribal healing approach works best: Rubbing your urine onto the affected and surrounding areas once or twice daily and leaving it on all day and night usually subdues irritation and heals the condition. Urine, with its ammonia and proteins, helps dilute and neutralize the oils that have penetrated deep into skin. Fourthly, 1½-2 hours after urine has been on the skin, applying the Primal Facial Body Care Cream helps further neutralize the oils, and soothe and protect the skin from additional burn. For the Primal Facial Body Care Cream recipe, *see* the book The Recipe For Living Without Disease, Chapter 15.

POLIO is a viral detoxification of the spinal cord. Polio occurs in an individual who has an allergy to eating cooked green foods and cooked red fruits and vegetables. His or her digestion has not mutated to fractionate, assimilate or utilize those foods properly. Consequently, resins and residues collect in the spinal cord. However, most often polio has been caused by metal toxicity, especially from vaccines and household and agricultural pesticides that embed, contaminate and degenerate spinal tissue. In all cases of spinal cord contamination in which the body utilizes the poliomyelitis virus for detoxification, poor nutrition during that detoxification often results in massive nerve-cell destruction, resulting in partial paralysis. *See* If I Lack Enzyme-Mutations, What Foods Should I Avoid?, page 174.

Symptoms at the viral stage: nausea, fever, diarrhea, irritability and headache.

Eating raw greens, raw red fruits and vegetables, plenty of smoothies, unheated honey, raw fat and raw unpasteurized apple cider vinegar has helped remove the resins that have collected in the spine and nervous system (that the poliomyelitis detoxifies) without causing permanent paralysis. Eating raw meat often, including raw fish and/or raw fowl, restored nerve health. When a person already had paralysis from polio, eating those foods that were suggested above and avoiding those that should be avoided, gradually reversed some paralysis in every case.

POLLUTION FROM VEHICLES: *See* Asphyxiation, page 227, and Nausea, page 295.

PREMENSTRUAL SYNDROME (PMS): Low pyruvate (protein sugar) level in the blood is the main problem in PMS. Coffee and substances with caffeine, such as sodas, aspirin, and chocolate, irritate glands and nerves, creating toxicity, low blood sugar and irritability. (If you eat or drink a substance with caffeine during PMS, you are likely to hate everyone.) Also, avoiding processed, cooked and even raw sweets (unless it is raw unripe fruit with raw fat) helps prevent hormonal imbalances associated with PMS. Avoid eating cooked meats because, they create too many volatile toxins, drying and irritating the entire body. Women with too high adrenaline levels should eat mostly white raw meats during PMS.

Eating raw unripe fruit, raw green vegetable juices, and unheated honey encourages alkalinity and psychological stability. Drinking full-fat raw milk (when available), and eating fresh raw fish, raw mushrooms, and a diet that is high in raw fat works wonders. Women who get listless during and after menstruation develop a type of anemia during their cycle. Eating plenty of raw meat alleviates that condition. Eating white with red meat helps prevent irritability. For a balanced diet, *see* the book The Recipe For Living Without Disease, Chapter 12. *See* Menstrual Cramps, page 290.

PROSTATITIS is a detoxification of the prostate gland. This is primarily related to the lack of enzyme-mutations for eating cooked and processed greens; the resins and residues have collected in the prostate. *See* If I Lack Enzyme-Mutations, What Foods Should I Avoid?, page 174. When prostatitis is compounded with pollution, prostate cancer often results.

Symptoms: pain between the scrotum and rectum, frequent urination accompanied by a burning sensation, blood or pus in the urine and fever. Add the following symptoms for long term prostatitis: lower back pain, premature ejaculation, or loss of potency.

Drinking 8-12 ounces raw green vegetable juices with ½ teaspoon raw unpasteurized apple cider vinegar once or twice daily helps cleanse resins and residues that have collected in the prostate over many years of eating cooked greens. Eating zucchini, pumpkin seeds, and unheated bee pollen helps to revitalize the prostate gland.

PSORIASIS is characterized by patches of red eruptions on the skin that are sometimes covered with dry, silvery scales. These sores usually grow in size without healing. Psoriasis is mainly from lack of enzyme-mutations for eating cooked red fruits and vegetables; those resins congest the lymphatic system. *See* If I Lack Enzyme-Mutations, What Foods Should I Avoid?, page 174.

Allergies to volatile toxins is also a factor in many cases. *See* Preservatives and Pesticides, page 196, Edema, page 260, *and* Overweight, page 296.

Eating plenty of raw fat, fresh raw tomato puree and other raw red and orange foods (like strawberries, cherries, red bell peppers, oranges and carrot juice) along with a balanced raw diet reverses this condition in time. *See* the book The Recipe For Living Without Disease, Chapter 12.

PYORRHEA is most often a detoxification of the brain and glands in the mouth that eliminates through the gums, often forming pus and causing loosening of teeth. Some times that condition is caused by lactose intolerance. Pyorrhea can be controlled by improving mineral absorption. *See* Mineral Deficiency, page 291.

Avoiding pasteurized dairy is essential. When drinking raw milk (preferably with extra cream), blending in unheated honey usually promotes lactose digestion. However, if there is still some upset from drinking milk, avoiding milk altogether and eating plenty of raw fish settles pyorrhea.

Drinking juices too quickly can cause blood pressure to rise too quickly and make teeth and gums more sensitive. Therefore it is better to sip juices. Or eating no-salt-added raw cheese with raw juices prevents the blood pressure problem, and this combination supplies added raw minerals that are so lacking in pyorrhea.

Drinking fresh raw ginger root and unheated honey mixed in good mineral water or fresh raw vegetable juices soothes and promotes healing of the gums. The ginger may be pressed with a garlic press, juiced or shredded, and set to stand in water or in juice for an hour or more.

Because of the solidity of gums and associated nerves, it takes at least three months to stabilize this condition. Having patience and eating properly will see a person through without having to have teeth extracted.

Inflammation usually prevents chewing, so blending raw foods and making raw meat into pâté makes eating easier. *See* Pâté, page 211. For a balanced diet, *see* the book The Recipe For Living Without Disease, Chapter 12.

General gum sensitivity is most often the result of low blood protein level accompanied by low blood sugar level. General gum sensitivity should not be confused with pyorrhea. *See* Pain, Gum Sensitivity, page 298.

RADIATION BURN: Topically, applying a poultice made of 1 cup raw coconut cream, unheated-above-96° Fahrenheit fermented coconut oil or stone-pressed olive oil, ½ cup fresh raw tomato puree, 1 raw fertile egg and ½ tablespoon of sun-dried powdered clay on radiation burn, covering with a white cotton or silk cloth, for at least 1 hour 4 times daily soothes and promotes healing. Fresh raw aloe vera gel, taken directly from a leaf, may be added to that formula for better results.

Drinking within 4 hours of making a mixture of 15 raw eggs, 2 unripe bananas, and ½ cup unheated honey blended together helps heal and strengthen burned cells. Adding fresh raw aloe vera gel to that recipe improves results. For the rest of the day, eating plenty of raw full-fat milk and honey, or raw fresh unripe fruit and raw fish, and getting plenty of fresh air in the shade soothes and refreshes the body. *See* Burns, page 235.

RADIATION-POISONING: *See* Detoxification of Radiation, page 257.

RAGE: *See* Anger, page 224, *and* Hypoglycemia, page 274.

RASH is a detoxification of or through the skin, often involving yeast. The remedies for burns usually effect immediate relief from itching and aid healing. Another effective salve can be made by blending ½ tomato, 1 teaspoon unheated-abovve-96° Fahrenheit fermented coconut oil, or raw coconut cream or stone-pressed olive oil, ¼ teaspoon sun-dried clay and 1/8 teaspoon royal jelly. Alternating these two salves speeds detoxification and usually prevents thickened and hardened tissue (scarring). *See* Infant Problems, Diaper Rash, page 277.

RECTAL ITCHING is most often unidentified yeast cleaning the area. Soak a cotton or silk cloth in a mixture of equal portions of plain raw kefir and raw unpasteurized apple cider vinegar, and slightly tuck the cloth into the rectum. Let it stay over night and all day for constant relief until the rectal detoxification stops. For longer-lasting relief with only nightly insertion of the cloth, add to that mixture, unheated-above-96° Fahrenheit fermented coconut oil or cold-pressed-below-96° Fahrenheit peanut oil. Either oil may be used by itself but itching may be persistent. The most effective remedy for speeding detoxification and healing the rectum has been to insert a small-finger-sized slice of raw beef into the rectum, leaving only $^{1}/_{8}$ inch protruding from the anus all day and night.

RHEUMATIC FEVER is a detoxification of connective tissue linking muscles, cartilage, and bone. It occurs mainly in children, ages 4-18, whose lymph systems are impaired. Rheumatic fever is characterized by fever, swelling and pain in joints, sore throat, and heart complications, and often is caused by vaccines, antibiotics, medications, or toxins consumed by the mother during fetal development. When a wholesome raw diet had not been adhered to during this process, the RNA and DNA were further damaged, causing residual problems, such as heart disease, arthritis, chorea, tissue and skin problems. Rheumatic fever occurs in people who lack enzyme-mutations for eating cooked green and cooked red fruits and vegetables, causing acidity and other volatile toxins that damage cells. Usually, molds are active in this condition, affecting connective tissue and the heart. Avoiding cooked green and cooked red fruits and vegetables is a start. *See* If I Lack Enzyme-Mutations, What Foods Should I Avoid?, page 174.

Eating plenty of fresh raw alkalizing foods most often relaxed symptoms within three weeks. However, the energy level often remained low until the heart was repaired. Eating a balanced raw diet, including raw meat at least 5 days weekly, usually stabilized the heart within six months. Complete healing takes many years.

RHEUMATISM is acute and chronic stiffness of the muscles with pain in the joints. Usually, that results from low blood protein sugar accompanied by lack of enzyme-mutations for eating cooked green and yellow foods. *See* If I Lack Enzyme-Mutations, What Foods Should I Avoid?, page 174. Avoiding cooked green and cooked yellow foods, and eating raw foods, including raw pineapple with raw meat and raw fat usually resolve rheumatism.

RHEUMATOID ARTHRITIS: *see* Rheumatism, above, *and* Arthritis, page 226.

RHINITIS is a detoxification of the nasal mucosa that causes increased mucous secretions and nasal congestion. That condition is related to brain toxicity and lack of enzyme-mutations for eating cooked red fruits and vegetables and sometimes cooked yellow foods. *See* If I Lack Enzyme-Mutations, What Foods Should I Avoid?, page 174. Avoiding cooked red and cooked yellow fruits and vegetables stops the build-up of cooked resins and residues, reducing damage from detoxifying through the nasal passages. The flow of mucus is necessary to free the body of toxins. Eating smoothies and raw red and raw yellow fruits and vegetables, including juices, helps to soothe nasal passages.

Poor thyroid function usually accompanies rhinitis. *See* Thyroid Problem, page 315.

RICKETS is severe malnutrition characterized in children by soft weak bones causing malformations like: bowlegs, knock-knees, narrow rib cage, bony beads along the ribs and protruded breast plate. In adults it occurs during severe bodily stress such as pregnancy and breast-feeding, and is accompanied by weakness and aching joints. Generally, rickets is caused by the same mineral toxicity and deficiency that creates low thyroid production. *See* Thyroid Problem, Underactive, page 315.

SALT CRAVING: Generally, a craving for salt is caused by poor thyroxin production (a thyroid hormone). *See* Thyroid Problem, page 315, Appendix I, page 139, *and* Appendix M, page 143.

Raw glandular thyroid supplements are helpful, enabling the thyroid to relearn the chemical structure of thyroxin so that it can produce it. Eating raw deep sea fish (tuna, salmon, swordfish), raw oysters, raw scallops, raw clams, no-salt-added raw cheese, unripe melons with an equal quantity of raw fat, plenty of raw tomatoes, and fresh raw celery, supply the body with minerals necessary to stabilize mineral balance and for the thyroid to produce thyroxin. *See* Mineral Deficiency, page 291.

However, about .5% of the human population needs salt once weekly. Therefore, if after two months of eating the foods suggested above, you continue to have an unusual craving for salt, eating only two grains of unprocessed salt once or twice weekly usually satisfies and calms the system and settles the craving with little or no cellular destruction.

SCIATICA is characterized by tenderness or pain in the sciatic nerve that runs from the back at the waist, down the hip and thigh to the ankle. Tenderness or pain can occur at any point along the sciatic nerve.

Drinking full-fat raw milk is very helpful for people with spinal problems. I suggest adding 3-4 tablespoons raw cream and 2 tablespoons unheated honey to each quart of milk.

Often, sciatica is associated with liver problems. When functions of the liver improve, symptoms of sciatica usually disappear. *See* Liver Problems, page 285 (the remedy suggestions are the same for sciatica, even if you don't have a liver problem).

Most sciatica problems result from metal or chemical toxicity in the bones and/or tendons in the spine and sciatic nerves. That toxicity enters the sciatic nerves, causing cellular damage and swelling. Usually, infection results to remove cellular decay. Drinking any of the remedies for pain every 2-3 hours mitigates pain. Soaking for about an hour in a hot bath helps relax the back. Following a balanced raw diet as suggested under Mineral Deficiency (page 291) will cleanse and strengthen the sciatic nerves.

Enjoying hot baths for up to 8 hours helps discharge electricity from back pain into the water instead of into the brain. *See* Bath, page 326.

SCOLIOSIS is curvature of the spine that sometimes causes pinched nerves and pain.

On a balanced raw diet with Nut Formula (page 194) or a little cooked starches, the spine straightens itself over a period of several years. Although completely straightening of the spine can't always be expected, you can eliminate the pain that periodically accompanies scoliosis. Eating raw meat, including raw fish and/or raw fowl, helps to relax the tension and discomfort, and rebuild the spine.

SCURVY is a form of malnutrition, characterized by swollen and bleeding gums, rough dry discolored skin, tenderness of joints and muscles, bruising easily, poor healing of wounds, and susceptibility to frequent detoxification (infections, parasites, virus, etc.). Scurvy occurs in individuals who lack the ability to assimilate cooked sugars and cooked fat properly. A lack of enzyme-mutations for eating cooked yellow foods is sometimes also a factor in scurvy. (Cooked yellow foods in some people rob blood sugars that are needed throughout the body.)

Avoiding cooked and processed sugars and fat and cooked yellow foods settles scurvy. Eating plenty of fresh unripe fruit and fresh parsley leaves usually relaxes symptoms in a few days. Eating plenty of unheated honey helps the utilization or elimination of stored processed sugars (such as glycogen). Then eating a balanced raw diet that includes raw meat corrects scurvy. *See* the book The Recipe For Living Without Disease, Chapter 12.

The SHAKES are a sensation of inner or outer trembling that often makes a person feel uncontrollable. Usually this is a condition resulting from low blood protein.

Eating raw meat with raw fat usually calms the shakes within 30 minutes. However, some people need to eat 1-4 raw eggs without any other foods for a period of ½-1 hour. If you have a protein assimilation problem, regularly eating raw mushrooms and unheated honey with raw meat usually resolves it.

SHINGLES is a detoxification of the skin's nerve endings, resulting in blisters, crustiness, and pain that can last for weeks. Shingles directly relates to a lack of enzyme-mutations for eliminating cooked and processed sugars. Those sharp crystallized toxins then store in the skin, irritating nerve endings, causing shingles.

Avoiding cooked and processed sugars, and eating plenty of unheated honey (1-1½ cups daily for 2-3 weeks), and fresh unripe fruit, especially bananas, resolve this condition within a few days. Eating plenty of raw meat gradually heals the damage done by the cooked and processed radical sugars. If the nerves are scarred, eating cucumber with coconut meat or raw coconut cream gradually dissolves scars.

SINUSITIS is a mild detoxification of the sinus passages, causing mucus congestion and discharge, earache, headache, pain in or around the eyes, fatigue, cough, low fever and susceptibility to other detoxification (infections).

Avoiding coffee, teas and all substances that contain caffeine eliminates ½ of the toxins being discharged during sinusitis. Sunshine helps heal this condition. Eating plenty of raw fish, plenty of fresh raw lemon juice, 3-6 raw eggs daily, and not drinking much milk until the condition clears, speeds this detoxification. Eating equal portions of grated raw horseradish root, fresh raw lemon juice and unheated honey helps thin mucus.

See suggestions for Thyroid, Underactive, page 315.

SLEEPLESSNESS: *See* Insomnia, page 280.

SMOKING ADDICTION is rarely an addiction to nicotine. It is always a need for enzymes and blood sugar. Smoking causes a toxic response in the body that forces the liver to produce hormones that call for stored sugars. The preferred blood sugar glycogen is made of the protein sugar pyruvate that is best obtained from eating raw meat. It can enter the blood to help arrest monoxides and tars. The raised blood sugar level causes a rush of energy. The rush from smoking is not a healthy way to raise blood sugar and enzymes to increase energy because monoxides and tars poison and kill cells and clog the body. Over many years, if those tars remain in the body, they crystallize and clog and dry many bodily systems, especially kidneys and lungs.

A raw diet high in unheated honey, raw unripe fruit, raw fat, and raw meat is a preferable way to keep blood sugar levels and energy high. Eating unripe melons and pink grapefruit help the body remove tars from membranes and blood. Drinking a blended mixture of ½-1 cup fresh unripe pineapple or apple, ½-1 cup peeled cucumber, ¼-½ cup unheated honey, ½ teaspoon raw unpasteurized apple cider vinegar and 4 tablespoons raw coconut cream 3 days weekly helps dissolve tars and tar crystals. Drinking that mixture and eating fresh raw fruit in combination with raw fat every 3-4 hours, and whenever you crave a smoke, and taking deep breaths of air, especially fresh air, usually alleviate the craving for a smoke.

SORE THROAT: Drinking a mixture of 4 ounces warm good mineral water, 1-2 tablespoons raw unpasteurized apple cider vinegar, 2-3 tablespoons fresh raw lemon juice, and 2-4 tablespoons unheated honey several times daily usually relieves sore throat in minutes and keeps the symptoms relatively unnoticeable. If not, *see* Pain, page 297. *See* the book The Recipe For Living Without Disease, Chapter 15.

SPINAL MENINGITIS: *see* Meningitis, page 289.

SPRAIN: Warmth increases circulation and healing. Cold compresses reduce circulation and healing. Therefore, to promote healing to the area, apply warm compresses over a liniment made of leek.

To make the liniment, juice 1 leek and 1 tablespoon fresh raw ginger root (or blend and strain), and mix with either 4 tablespoons of raw coconut cream, or unheated-above-96° Fahrenheit fermented coconut oil, peanut oil or olive oil. For preferred healing, wrap the sprain in thinly sliced warm raw steak. To warm the steak, place it in a closed glass jar and immerse in a hot bowl of water (not too hot).

Following the same suggestions for bruises will heal sprains (*see* Bruise, page 235).

STIFFNESS: The Drink for Moisturizing and Lubrication relaxes the body (*see* page 210). Drinking that before bedtime has produced the best results.

If a person is chronically stiff, most often she or he lacks enzyme-mutations for eating cooked red fruits and vegetables that results in toxicity and mineral deficiency. Avoiding cooked red fruits and vegetables and having the raw egg/butter/honey/lemon drink (given in the preceding paragraph) at least once daily relieves stiffness. *See* If I Lack Enzyme-Mutations, What Foods Should I Avoid?, page 174. *See* Mineral

Deficiency, page 291.

STOMACH, ACID: Eating no-salt-added raw cheese, or raw fresh coconut, or bread (unbleached and nonfortified), and sipping honey usually absorbs stomach acidity. Drinking a mixture of 1 cup good mineral water with ¼ teaspoon sun-dried powdered clay, 2 tablespoons of honey and the juice of 1-2 lemons (or limes) neutralizes stomach over-acidity. Sometimes it is best to neutralize the acidity first and then absorb it with no-salt-added raw cheese or bread.

STRESS: Eating a Nut Formula (page 194) or cooked starch with raw fat and fresh unripe fruit raises blood sugar and neutralizes overproduction of hormones that accompany stress. Eating raw meat supplies the proteins, and drinking fresh vegetable juice supplies the concentrated vitamins and minerals needed during stress. Drinking 4-8 ounces of raw cream helps immediate relaxation. Doing something that is fun or relaxing stimulates confidence and creative problem-solving. For suggestions on reducing stress and enjoying life, first *see* Awareness, page 325, then *see* Depression, page 254, *and* Mental Illness, page 290.

STROKE: A stroke results when blood is blocked from some part of the brain, killing cells in the area. Strokes occur when heterocyclic amines and other residues from eating cooked meat accumulate in the brain, usually caused by a lack of enzyme-mutations for eating cooked meat.

Symptoms warning of this condition are low blood pressure (not high, as the myth states) accompanied with severe sluggishness and irritability, anxiousness, chronic fear, constant stress, poor muscle tone, and general debilitating health.

Eating plenty of fresh raw meat, raw mushrooms and an alkalizing raw diet usually prevents stroke or corrects the results of stroke. *See* Alkalizing Food, page 178.

SUNBURN: *See* Burns, page 235. Also, avocado or raw milk rubbed on the skin is healing. (Caution: avocado stains clothes.)

SURGERY: Eating plenty of unheated honey and getting into fresh air and sunshine facilitate healing. For at least 10 days, drinking plenty of smoothies has helped to arrest toxic medication and anesthesia. Eating 3 smoothies daily for one week before surgery, each consisting of 3 eggs, reduced damage from medication and anesthesia. Eating raw meat facilitated healing.

SWOLLEN GLANDS is a condition from accumulated volatile toxins and resins in lymph glands. Drinking plenty of unheated honey, fresh raw orange or lemon juices and tomato puree alkalizes the blood. If a person suffers chronically with swollen glands, he or she probably lacks enzyme-mutations for eating cooked green foods. Avoiding cooked greens and eating raw greens help eliminate stored resins and residues caused by eating cooked greens. *See* If I Lack Enzyme-Mutations, What Foods Should I Avoid?, page 174.

SYPHILIS is a viral detoxification affecting almost any organ or tissue in the body, especially genitals, skin, mucous membranes, aorta, brain, liver, bones and nerves, and is caused by the inability to utilize caffeine and cooked green foods. Extreme acidity and accumulation of volatile toxins deteriorate cells, forcing the body to manufacture this virus en masse. *See* If I Lack Enzyme-Mutations, What Foods Should I Avoid?, page 174.

Strictly adhering to the following regime for at least 8 days has worked the best without having to use harmful drug therapy. Drinking a blend of 18 tomatoes (Roman variety work a little more quickly) with at least 5 tablespoons of unheated honey and 5 teaspoons fresh raw lemon juice neutralizes toxins and has eliminated the body's need for the virus. Eating other foods that are alkalizing reinforced the effects of the tomato/honey/lemon drink. Eating very little meat during the eight-day period prevented the blood from getting acidic, which would have irritated the condition. *See* Alkalizing Food, page 178.

After the eight days, eating plenty of raw meat, including raw fish, and raw eggs gradually healed the deterioration and breakdown from this severe detoxification. *See* Appendix Q, page 151.

TEETH: *See* Tooth And Gum Disorders, page 316.

THYROID PROBLEM:

Underactive: Symptoms: poor-looking hair, low energy level, fearful nature.

Eating unsulfured non-steamed dates with no-salt-added raw cheese with an equal quantity of raw fat energizes the thyroid. Eating plenty of alkalizing foods (like tomato) cleanses the thyroid, especially of toxic minerals, including those caused by table salts. *See* Alkalizing Food, page 178. For a balanced diet, *see* the book The Recipe For Living Without Disease, Chapter 12.

Eating no-salt-added raw cheeses, fresh raw ocean fish (including scallops, oysters or clams), whole raw milk, Nut Formula (page 194) and, occasionally, ¼ teaspoon of sun-dried clay mixed in fresh raw vegetable juices or smoothies supplies the thyroid with minerals it needs to properly function and produce hormones. Mixing 5 drops of organically grown vanilla extract into fresh raw juice or smoothies helps stimulate the thyroid. *See* Vanilla Extract, page 201.

If headaches are experienced, tomatoes should not be eaten for a week or more. In that circumstance, tomatoes may produce too heavy of detoxification, causing the blood to become too toxic and raising blood pressure.

If this diet doesn't correct the condition within eleven weeks, eating a natural raw thyroid glandular supplement may be necessary. However, if neither the diet nor the glandular supplement helps, going to a doctor for prescription thyroid hormones may be required for proper hormonal balance.

Overactive: *See* Hyperactive, page 272, *and* Hyperthyroid, page 273.

TONSILLITIS is a detoxification of the tonsils, causing reddened and swollen tonsils and throat, hoarseness, difficulty swallowing, coughing, fever, headache, earache, nausea, vomiting, sinus congestion and discharge, and swollen lymphatic glands throughout the body. Tonsils mainly protect the brain by dissolving and neutralizing degenerative brain cells. Therefore, it is preferable to keep your tonsils. If the brain cells are toxic with metals or other toxins, the tonsils may frequently inflame and are damaged. Tonsillitis usually occurs in individuals lacking enzyme-mutations for eating cooked red fruits and vegetables. *See* If I Lack Enzyme-Mutations, What Foods Should I Avoid?, page

174.

Eating salt or caffeine interferes with and irritates this detoxification. Avoiding salt, anything with caffeine, including soft drinks and chocolate, and cooked red fruits and vegetables minimizes tonsil infections.

Drinking a blend of 3 cups fresh raw tomatoes and 4 tablespoons fresh raw lemon juice has helped neutralize the volatile toxins. Best results have come from drinking the mixture within one hour of making it, and then 4 hours later making and drinking another of the same mixture. Eating other raw foods, if desired, is fine. That regime followed for one day usually relieved tonsillitis on the third day.

For an accompanying sore throat, drinking unheated honey mixed with a good mineral water ("Naturally Sparkling" water is best) usually brings relief. If not, *see* Pain, page 297.

TOOTH AND GUM DISORDERS usually occur from poor assimilation of minerals. Processed minerals, including metallic, from canned food, Novocain, vaccines, medical or recreational drugs, chlorinated and fluorinated waters, processed cheese, and caffeine (including chocolate) are especially harmful for, and often causative in, tooth and gum conditions.

Root canals sometimes result in large deep abscesses that affect the entire body. Those abscesses can cause general fatigue, neck and shoulder soreness and stiffness, and reddened eye(s). I have seen very debilitating conditions as a result of the body trying to dissolve and remove nerve and bone toxicity around teeth, especially root canals. Fatigue that results may continue for years as long as the infection continues. Even on a healthy diet, the toxicity around the teeth may require more nutrients than most people can eat. Therefore, if persistent infection occurs, it may be preferable to have a root-canal tooth extracted.

Amalgam fillings, called silver fillings, contain large quantities of toxic mercury and should not be used to fill teeth. The best dental filling material is porcelain or ceramic inlays. For crowns and bridges, I suggest using those that are reinforced with gold because so much more of your tooth will remain. I have seen gold-reinforced crowns last 30 years. If you use only ceramic or porcelain crowns or bridges, each tooth must be severely ground to a small post. That little post of a tooth that remains may easily break in 1-5 years. Then, if you want to have a stable tooth, you must have a root canal or an artificial tooth must be drilled and screwed into the jaw bone.

Drinking plenty of full-fat raw milk begins reversing those problems. If raw milk is not available, eating raw fish works almost as well. Drinking raw milk and eating raw fish speed the healing process in most people. *See* Pyorrhea, page 305. *See* Mineral Deficiency, page 291.

TOOTHACHE: *See* Pain, page 297. *See* Tooth And Gum Disorder, page 316.

TRAUMA: Making yourself warm and comfortable, having a good cry, and staying away from demands for awhile nurture you back to normal. Thinking about successes and better times help put a difficult experience behind you. Whether you have a good voice or not, singing encouraging songs is healing. Watching stand-up or other comedy with the intent to enjoy it can bring about speedy relief. Eating raw meat helps produce calm determination.

Eating plenty of unheated honey, and a Nut Formula (page 194) or cooked starch with raw fat and fresh raw unripe fruit helps restore and maintain hormonal balance and blood sugar. Eating a raw egg every 1-1½ hours usually speeds relaxation. Drinking ½-1 cup raw cream immediately soothes the body and mind.

TUBERCULOSIS is a severe detoxification of very volatile toxins that are hormone-related and discharged from the lungs. These toxins may affect other glands, organs and tissues as the toxins travel through the blood. The volatile toxins are mainly formed from cooked green foods in people who lack enzyme-mutations for eating cooked greens, including smoking tobacco or herbs. *See* If I Lack Enzyme-Mutations, What Foods Should I Avoid?, page 174.

Avoiding cooked greens, plus eating plenty of raw green salads, and plenty of hearty foods (like pasta with raw fat and raw beef, or raw beef sandwiches) has strengthened and healed tubercular sufferers without permanent damage and without medication.

ULCERS are open sores on the mucous membranes or skin. Ulcers occur in people who lack enzyme-mutations for eating cooked and processed red fruits and vegetables. *See* If I Lack Enzyme-Mutations, What Foods Should I Avoid?, page 174.

Skin ulcers occur in people who have an allergy to cooked and processed red fruits and vegetables, and cannot assimilate minerals. Avoid anything with caffeine, including chocolate and sodas. Caffeine interferes with mineral assimilation.

Drinking good mineral water and unheated honey, and being active, flush the skin with minerals to bind with toxins and neutralize them. Eating no-salt-added raw cheese helps to heal.

Intestinal and stomach (mucous membrane) ulcers: Drinking plenty of smoothies for one week, and eating raw butter, unripe papaya and other unripe fruit (but no tomato or citrus) bind toxins and revitalize the tissues. After one week, the following regime detoxifies toxins that are stored in stomach and intestinal membranes: plenty of fresh raw white cabbage juice and tomato purees, some raw milk with raw fertile egg(s) and unripe banana, plain raw kefir with a little fresh unripe pineapple, plenty of butter and unheated honey. Best results have been achieved by eating very little raw meat, and no cooked meat or pasteurized milk for two weeks. After the two weeks (the time it usually takes for ulcers to cleanse, close, and enter the first stages of healing) eating plenty of raw meat, ½ cup white cabbage juice (for 4 weeks) and alkalizing foods daily heals and strengthens mucous membranes.

UNDERWEIGHT: Gaining weight sometimes requires correcting an underactive thyroid. *See* Thyroid Problem, Underactive, page 315. Otherwise, it is an indication that not enough protein and fat are being eaten together, or that protein is not assimilated. Eating plenty of raw meat with plenty of raw fat usually reverses this condition within a month. The quickest way to gain weight is to add 3 ounces of raw cream and 2-3 tablespoons unheated honey to 32 ounces of raw milk and drink that throughout each day. That mixture should be in addition to all other foods on a balanced raw diet. *See* the book The Recipe For Living Without Disease, Chapter 12 for a balanced raw diet.

URETHRA INFECTION OR PAIN: Most often, urethra problems stem from kidney or gall bladder stones that scrape and irritate the urethra as stones pass through the urethra. Most cases readily responded to the suggestion for kidney stones. *See* Kidney Stones, page 282. James suffered with this problem for weeks. I suggested long hot baths that helped when he could get them. (His home was equipped with a shower but not bathtub.) Finally after many weeks, he began eating a raw milk diet only. Within 24 hours, all of his pain subsided. I suggest adding 4-6 tablespoons raw cream and 2 tablespoons unheated honey to every 28 ounces of milk.

VACCINE-INDUCED DISEASES (VID) can be mitigated or reversed by eating 1-2 raw eggs every 1-2 hours until symptoms are alleviated enough, which may take weeks. Then, I suggest eating a balanced raw diet with plenty of raw fat and raw meat. Those suggestions are for the time period within 10 days after injection. For people who can acquire raw butter and unheated honey, they can mix 7 tablespoons of raw butter with 1 tablespoon unheated honey, and eat 1 teaspoon of that mixture after each egg.

For those who suffer VID from vaccines injected further in the past, I suggest a balanced diet as given in the book The Recipe For Living Without Disease, pages 40-42. For the afternoon fruit meal, I suggest eating ½-1 cup raw berries (raspberries, blackberries, boysenberries, or cranberries) blended with 3-8 tablespoons raw coconut cream, 1-2 tablespoons unsalted raw butter, and 1-2 tablespoons raw cream to help remove the mercury and aluminum that are common ingredients used in vaccines. Those two toxins cause blood and neurological serums to become high in sediment and cause excessive clotting, resulting in strokes, seizures and many other neurological VID's.

For more information on the dangers of vaccines, read the book by Dr. Rebecca Carley, M.D., Inoculations: The True Weapons of Mass Destruction; and, Causing VIDs; An Epidemic of Genocide. Dr. Carley is a court-qualified expert in VIDS and Legal Abuse Syndrome.

VAGINITIS: *See* Yeast Infection, page 322.

VARICOSE VEINS are veins that have become swollen, enlarged and twisted (vascular flabbiness). (A friend calls these "very close" veins - close to the surface.) Caffeine is the greatest cause of flabby veins in most people. Bodies that have varicose veins have irritating storages of caffeine or other toxins in the veins making them water-bloated and sluggish. Oral (birth control pills) and injected contraceptives also cause varicose veins. Avoiding caffeine in beverages and medications, and dried peppers (including black and cayenne) is important to healing.

Eating raw unripe pineapple with raw cream, when available, or stone-pressed olive oil, and taking plenty of warm baths, soothe and strengthen varicose veins. Eating plenty of raw meat, including fish, helps regenerate veins, making them strong and perky over a period of many years.

VENEREAL DISEASE is a detoxification of the genitals usually caused by the inability to utilize caffeine and cooked green foods. *See* If I Lack Enzyme-Mutations, What Foods Should I Avoid?, page 174.

Avoiding caffeine and cooked green foods, and drinking plenty of raw milk with added raw cream and unheated honey soothe the tissues and make those detoxifications easier.

See Gonorrhea, page 266.

See Syphilis, page 314, *and* Appendix Q, pages 151-153.

VERTIGO is a condition in which a person or his surroundings seem to whirl. Excess adrenaline is usually a factor. In vertigo, adrenaline utilized all blood sugar, fat and protein, and saturated nerves relating to balance with acidity. In every case I have seen, some type of industrial chemical, including medication, poisoned those nerves. If the DNA was damaged before the toxicity was removed, reversal was extremely slow or did not occur.

Eating raw meat and unheated honey, small amounts of Nut Formula (page 194) frequently, or a small amount of cooked starch in combination with plenty of raw fats and raw fruit re-supplies the blood with nutrients, and usually vertigo subsides.

VISION AND FOCUS DISORDERS are characterized by blurred vision, eye fatigue, inability to see far or near, squinting, light sensitivity, itchy, bloodshot or burning eyes and lids.

Caffeine in any form, including chocolate, coffee, tea and soda, damages nerves and brain. In many people it damages eyes. Caffeine consumed by a mother during pregnancy and breast-feeding can cause poor vision in her child. Excess adrenaline causes dryness, nerve damage, and in some people creates poor vision. Medicinal insulin also causes vision disorders. *See* Cataracts, page 244.

Eating plenty of live foods, especially raw fats with foods that are red or orange (indicating abundant vitamin A content), such as carrot juice, apricots, watermelon and raw tuna, soothes and nourishes eyes. As a result of eating a raw diet, especially raw red meat, most vision disorders have stopped the "normal" progression toward poorer vision. I have seen few instances where vision disorders completely reversed. Adding 1-2 drops of raw egg white (from antibiotic-free and hormone-free chickens) to the eyes once or twice daily gradually and continuously improved vision. Those who continued to consume caffeine on a predominantly raw diet did not improve their vision. Either their eyesight remained poor or it continued a slower progression toward poorer eyesight.

VITAMIN DEFICIENCIES, when severe, are indicated by dark circles under eyes, pallid face, poor energy, sleeplessness for people who are usually able to sleep, and fearful attitudes.

Eating plenty of fresh raw unripe fruits, unheated honey, vegetable juices and sometimes salads supplies naturally bioactive, enzyme-bound vitamins for proper assimilation and utilization.

Symptoms of chronic vitamin deficiency are powdery tongue in the morning, loss of peripheral vision, flatulence, nervous and fearful thoughts about the future and related psychological complications (like making difficulties where none exist). A chronic vitamin deficiency is often misdiagnosed as a severe potassium deficiency. Ironically, consuming vitamin supplements increase those symptoms rather than mitigate symptoms.

Eating plenty of fresh raw vegetable juices, raw unripe fruit, especially banana and melon, and frequently eating small amounts of

Nut Formula (page 194), or a little cooked starch with plenty of raw fat (e.g., unsalted raw butter, avocado, stone-pressed olive oil) and sometimes a fresh raw salad gradually replenishes missing vitamins. Avoid eating salads with oils of any kind (olive, peanut, etc.) - the combination prevents the vitamins in salads from being digested. However, raw oils may be eaten with cooked starches at the same meal with a salad.

WARTS: The same remedy for corns. *See* Corns, page 265.

WATER RETENTION: *see* Edema, page 260.

WORMS, *see* Parasites, page 299.

X-RAYS: *See* Detoxification of Radiation, page 257, *and* Radiation Burn, page 306.

YEAST INFECTION is characterized by swollen, inflamed and itchy skin. Yeast eat tissue toxins and alkalize the system. Yeast are helpful and should be allowed to run their cycle. Medication poisons the already toxic and hardened tissue, causing it to remain toxic and hardened. If your goal is to improve your health, the worst thing you can do is to destroy a yeast infection with medications.

Alcohol, coffee, teas, aspirin, soft drinks with caffeine and salt consumed in large quantities over years are all poisonous, overstimulating adrenals and pancreas. The high levels of adrenaline and insulin create toxic conditions and dryness that cause lesions, thereby creating conditions where yeast are necessary for cleansing.

Eating a raw diet that contains regular meals, small quantities of Nut Formula (page 194) or some cooked starch with plenty of raw fat eliminates the excess adrenaline and insulin levels. Eating raw tomatoes, nonsteamed figs, fresh vegetable juices, especially green, and raw unpasteurized apple cider vinegar alkalizes and soothes tissues and reverses the toxic condition.

Vaginal yeast infection: All of the above applies. Drinking 2-3 raw eggs blended with 2-3 tablespoons unheated honey and ½ unripe banana provides the vagina with a constant supply of healthy nutrients to build mucus that flushes and removes toxicity with the help of smaller colonies of yeast (less itching, too). Eating raw fish and/or raw fowl 3-4 times weekly strengthens the tissues and replaces destroyed nerve tissue and skin, increasing sensuality.

Douching with one of the following eliminates discomfort: ½ tablespoon raw apple cider vinegar mixed in 4 ounces of water, or 4 ounces plain raw kefir, or 3 ounces of your own urine.

A woman who had suffered vaginal yeast infections every time she had sex throughout her life had tried everything suggested above. Those mitigated the yeast infections, but she still experienced pain after sex. As a last resort, she tried an Ayurvedic medical method: she drank her first urine of each day for several weeks. Within two weeks, the recurring infections completely ceased.

POSTSCRIPT

I have been very limited in financial resources to fund my experiments and research over the years. But I did them. Although my results with reversing disease have been extraordinary, I know that my work has the potential to achieve even more remarkable results by incorporating fresh raw herbs. I will continue my work in this direction. That involves obtaining funding, seeds, bulbs and rooted cuttings, to grow therapeutic herbs so that we may use them fresh and raw. If anyone has access to funding, herbal seeds, bulbs and rooted cuttings, please contact me at: Optimal Ways of Living, P.O. Box 176, Santa Monica, CA 90291. Your donations will be utilized well and appreciated. Thank you.

Health Methodologies; Opinions And Tips

ACUPRESSURE is the application of pressure by fingers, thumbs, hands and elbows to specific points on the body that have been found to directly affect glands, organs and nerve centers, with the intent to stimulate healing of malfunctioning or pained glands, organs, and nerve centers. Some acupressurists work on a person's hands and feet only. Some acupressurists like to dig deeply to break free what they call crystals, deposits and other blockages. Acupressure is often effective. However, the consequential bruises, internal lacerations, fluid leakages and the quantity of toxins that are released are often a problem, creating damage locally and throughout the body, including the heart.

If gentle acupressure is applied while plenty of raw fats are suspended in the blood, a certain amount of released toxins will be arrested and eliminated properly. Therefore, eating a raw diet that is high in raw fat 5 days before and 10 days after having treatments is beneficial. Treatments that are intended to gradually remove blockages with gentle pressure promote healing and cleansing more easily occurs.

ACUPUNCTURE is the application of needles inserted into and through the skin in specific nerve points on the body that have been found to directly affect glands, organs, and nerve centers, with the intent to stimulate healing of malfunctioning or pained glands, organs, and nerve centers. Acupuncture is often effective. However, the needles lacerate skin and nerve cells, leaving them susceptible to scarring. Scarring is often the case. Scars increase with each treatment and lead to eventual desensitization to pleasure as well as pain. Therefore, I have mixed conclusions about acupuncture. I would favor it over Western medical methods.

AWARENESS: Asking yourself questions about your individual needs and what you enjoy, leads to answers that promote happiness and self-esteem. Listening to your body's needs and enjoyments are part of that questioning. Instead of dwelling on all the possible things that could go wrong, or that already have gone "wrong", living in the moment and choosing which dreams you wish to follow give you power to create a more desirable future. Imagining the worst things that can happen, so that you will be ready and prepared just in case they happen, creates tension, criticism and cynicism. It is useless to waste time considering infinite negative possibilities. It is helpful to consider negative probabilities but it is futile and debilitating to dwell on negative probabilities and possibilities. If negative probabilities exist, make the best plans of action to change those directions. Tension and criticism/cynicism attract tense, cynical, critical people and experiences; a stressful and exhausting cycle. Are you as prepared for the best possibilities? Preparing for the best experiences creates hope and joy. Hope and joy attract happier, creative people and experiences to you, and synchronicity; a delightful cycle. Therefore, imagining and fantasizing positive experiences with the belief that they are probable creates a happier and more fulfilling life. If you quit, whose life do you surrender? Ecological considerations and compassion create healthier environments, and consequently healthier and happier people.

BATHS/SAUNA/STEAM promote circulation and health. However, chlorinated water vapor is toxic because it kills cells and bacterium necessary for good health. Chlorine vapors are toxic to sinuses, bronchi, lungs, blood, brain and nervous system. Baths, including Jacuzzi, are preferable because the toxins that are perspired drift into the water, away from the skin. I suggest adding 2-3 cups raw milk, 3 tablespoons raw unpasteurized apple cider vinegar, and 2 tablespoons sun-dried sea salt to the water. Or add ½ cup sun-dried clay, 2 ounces raw unpasteurized apple cider vinegar and 3 tablespoons raw coconut cream. The coconut cream is optional but it is beneficial because it keeps the skin from drying as a result of the clay. Those ingredients in both bath formulas will help pull toxins from the skin and hold them in the water so they are not reabsorbed into the skin during the bath. Also, they will bind with toxins in municipal water and prevent them from entering the skin and body. Municipal waters contain many harmful chemicals. One example is the water in Los Angeles that contained 192 toxins when I had it analyzed in 2003. When fluoride was added to the water, the chemical toxins rose from 157 to 192. As you can surmise, there are many compounds that are part of fluoride. Fluoride is a toxic byproduct of industrial processes including the manufacturing of aluminum.

When using saunas to perspire toxins from the body, it is healthier to shower and rinse toxic perspiration every 3-4 minutes so that perspired toxins are not reabsorbed into the skin, eventually reentering the body.

Steam baths are the least desirable form to evoke perspiration of toxins from the body. Steam burns mucous membranes, including those in the lungs, bronchi and sinuses. If using steam baths, use good mineral water to produce the steam. Do not use municipal water. Shower and rinse often.

When showering with municipal city water that is chlorinated, it is best to have non-chemical filters installed that will eliminate chlorine and some other chemicals. Chlorine vapors (chloroform) gradually weaken and damage lungs, blood, thyroid and brain, predisposing people to pneumonia, other respiratory conditions, and meningitis of spine and brain.

The spleen mainly regulates the body's adaptability to cold and hot temperatures. It removes red blood cells from the blood stream to thin the blood and cool the body. It adds red blood cells to the blood to thicken the blood and heat the body. People who do not have spleens should ease into hot baths and drink more fluids immediately prior to entering a hot bath.

BEAUTY TIPS: Several times a week, applying onto the skin, a thin paste made of 1 teaspoon sun-dried powered clay mixed with 1½ tablespoons raw unpasteurized apple cider vinegar, or clay mixed with 1 fertile raw egg, or clay mixed with 1 tablespoon fresh raw papaya juice with ½ tablespoon good mineral water, attracts and absorbs toxins. Alternating apple cider vinegar, then egg, then papaya in the paste is healthiest for skin. Papaya helps remove scars, such as acne.

All skin oils, soaps and lotions are made with processed oils, "natural" or not, that smother and make skin toxic as well as lubricate it. If you can't eat it, why would you feed it to your skin? Applying a cold-pressed-below-96° Fahrenheit oil, especially coconut and peanut oils, or raw unsalted butter mixed with a drop of unheated honey or raw royal jelly feeds and protects the skin without smothering and poisoning it. After fifteen minutes, wipe any excess. It is healthier for the skin to be allowed to breathe every few days without oils, even if oils are cold-pressed. *See* Primal Facial Body Care Cream in the book The Recipe For Living Without Disease, Chapter 15. *See* Sleep and Rest, page 327.

BIOFEEDBACK machines can help us become familiar with our mental and emotional states of illness and health. By achieving that awareness, we can learn to alter undesirable mental and emotional states to those that are relaxed and life-changingly positive.

Electro Dermal Screening Devices can cause serious ill effects. *See* page 332.

BIRTH CONTROL: In all fairness and logic, since it is the man's sperm that impregnates a woman, it is the man's responsibility. It is up to the man to calculate fertile times. He should not rely on anyone else's calculations, including the woman's. If a man wants to be certain that he does not impregnate a woman, he must not ejaculate inside her. If a woman cannot trust a man to withhold ejaculation, during intercourse use a diaphragm or cervical cap eight days before and during ovulation (ten days total). If you failed to practice birth control eight days before and during ovulation, douche with apple cider vinegar immediately after intercourse. Drinking the pepper-tasting blended combination of 6 tablespoons fresh papaya seeds and ½ cup good drinking water 1-3 hours before sex or within 20 minutes after sex usually prevents pregnancy. When using a prophylactic, sensation can be increased by lubricating the penis with unheated-above-96° Fahrenheit fermented coconut oil, or peanut oil or stone-pressed olive oil and lubricating, thoroughly, the penis and outside of the condom after it is on the penis. It feels the closest to not wearing anything.

BIRTHING: Using any or all of the pain remedies reduces pain and bruising, especially the unheated honey/raw unsalted butter mixture, and the bee pollen mixed with raw milk or carrot/green vegetable mix. *See* Pain, page 297. Drinking the Drink For Moisturizing and Lubrication (page 210) daily 3 weeks before baby is due helps ease birth and prevent tearing of tissue during birth. The prone position for birthing makes birthing more difficult and painful, working against gravity. The prone position is for the convenience of doctors and medical personnel. Kneeling or squatting works with gravity, causing milder contractions and less stress. Birthing in a warm bath with 2 cups milk, 3 tablespoons coconut cream (optional but keeps the skin from drying) and 3 tablespoons raw unpasteurized apple cider vinegar helps prevent muscle cramps, keeps muscles as relaxed as possible, and eases bruising. Remaining in the bloody warm bath, lying back and holding child for at least 45 minutes soothes and relaxes the mother and eases baby's entrance into the dry world. *See* Pregnancy, page 336. Many women who were on the Primal Diet for at least 2 years, experienced only two major contractions during labor. The first pushed the baby's head through and the second pushed the rest of the baby free and into the arms of the father or midwife. That is relatively easy birthing.

Caesarean section, that is, surgical removal of child through the abdomen, severs the connections between the mother's spinal cord and her brain, and severs the blood and lymph circulation to vital abdominal areas, including uterus, while scarring nerves, veins, lymph, muscles and skin. Consequently, sensation for sexual pleasure and control over motor responses and hormone productions are drastically reduced, usually ill-effecting a woman for the remainder of her life. Too often this adversely affects the tone and shape of a woman's constitution and figure. In many cases when caesarean section was administered, a spinal injection and/or muscle relaxant given to the mother during an earlier stage of the birthing process prevented proper contractions. Birthing was slowed or even stopped, resulting in caesarean section. In 94% of caesarean sections, doctors chose caesarean birth because they didn't want to wait around countless hours for delivery to occur. In only 6% of caesarean sections has mother or child been in danger and benefited from caesarean surgery.

See Hemorrhage, page 270, about preventing excessive bleeds.

BREATHING supplies oxygen to every cell in the body. Oxygen is as important as nutrition. Learning to breath properly from the diaphragm slowly and fully, increases mental clarity, physical energy, and emotional balance. Hatha yoga utilizes excellent breathing exercises.

CHELATION THERAPY uses chemicals to attract heavy metals, such as mercury, cadmium and lead, and plaque from soft tissues, such as glands, organs, veins and arteries, for elimination. In over 200 cases, I have witnessed that the body does not excrete or secrete most of those toxins. Along with the various chemicals used in chelation therapies, the metals and plaque re-store in the body, that is, in the bones, bone-marrow, lymph, connective tissue and skin. In the long-term, chelation therapies are the most harmful therapy, next to medical chemotherapies. Factually, chelation therapies are chemotherapy. The body needs tremendous amounts of fats to bind with and excrete concentrations of any toxin, especially free-radicals (metals). No one could eat enough fat to make chelation therapies safe.

CHIROPRACTICS is the manipulation of the body to place bones in their joints properly so that nerves are not pinched and circulation flows more easily. Pinched nerves can cause anything from indigestion to impotency by cutting off circulation, as well as block communication to the brain. In youth, it can cause spinal compression, resulting in scoliosis. Accompanying a healthy diet, chiropractic adjustments can assist a body to better health when needed.

COLONIC is a radical flushing of the colon; that is, it is an extreme form of enema. Colonics may flush impacted matter from the colon but they force enormous amounts of toxins into the blood stream where they cause heart and brain damage. Another side effect of colonics is that they strip the colon for up to 45 days of friendly E.coli bacteria that are necessary for the body to synthesize proteins and B vitamins. That can result in indigestion, hypoglycemia, fatigue, anemia, depression, irritability and backaches.

Cleansing impacted matter from the colon can be done gradually on a raw diet that includes plenty of raw fats eaten with raw citrus, especially unripe pineapple, raw vegetable juices and some raw vegetables.

CONTAGIOUS is an overused, manipulative word/concept that incites fear, driving people to go to war within themselves and their bodies. Natural microbes are all beneficial. With most people, eating cooked foods and exposure to pollution creates toxicity that causes the body to weaken and deteriorate. Eating a raw diet prevents further accumulations of toxic matter in the body, and through many years, cleanses old accumulations. A person suffers bacterial and/or parasitical and/or viral infection because he or she has toxins in the body that need to be detoxified, not because someone has given him or her an unnecessary plague. Just as termites do not eat a healthy living tree, natural microbes will not eat healthy tissue. *See* Common Cold, page 249.

EATING BEFORE SLEEP is very healthful when on a raw diet because raw food is easy to digest, and the body doesn't have to go too many hours without a good supply of fresh nutrients during sleep. After five hours, there is a blood-protein deficiency resulting in red blood cells eating other red blood cells. That cannibalism causes tremendous toxicity that makes many people feel drained and lethargic even after 8-10 hours of sleep. Therefore, it is healthiest to wake after 5 hours to drink ½-1 cup of room-temperature raw milk, or raw milk shake, or 2 raw eggs. Food may be kept at your bedside. Then immediately return to sleep. Do not eat fruit or drink a smoothie when waking to eat, because you may not be able to immediately return to sleep.

ECOLOGY: Records and statistics kept by the Price-Pottenger Foundation (*see* Bibliography, page 340) include documentation supporting the findings that eating raw foods is ecologically conscientious. Dr. Francis Pottenger's logs document the effects of animal excrement on plant growth. Three control groups of cats were employed in the following experiment: All animals were fed the same foods but the foods were prepared differently for each group. Group #1 was fed raw foods, Group #2 was fed cooked foods, and Group #3 was fed processed, cooked and packaged foods. Plants fertilized with excrement from Group #1 grew lush, green and healthy. Plants fertilized with excrement from Group #2 grew half as well as Group #1. Plants fertilized with excrement from Group #3 grew sparse, baring few leaves and coarse rigid stalks.

ELECTRO DERMAL SCREENING DEVICES (EDSD, or EDD): Using biofeedback, computerized electrical devices attempt to diagnose health problems. However, when electricity is used to rebalance the body, there can be serious repercussions. In the case of EDSDs, the computer sends electrical signals to the brain and body that are believed to be the frequencies of a healthy person. But those idealized frequencies are relative to the programmer's understanding of health, which may be biased or prejudiced against important bodily functions or substances, such as the production of mucus, bacteria, parasites and virus. The fact that every human body is different and emits varied electrical frequencies negates the ideological validity of EDSD. The electrical signals supplied by the EDSD machine may or may not give the body false ideas about its needs and state of well being. Consequently, the body's systems might fail to respond properly, healthfully.

The epoxy-detoxification and cancerous burn that I mentioned earlier on pages 213-214, was forced by an EDSD treatment. Hindsight is too late, as we all know, and I regret having agreed to be electrically treated with the EDSD.

Is EDSD an electrical brainwashing (reprogramming) of bodily functions? I don't know enough about it, and I was under the impression that the therapist was simply diagnosing me, not treating me with EDSD. People defending EDSD said that the therapist treated me on the machine for too long and therefore I experienced violent side effects. One of those many side effects was that my body stopped producing protective and cleansing mucus that would have bound and flushed the epoxy without having caused cancer and the severe third-degree burns to my skin and eye and the excruciating pain. Another side effect of the EDSD is that I felt hyperactive and anxious, making it difficult for me to relax or sleep more than three hours at a time. If I wanted to sleep longer, I had to sleep in a hot bath for 1-3 hours and then sleep in bed for 2-3 hours. I had to lie on grass and ground for 40 minutes per day to reduce the feeling that I was constantly being exposed to excessive electrical charge. The EDSD computer diagnosed me as having many problems that I didn't have until after it treated me for them. In one case, the EDSD machine diagnosed me as having sensitivity to sunlight. Until then, I was able to sun-gaze easily and enjoy intense sunlight into my brain for long periods. After EDSD treatment, I experienced an uncanny sensitivity to sunlight that affects me to this day (2005). It has caused an intense furrowing of my brow that has caused many lines to develop. Still, I cannot stare into the sunlight for more than a few seconds. The EDSD also diagnosed and treated me for allergies I did not have but developed immediately after the EDSD treatment. Like medicine, EDSD seems to be very risky.

EXERCISE increases circulation and sometimes releases and spends difficult-to-utilize stored cooked fats; therefore exercise is healthy. However, when the combination of a raw diet and exercise is not appealing, exercise is not necessary. Exercising when feeling anxious, or feeling a need to be active, is healthful. Exercise spends excess hormones that cause such restlessness. Hatha yoga postures are good for stretching when one is feeling tight but not wanting strenuous exercise.

Proper breathing is very often the most important exercise. Breathing exercises increase oxygen and carbon dioxide utilization. Therefore, breathing exercises increase health of body and mind.

EXPRESSION: Expressing ourselves with the goal of creating a happier future attracts a happier future. Health automatically inspires creativity, more positive outlook and happiness.

FAMILY PLANNING: Drinking 8 tablespoons of fresh papaya seeds blended with ½ cup good drinking water twice daily for 18 days has caused miscarriage in up to 8 weeks of pregnancy. Eating plenty of fresh raw horseradish root increased the incidence of miscarriage but had a tendency to make women irritable. Eating 1 cup whole moldy blackberries blended with ½ cup good mineral water sometimes caused miscarriage, usually within 2 weeks of eating them. (Blackberries had been molding for no more than, and no less than, 4 weeks.) Inserting 1 teaspoon cold-pressed pennyroyal (an herb) tincture through the cervix and rubbing it vigorously on to the uterus, usually caused abortion in up to 6 months of pregnancy. (It took up to 21 days with mild cramping before abortion was complete). Inserting a mixture of 2 tablespoons pennyroyal tincture and ¼ cup good mineral water into the uterus, and lying on your back with buttocks raised and holding it in the uterus for at least 2 hours, usually caused abortion in the same manner. That procedure was best performed at bedtime.

Vigorously rubbing 4 drops of cold-pressed pennyroyal oil (instead of tincture) directly onto the cervix, usually caused abortion within 3 days, usually with intense labor pains.

Regardless how miscarriage may occur, have remedies for hemorrhage ready (*see* Hemorrhage, page 270). At first signs of miscarriage, begin taking hemorrhage remedies to prevent radical infection and excessive bleed.

FASTS, that is, not eating or drinking food, starve healthy cells as well as weak cells. After 5 hours of not eating or drinking food, cells become cannibalistic and eat each other, causing extreme systemic toxicity. (*See* Eating Before Sleep, page 331) I do not recommend fasting for anyone. Gradually detoxifying the body through good nutrition is a more loving way to care for our bodies. *See* Detoxification, page 255. My next book will discuss and suggest many effective methods to healthfully inspire and speed detoxification.

FRESH AIR AND SUNSHINE: Getting as much of those as you can reduces the need for lengthy detoxification, and makes detoxification easier.

Sunshine does not create skin cancer. A deficiency of utilizable fat in the skin prevents proper absorption of sun rays and prevents the skin's ability to transform sun rays into vitamin D. Resultantly, the skin burns and dries, creating vast amounts of dead cells that the body can't afford to discard. Skin cancer develops in people who are especially deficient in utilizable fat in the skin. The fat deficiency is from not eating fat, especially raw fat, or the inability to utilize cooked and processed fat, or the application of any skin lotion (including all suntan lotions) because skin lotions smother and poison the skin.

It is imperative that we do not shower or bathe the morning of a day of sunbathing. Washing removes the body's natural oils that are a natural sunblock. Rubbing a little unrefined cold-pressed-below-96° Fahrenheit coconut or peanut oil into the skin the night before sunbathing promotes tanning and reduces the likelihood of burn.

People who had normally sunburned easily before eating a raw diet (which included plenty of raw fat) were able to sunbathe without sunblocks and without burning after 1-5 months. It is best to start sunbathing in short periods (as much time as feels comfortable). Those who experience many months each year without sunbathing may have to burn a little each year. *See* Burns, page 235.

FRUITARIANISM is following a diet that consists of eating only fruit. A fruitarian diet cleanses the body but does not build and strengthen it. Bones, teeth, nerves, and tissue in general deteriorate when fed mainly fruit. Most people on mainly fruitarian diets lack focus and clarity, and are excessively emotional.

HAIR SPRAY SUBSTITUTE: Store-bought hair sprays damage hair and are very toxic to the sinuses, bronchi, lungs, blood, scalp, brain and entire body.

A natural hair spray can be easily made by mixing 1½ teaspoons unheated honey into 1 cup of good mineral water. Pour into a spray bottle and use as you would normally use hair spray. (That mixture will eventually ferment. In warm temperatures it may last as little as 3 days. If kept in a cool place, it will last as long as 10 days.)

HERBS AND HERBAL THERAPY are the use of plants as remedies for all maladies. The success rate of herbal therapies is double that of the medical profession. In conjunction with a healthy raw diet, fresh herbs stimulate and promote better health and ease detoxification. However, when herbs are steeped, cut, powdered or processed using heat above 90° Fahrenheit, they create as much toxicity as they supply healing properties. They cause an overly acidic digestive environment, blood and neural fluids. If digestion is impaired, all other bodily processes are impaired also, and health suffers.

If a person is in need of the effects of an herb, it would be best to eat or juice the fresh herb. But if the fresh herb cannot be obtained, steeping the dried herb in water in the sun for a long afternoon, or for 24 hours, then adding the raw juice of ¼ fresh lemon and 1-3 tablespoons unheated honey to each cup before drinking it minimizes toxicity.

HOMEOPATHY is treating disease by drugs, given in minute doses, which would produce in a healthy person symptoms similar to those of the disease. Homeopathic medicine has twice the success rate of Western medicine. However, too often I have seen that homeopathy is like Western medicine in that both are remedial and not curative. They arrest symptoms without eliminating the cause of disease.

METABOLIC TYPES AND METABOLIC TYPING consider that people who metabolize differently should eat different foods. That is, because some people are extremely athletic or non-physical, or somewhere in between, it is believed that each of those types should eat different foods. I have not found any long-term empirical evidence that supports those theories. All tribes contain individuals who metabolize differently, yet they consume the same foods daily without distress or disease. I have received many patients who developed serious disease or increased symptoms of their diseases by adhering to the suggestions postulated by people who promote Metabolic Typing. I strongly disagree with Metabolic Typing because it prohibits or restricts important foods from people who need those foods, especially raw meats and dairy, and advises foods that cause toxicity, and preferably should not be eaten.

PETS, like all creatures, have eaten raw foods for millions of years. Feeding pets dried, processed and cooked foods causes them to develop discomfort, illness and disease. Research documenting this is available through the Price-Pottenger Foundation (*see* Bibliography, page 340).

PREGNANCY, as every one knows, is the process of growing a child. How that child grows depends on genetics, what the mother eats, and what drugs the mother takes. Every drug alters the genetic structure or weakens the DNA and RNA of some young cells. Therefore, it is best not to take medication, especially during pregnancy.

The stress factors are tremendous during pregnancy. Not only is the mother responsible for carrying the extra being, her body also feeds the child and discards the child's wastes. If what the fetus needs is not present and freely available in the lymph and blood of the mother, the placenta calls for and leaches protein and other nutrients from the mother's cells, via the production of certain hormones. Many women nowadays age 2-8 years with each pregnancy, resulting from the leaching process.

To prove how important utilizable proteins are during pregnancy, take a look at how many women lose muscle tone during and shortly after pregnancy. Muscle tissue is not the only tissue that is leached from the mother if utilizable protein and fat aren't available in the blood and lymph. Also, glandular, nerve, brain, arterial and bone cells are leached. Eating plenty of raw meat and fat before and during pregnancy grows a strong healthy child (genetics allowing) and prevents the mother from sacrificing her body for her child.

Nausea during pregnancy indicates that the mother's system is too acidic and toxic. Eating red meat may cause more nausea and vomiting even if the red meat is raw. Therefore, if experiencing morning sickness, it is best to follow the suggestions in Alkalizing Food, page 178, and eat raw white meat, especially raw fish, and unripe pineapple or other unripe fruit with a raw fat.

Many women who cannot discard the accumulation of wastes - fetal and their own - during pregnancy, usually bloat with fluids, or get fat during or after pregnancy. They retain the wastes within their bodies, bound in difficult-to-discard cooked fat and fluids. Eating plenty of raw fat before and during pregnancy usually prevents bloating and fat retention. However, if bloating or fat retention occurs when eating raw fat, it usually gives women more strength. The fluid and fat can be more readily discarded within months after birthing when fat is eaten raw.

After bathing, daily massaging unheated-above-96° Fahrenheit fermented coconut oil, or peanut oil, or stone-pressed olive oil into thighs, buttocks, hips, abdomen and breasts, reduces or eliminates the formation of stretch marks (scars). Wipe off excess after 15-20 minutes.

Sexual intercourse with orgasm during the eighth month often makes the blood too rich in hormones for the fetus to properly establish brain functions. Kissing and petting without orgasm is good. (It might be a sensitive gesture for the man also to refrain from having orgasm for that month.)

See Miscarriage, page 292, *and* Overweight, page 296.

SLEEP AND REST are necessary for healing. Ninety percent of healing happens during very restful states. Most people only achieve those states during sleep. Therefore, most healing occurs during sleep. A nap daily is not only a beauty aid, it is rejuvenating physically, emotionally and mentally. When on a healthy raw diet, situations that seemed so complex, difficult, or futile before a nap are often magically reduced to something more solvable after a nap. To help yourself sleep better and become healthier, sleep, or at least nap, when tired.

STRETCH MARKS, SCARS AND WRINKLES result from poor healing because of poor nutrition. Eating raw meat, and raw fat like avocados, raw cream and butter, unheated-above-96° Fahrenheit fermented coconut oil, and stone-pressed olive oil, prevents or very gradually reduces stretch marks and scars. Applying raw red meat to wrinkles over night feeds and nourishes the skin and reduces wrinkles.

Topically, vigorously rubbing a mixture of 2 tablespoons fresh raw papaya and 1 tablespoon unheated-above-96° Fahrenheit fermented coconut oil or stone-pressed olive oil into the skin once weekly helps to gradually remove stretch marks and scars. The vigorous rubbing should not cause abrasions. Wipe off excess after 15-20 minutes. As some of the naturally embalmed dead cells (scar tissue) that are more toxic dissolve, some red spots and slight acne may result.

SUNSHINE: *See* Fresh Air and Sunshine, page 334.

TEAS that are steeped in the sun without ever having been cooked can supply certain minerals and provide obscure nutrients that an individual may be lacking. That is herbal therapy's claim to increase health. However, dried leaves, stems and roots are deficient in enzymes and turn overly acidic in the body. Digestion is impaired. If digestion is impaired, all other bodily processes are impaired and health suffers. *See* Herbs and Herbal Therapy, page 335.

WEIGHT AND DENSITY should be measured differently when eating a raw diet that includes raw meat. The body becomes denser and often gains about one pound each year without increasing girth. Consequently, present weight charts are inaccurate. Oversized people hoping to become trim should forget the scale. Measuring the dimensions of the body to see that the body is trimming is the only accurate measurement. *See* Overweight, page 296.

4BIBLIOGRAPHY
(very partial)

BÉCHAMP OR PASTEUR, E. Douglas Hume, England, The National Hygiene Press, available from Price-Pottenger Foundation, P.O.Box 2614, La Mesa, CA 91943-2614.

BIO-ATTACK ALERT, Theodore A. Strecker, LL.D., The Strecker Group, 1301 Colorado Bl, Eagle Rock, CA 90041 (reference of discoveries in medical literature regarding the creation of AIDS and other deadly viruses).

CANCER: DISEASE OF CIVILIZATION? AN ANTHROPOLOGICAL AND HISTORICAL STUDY, Vilhjalmur Stefansson, Hill and Wang, New York (1960), available at the Stefansson Collection, Dartmouth College. (This collection contains numerous reports and accounts by medical doctors, nurses, researchers and explorers that eating raw food, including raw meat, prevented disease.)

CONFESSIONS OF A MEDICAL HERETIC, Robert S. Mendelsohn, M.D., Contemporary Books, Inc., Two Prudential Plaza, Chicago, IL 60601-6790 (1990).

DON'T GET STUCK! THE CASE AGAINST VACCINATIONS, Hannah Allen, The American Natural Hygiene Press, P.O. Box 1083, Oldsmar, FL 33557.

THE FACTS ABOUT FATS, John Finnegan, Celestial Arts Publishing, P.O. Box 7123, Berkley, CA 94707 (1993).

FATS THAT HEAL, FATS THAT KILL, Udo Erasmus, Ph.D., Alive Books, 7436 Frasier Park Drive, Burnaby, B.C., Canada V5J5B9 (1993).

INOCULATIONS: The True Weapons of Mass Destruction; and, Causing VIDs; An Epidemic of Genocide, Carley, M.D., Rebecca (2004)

MAN'S CORRECT DIET, R.B. Pearson, Health Research, 70 Lafayette Street, Mokelumne Hill, CA 95245 (1921).

NATIVE NUTRITION, Ronald F. Schmid, N.D., Healing Arts Press, One Park Street, Rochester, Vermont 05767 (1994).

NUTRITION AND PHYSICAL DEGENERATION, Weston A. Price, M.S., D.D.S., F.A.C.D., The Price-Pottenger Foundation, P.O. Box 2614, La Mesa, CA 91943 (1989).

THE PERSECUTION AND TRIAL OF GASTON NAESSENS, Christopher Bird, H.J. Kramer, Inc., P.O. Box 1082, Tiburon, CA 94920 (1991).

POTTENGER'S CATS: A STUDY IN NUTRITION, Dr. Francis F. Pottenger Jr., M.D., F.A.C.D., The Price-Pottenger Foundation, P.O. Box 2614, La Mesa, CA 91943 (1995).

RACE DECLINE AND RACE REGENERATION, Weston A. Price, M.S., D.D.S., F.A.C.D., The Price-Pottenger Foundation, P.O. Box 2614, La Mesa, CA 91943 (1941).

SMALLPOX VACCINE AND AIDS, Pierce Wright, London Times, May 11, 1987.

VACCINATIONS - THE SILENT KILLER, A CLEAR AND PRESENT DANGER, Ida Honorof and E. McBean, Ph.D, N.D., Honorof, McBean, P.O. Box 5449, Sherman Oaks, CA 91403 (1977).

VACCINATION CONDEMNED, Elben, Better Life Research, P.O. Box 42002, Los Angeles, CA 90042.

~ INDEX ~

~ A ~

~ *D* ~

~ *E* ~

~ *F* ~

~ *G* ~

~ *H* ~

~ *I* ~

~ O ~

~ P ~

~ *W* ~

For information on individualized consultations and programs with Aajonus Vonderplanitz, please e-mail or leave a message:

e-mail: optimal@earthlink.net
Message: 310-226-7055

I have been very limited in financial resources to fund my experiments and research over the years. But I did them. Although my results with reversing disease have been extraordinary, I know that my work has the potential to achieve even more remarkable results by incorporating fresh raw herbs. I will continue to work in this direction. That involves obtaining funding, seeds, bulbs and rooted cuttings to grow therapeutic herbs so that we may use them fresh and raw. If anyone has access to funding, herbal seeds, bulbs and rooted cuttings, please contact me at:

Optimal Ways of Living
P.O. Box 176
Santa Monica, CA 90406-0176

Your donations will be utilized well and appreciated. Thank you.

PRODUCT-LIST ORDER FORM

Optimal Ways of Living
P.O. Box 176
Santa Monica, CA 90406-0176

Please send me your newest list of producers of raw food products.

I enclose a check or money order (not cash) for $15 to cover costs of service, materials and shipping.

(Allow 4-6 weeks for delivery, or much sooner by e-mail.)

Name ______________________________

Address ______________________________

City ____________________ State ______ Zip ______-_____

Phone #s ______________________________

E-mail Address ______________________________

Your information will not be sold or disclosed to any anyone, including an outside mailing list.